Nephrology

Editor

JOHN A. KELLUM

CRITICAL CARE CLINICS

www.criticalcare.theclinics.com

Consulting Editor
RICHARD W. CARLSON

October 2015 • Volume 31 • Number 4

ELSEVIER

1600 John F. Kennedy Boulevard • Suite 1800 • Philadelphia, Pennsylvania, 19103-2899

http://www.theclinics.com

CRITICAL CARE CLINICS Volume 31, Number 4
October 2015 ISSN 0749-0704, ISBN-13: 978-0-323-40078-7

Editor: Patrick Manley
Developmental Editor: Casey Jackson

Critical Care Clinics (ISSN: 0749-0704) is published quarterly by Elsevier Inc., 360 Park Avenue South, New York, NY 10010-1710. Months of issue are January, April, July, and October. Business and Editorial Offices: 1600 John F. Kennedy Blvd., Suite 1800, Philadelphia, PA 19103-2899. Customer Service Office: 6277 Sea Harbor Drive, Orlando, FL 32887-4800. Periodicals postage paid at New York, NY and additional mailing offices. Subscription prices are $210.00 per year for US individuals, $503.00 per year for US institution, $100.00 per year for US students and residents, $255.00 per year for Canadian individuals, $630.00 per year for Canadian institutions, $300.00 per year for international individuals, $630.00 per year for international institutions and $150.00 per year for Canadian and foreign students/residents. To receive student/resident rate, orders must be accompanied by name of affiliated institution, date of term, and the signature of program/residency coordinator on institution letterhead. Orders will be billed at individual rate until proof of status is received. Foreign air speed delivery is included in all Clinics subscription prices. All prices are subject to change without notice. POSTMASTER: Send address changes to Critical Care Clinics, Elsevier Periodicals Customer Service, 11830 Westline Industrial Drive, St. Louis, MO 63146. **Customer Service: 1-800-654-2452 (US). From outside of the US, call 1-314-447-8871. Fax: 1-314-447-8029. E-mail: journalscustomerservice-usa@elsevier.com (for print support) or journalsonlinesupport-usa@elsevier.com (for online support).**

Reprints. For copies of 100 or more of articles in this publication, please contact the Commercial Reprints Department, Elsevier Inc., 360 Park Avenue South, New York, NY 10010-1710. Tel.: 212-633-3874; Fax: 212-633-3820; E-mail: reprints@elsevier.com.

Critical Care Clinics is also published in Spanish by Editorial Inter-Medica, Junin 917, 1er A, 1113, Buenos Aires, Argentina.

Critical Care Clinics is covered in MEDLINE/PubMed (Index Medicus), EMBASE/Excerpta Medica, Current Concepts/Clinical Medicine, ISI/BIOMED, and Chemical Abstracts.

Contributors

CONSULTING EDITOR

RICHARD W. CARLSON, MD, PhD
Chairman Emeritus, Director, Medical Intensive Care Unit, Department of Medicine, Maricopa Medical Center; Professor, University of Arizona College of Medicine; Professor, Department of Medicine, Mayo Graduate School of Medicine, Phoenix, Arizona

EDITOR

JOHN A. KELLUM, MD, FACP
Professor of Critical Care Medicine, Medicine, Bioengineering, and Translational and Clinical Science; Director, Center for Critical Care Nephrology, The CRISMA Center, University of Pittsburgh Medical Center, University of Pittsburgh School of Medicine, University of Pittsburgh, Pittsburgh, Pennsylvania

AUTHORS

SEAN M. BAGSHAW, MD, MSc, FRCPC
Division of Critical Care Medicine, Faculty of Medicine and Dentistry, University of Alberta, Edmonton, Alberta, Canada

RINALDO BELLOMO, MD, FRACP, FCICM
Department of Intensive Care, Austin Hospital; Department of Epidemiology and Preventive Medicine, Australian and New Zealand Intensive Care Research Centre, School of Preventive Medicine and Public Health, Monash University, Melbourne, Victoria, Australia

AZRA BIHORAC, MD, MS
Departments of Medicine and Anesthesiology, University of Florida, Gainesville, Florida

JOSEPH A. CARCILLO, MD
Department of Critical Care Medicine and Pediatrics, University of Pittsburgh School of Medicine, Pittsburgh, Pennsylvania

LAKHMIR S. CHAWLA, MD
Divisions of Intensive Care Medicine and Nephrology, Associate Professor, Department of Medicine, Washington DC Veterans Affairs Medical Center, Washington, DC

LING-XIN CHEN, MD
Nephrology Fellow, Section of Nephrology, Department of Medicine, University of Chicago, Chicago, Illinois

MIGUEL A. CRUZ, PhD
Department of Medicine, Baylor College of Medicine, Center for Translational Research on Inflammatory Diseases (CTRID), Michael DeBakey VA Medical Center, Houston, Texas

JAMES F. DOYLE, MBChB, MFICM
Intensive Care Unit, Senior Clinical Research Fellow; Department of Intensive Care Medicine, Surrey Peri-Operative Anaesthesia and Critical Care Collaborative Research Group, Royal Surrey County Hospital, NHS Foundation Trust, Surrey, United Kingdom

FRANCOIS DURAND, MD
Professor of Hepatology, Service d'Hépatologie et Réanimation Hépatodigestive, Hepatology and Liver Intensive Care Unit, INSERM U773, Université Paris VII Hôpital Beaujon, Clichy, France; INSERM U1149, University Paris VII, Denis Diderot, Paris, France

LUI G. FORNI, BSc, MB, PhD
Intensive Care Unit, Professor, Department of Intensive Care Medicine, Surrey Peri-Operative Anaesthesia and Critical Care Collaborative Research Group, Royal Surrey County Hospital, NHS Foundation Trust; Faculty of Health and Medical Sciences, University of Surrey, Surrey, United Kingdom

STUART L. GOLDSTEIN, MD
Director of the Center for Acute Care Nephrology, Department of Pediatrics, Cincinnati Children's Hospital Medical Center; Professor, University of Cincinnati College of Medicine, Cincinnati, Ohio

HERNANDO GOMEZ, MD, MPH
Department of Critical Care Medicine, Center for Critical Care Nephrology, The CRISMA Center, University of Pittsburgh, Pittsburgh, Pennsylvania

CHARLES HOBSON, MD, MHA
Department of Surgery, Malcom Randall VA Medical Center, NF/SG VAMC; Department of Health Services Research, Management, and Policy, University of Florida, Gainesville, Florida

JACOB C. JENTZER, MD
Fellow, Department of Critical Care Medicine, UPMC Presbyterian Hospital, University of Pittsburgh Medical Center, Pittsburgh, Pennsylvania

MICHAEL JOANNIDIS, MD
Professor of Intensive Care and Emergency Medicine, Division of Intensive Care and Emergency Medicine, Department of Internal Medicine, Medical University Innsbruck, Innsbruck, Austria

SANDRA L. KANE-GILL, PharmD, MS
Associate Professor, Department of Pharmacy and Therapeutics, University of Pittsburgh School of Pharmacy; Faculty, Center for Critical Care Nephology, University of Pittsburgh Medical Center, University of Pittsburgh School of Medicine, Pittsburgh, Pennsylvania

CONSTANTINE J. KARVELLAS, MD, SM, FRCPC
Assistant Professor (Critical Care/Hepatology), Division of Critical Care Medicine; Division of Gastroenterology, Faculty of Medicine and Dentistry, University of Alberta, Edmonton, Alberta, Canada

JOHN A. KELLUM, MD, FACP
Professor of Critical Care Medicine, Medicine, Bioengineering, and Translational and Clinical Science; Director, Center for Critical Care Nephrology, The CRISMA Center, University of Pittsburgh Medical Center, University of Pittsburgh School of Medicine, University of Pittsburgh, Pittsburgh, Pennsylvania

JAY L. KOYNER, MD
Associate Professor of Medicine, Section of Nephrology, Department of Medicine, University of Chicago, Chicago, Illinois

JOHAN MÅRTENSSON, MD, PhD, DESA
Department of Intensive Care, Austin Hospital, Heidelberg, Victoria, Australia; Department of Physiology and Pharmacology, Section of Anaesthesia and Intensive Care Medicine, Karolinska Institutet, Stockholm, Sweden

ETIENNE MACEDO, MD, PhD
Department of Medicine, University of California San Diego, San Diego, California; Nephrology Division, University of Sao Paulo, Brazil

RAVINDRA L. MEHTA, MD
Professor of Clinical Medicine; Associate Chair for Clinical Research, Department of Medicine, University of California San Diego, San Diego, California

MITRA K. NADIM, MD
Associate Professor of Medicine, Division of Nephrology, Department of Medicine, Keck School of Medicine, University of Southern California, Los Angeles, California

TRUNG C. NGUYEN, MD
Section of Critical Care Medicine, Department of Pediatrics, Baylor College of Medicine/ Texas Children's Hospital, Center for Translational Research on Inflammatory Diseases (CTRID), Michael DeBakey VA Medical Center, Houston, Texas

MICHAEL E. O'CONNOR, MBBS, BSc, MRCP, FRCA
Adult Critical Care Unit, The Royal London Hospital, Barts Health NHS Trust; William Harvey Institute, Barts and The London School of Medicine and Dentistry, Queen Mary University of London, London, United Kingdom

MARLIES OSTERMANN, PhD, MD, FRCP, EDIC
King's College London, Guy's and St Thomas Hospital, Department of Critical Care, London, United Kingdom

PAUL M. PALEVSKY, MD
Chief, Renal Section, VA Pittsburgh Healthcare System; Professor of Medicine and Clinical and Translational Science, Renal-Electrolyte Division, University of Pittsburgh School of Medicine, Pittsburgh, Pennsylvania

JOHN R. PROWLE, MA, MB BChir, MSc, MD, FRCP, FFICM
Honorary Clinical Senior Lecturer, Consultant in Intensive Care and Renal Medicine, Adult Critical Care Unit, The Royal London Hospital, Barts Health NHS Trust; Centre for Translational Medicine and Therapeutics, William Harvey Research Institute, Queen Mary University of London; Department of Renal and Transplant Medicine, The Royal London Hospital, Barts Health NHS Trust, London, United Kingdom

OLEKSA REWA, MD, FRCPC
Division of Critical Care Medicine, Faculty of Medicine and Dentistry, University of Alberta, Edmonton, Alberta, Canada

ZACCARIA RICCI, MD
Pediatric Cardiac Intensive Care Unit, Staff, Department of Cardiology and Cardiac Surgery, Bambino Gesù Children's Hospital, IRCCS, Rome, Italy

CLAUDIO RONCO, MD
Head, Department of Nephrology, Dialysis and Transplantation, San Bortolo Hospital; Head, International Renal Research Institute, San Bortolo Hospital, Vicenza, Italy

KAI SINGBARTL, MD, MPH, FCCM
Donald E. Martin Professor of Anesthesia and Pain Medicine, Department of Anesthesiology, Penn State College of Medicine, Milton S. Hershey Medical Center, Hershey, Pennsylvania

GIRISH SINGHANIA, MD
Department of Medicine, University of Florida, Gainesville, Florida

MATT VARRIER, MBBS, MRCP
King's College London, Guy's and St Thomas Hospital, Department of Critical Care, London, United Kingdom

GIANLUCA VILLA, MD
Section of Anaesthesiology and Intensive Care, Staff, Department of Health Science, University of Florence, Florence, Italy

STEVEN D. WEISBORD, MD, MSc
Staff Physician, Renal Section, VA Pittsburgh Healthcare System; Associate Professor of Medicine and Clinical and Translational Science, Renal-Electrolyte Division, University of Pittsburgh School of Medicine, Pittsburgh, Pennsylvania

Contents

Preface: Critical Care Nephrology   xiii

John A. Kellum

Diagnostic Criteria for Acute Kidney Injury: Present and Future   621

John A. Kellum

Acute kidney injury (AKI) is a clinical diagnosis guided by standard criteria based on changes in serum creatinine, urine output, or both. Severity of AKI is determined by the magnitude of increase in serum creatinine or decrease in urine output. Patients manifesting both oliguria and azotemia and those in which these impairments are persistent are more likely to have worse disease and worse outcomes. Short- and long-term outcomes are worse when patients have some stage of AKI by both criteria. New biomarkers for AKI may substantially aid in the risk assessment and evaluation of patients at risk for AKI.

Biomarkers in Acute Kidney Injury   633

Ling-Xin Chen and Jay L. Koyner

Acute kidney injury (AKI) is a common and often lethal complication that is also associated with severe morbidity in hospitalized patients. During the last decade, the standardization of AKI diagnostic criteria has helped to facilitate several large-scale investigations of biomarkers of AKI. These studies have led to the international clinical implementation of several biomarkers of renal injury. This review summarizes the results of many of these multicenter investigations and discusses the clinical utility and interpretation of several of these new clinical tests. The merits of combining biomarkers of kidney function is also discussed.

Sepsis-Induced Acute Kidney Injury   649

Johan Mårtensson and Rinaldo Bellomo

Acute kidney injury (AKI) is a serious yet potentially reversible complication of sepsis. Several molecular mechanisms involved in the development of septic AKI have been identified. These mechanisms may be important targets in the development of future therapies. This review highlights the role of the innate immune response to sepsis and its downstream effects on kidney structure and function with special reference to the adaptive cellular response and glomerular hemodynamic changes. In addition, current evidence surrounding the management of patients with septic AKI is summarized. Finally, potential novel therapies for septic AKI are presented.

Thrombocytopenia-Associated Multiple Organ Failure and Acute Kidney Injury   661

Trung C. Nguyen, Miguel A. Cruz, and Joseph A. Carcillo

Thrombocytopenia-associated multiple organ failure (TAMOF) is a clinical phenotype that encompasses a spectrum of syndromes associated with disseminated microvascular thromboses, such as the thrombotic microangiopathies thrombotic thrombocytopenic purpura/hemolytic uremic syndrome (TTP/HUS) and disseminated intravascular coagulation (DIC). Autopsies findings in TTP, HUS, or DIC reveal specific findings that can differentiate these 3 entities. Von Willebrand factor and ADAMTS-13 play a central role in TTP. Shiga toxins and the complement pathway are vital in the development of HUS. Tissue factor is the major protease that drives the pathology of DIC. Acute kidney injury (AKI) is a common feature in patients with TAMOF.

Drug-Induced Acute Kidney Injury: A Focus on Risk Assessment for Prevention   675

Sandra L. Kane-Gill and Stuart L. Goldstein

Drugs are the third to fifth leading cause of acute kidney injury (AKI) in critically ill patients following sepsis and hypotension. Susceptibilities and exposures for development of AKI have been identified, and some are modifiable allowing for the possibility of AKI prevention or mitigation of AKI severity. Using drug therapies for prevention of AKI has been attempted but with little success in human studies, so we must rely on risk-assessment strategies for prevention. The purpose of this article is to review the risk factors, risk-assessment strategies, prevention, and management of drug-induced AKI with emphasis on risk assessment.

A Clinical Approach to the Acute Cardiorenal Syndrome   685

Jacob C. Jentzer and Lakhmir S. Chawla

Acute kidney injury is a frequent complication of acute heart failure syndromes, portending an adverse prognosis. Acute cardiorenal syndrome represents a unique form of acute kidney injury specific to acute heart failure syndromes. The pathophysiology of acute cardiorenal syndrome involves renal venous congestion, ineffective forward flow, and impaired renal autoregulation caused by neurohormonal activation. Biomarkers reflecting different aspects of acute cardiorenal syndrome pathophysiology may allow patient phenotyping to inform prognosis and treatment. Adjunctive vasoactive, neurohormonal, and diuretic therapies may relieve congestive symptoms and/or improve renal function, but no single therapy has been proved to reduce mortality in acute cardiorenal syndrome.

Acute Kidney Injury in the Surgical Patient   705

Charles Hobson, Girish Singhania, and Azra Bihorac

Perioperative acute kidney injury (AKI) is a common, morbid, and costly surgical complication. Current efforts to understand and manage AKI in surgical patients focus on prevention, mitigation of further injury when AKI has occurred, treatment of associated conditions, and facilitation of renal recovery. Lesser severity AKI is now understood to be much more common, and more morbid, than was previously thought. The ability to detect AKI within hours of onset would be helpful in protecting the kidney and in preserving renal function, and several imaging and biomarker modalities are currently being evaluated.

Contrast-associated Acute Kidney Injury   725

Steven D. Weisbord and Paul M. Palevsky

Contrast-associated acute kidney injury (CAAKI) is a common iatrogenic condition. The principal risk factors for CAAKI are underlying renal impairment, diabetes in the setting of kidney disease, and intravascular volume depletion, effective or absolute. CAAKI is associated with serious adverse short-term and long-term outcomes, including mortality and more rapidly progressive chronic kidney disease, although the causal nature of these associations remains unproved. Patients with chronic kidney disease and other risk factors for CAAKI who present with acute coronary syndrome should undergo indicated angiographic procedures.

Acute Kidney Injury in Cirrhosis   737

Constantine J. Karvellas, Francois Durand, and Mitra K. Nadim

Acute kidney injury (AKI) is a frequent complication of end-stage liver disease, especially in those with acute-on-chronic liver failure, occurring in up to 50% of hospitalized patients with cirrhosis. There is no specific blood or urine biomarker that can reliably identify the cause of AKI in cirrhotic patients. This review examines studies used to assess renal dysfunction in cirrhotic patients including new diagnostic criteria and potential novel biomarkers. Although biomarker development to differentiate the cause of AKI in cirrhosis has promise, the utility of biomarkers to determine irreversible renal dysfunction with liver transplant remains lacking, warranting further investigation.

Short-term Effects of Acute Kidney Injury   751

Kai Singbartl and Michael Joannidis

Acute kidney injury (AKI) is associated with significant short-term morbidity and mortality, which cannot solely be explained by loss of organ function. Renal replacement therapy allows rapid correction of most acute changes associated with AKI, indicating that additional pathogenetic factors play a major role in AKI. Evidence suggests that reduced renal cytokine clearance as well as increased cytokine production by the acutely injured kidney contribute to a systemic inflammation state, which results in significant effects on other organs. AKI seems to compromise the function of the innate immune system. AKI is an acute systemic disease with serious distant organ effects.

Long-Term Follow-up of Acute Kidney Injury   763

James F. Doyle and Lui G. Forni

In the general hospital setting, approximately 15% of inpatients sustain an episode of acute kidney injury (AKI) but in the critical care environment this can increase to over 25%. An episode of AKI increases the risk for both future chronic kidney disease and associated cardiovascular complications. Discharge of patients who have suffered a renal insult resulting in AKI should include consideration of longer-term follow-up, which may require nephrology input. This increase in health care burden and economic costs may be quantified and justifies the need to develop robust quality-improvement projects aimed at AKI prevention, identification, and improved management.

Preventing Acute Kidney Injury   773

Etienne Macedo and Ravindra L. Mehta

Epidemiologic studies applying the acute kidney injury (AKI) classification system have confirmed the increasing incidence of AKI in different settings and its association with adverse outcomes. AKI is now a recognized important risk factor for new-onset chronic kidney disease, determining acceleration in progression to end-stage renal disease, leading to poor quality of life, disability, and long-term costs. AKI has been associated with high mortalities; however, it is likely that a significant number of deaths associated with AKI could be avoided. This article reviews the key aspects of the 0by25 initiative and its application in critically ill patients.

Principles of Fluid Management   785

Oleksa Rewa and Sean M. Bagshaw

Fluid therapy is the most common intervention received by acutely ill hospitalized patients; however, important questions on its optimal use remain. Its prescription should be patient and context specific, with clear indications and contradictions, and have the type, dose, and rate speci-fied. Any fluid therapy, if provided inappropriately, can contribute unneces-sary harm to patients. The quantitative toxicity of fluid therapy contributes to worse outcomes; this should prompt greater bedside attention to fluid prescription, fluid balance, development of avoidable complications attrib-utable to fluid overload, and for the timely deresuscitation of patients whose clinical status and physiology allow active fluid mobilization.

Fluid Overload   803

Michael E. O'Connor and John R. Prowle

Most critically ill patients experience external or internal fluid shifts and hemodynamic instability. In response to these changes, intravenous fluids are frequently administered. However, rapid losses of administered fluids from circulation and the indirect link between the short-lived plasma vol-ume expansion and end points frequently result in transient responses to fluid therapy. Therefore, fluid overload is a common finding in intensive care units. The authors consider the evidence of harm associated with fluid overload and the physiologic processes that lead to fluid accumulation in critical illness. The authors then consider methods to prevent fluid accu-mulation and/or manage its resolution.

Fluid Composition and Clinical Effects   823

Matt Varrier and Marlies Ostermann

The range of intravenous fluids available for therapeutic use and the differing indications are diverse. A solid understanding of the composition of different types of fluids is essential to understanding the physiologic effects following administration and the appropriate clinical application.

In this review, the authors describe the different fluids commonly available and discuss the potential benefits and harms depending on the clinical circumstances.

Renal Replacement Therapy   **839**

Gianluca Villa, Zaccaria Ricci, and Claudio Ronco

Renal replacement therapy (RRT) is a cornerstone in the clinical management of patients with acute kidney injury. Results from different studies agree that early renal support therapy (aimed to support the residual kidney function during early phases of organ dysfunction) may reduce mortality with respect to late RRT (aimed to substitute the complete loss of function during the advanced kidney insufficiency). Although it seems plausible that a timely initiation of RRT may be associated with improved renal and nonrenal outcomes in these patients, there is scarce evidence in literature to exactly identify the most adequate onset timing for RRT.

Understanding Acid Base Disorders   **849**

Hernando Gomez and John A. Kellum

The concentration of hydrogen ions is regulated in biologic solutions. There are currently 3 recognized approaches to assess changes in acid base status. First, is the traditional Henderson-Hasselbalch approach, also called the physiologic approach, which uses the relationship between HCO_3^- and P_{CO_2}. The second is the standard base excess approach based on the Van Slyke equation. The third approach is the quantitative or Stewart approach, which uses the strong ion difference and the total weak acids. This article explores the origins of the current concepts framing the existing methods to analyze acid base balance.

Index   **861**

Nephrology
CRITICAL CARE CLINICS

FORTHCOMING ISSUES

January 2016
Obstetric and Gynecologic Emergencies
Peter Papadakos and Susan Dantoni,
Editors

April 2016
Gastrointestinal Issues in Critical Care
Rahul Nanchal and Ram Subramaniam,
Editors

July 2016
Hepatology and Critical Care
Rahul Nanchal and Ram Subramaniam,
Editors

RECENT ISSUES

July 2015
Sleep and Circadian Rhythms in the ICU
Vipin Malik, *Editor*

April 2015
Telemedicine in the ICU
Richard W. Carlson and Corey Scurlock,
Editors

January 2015
Advances in Hemodynamic Monitoring
Michael R. Pinsky, *Editor*

ISSUE OF RELATED INTEREST

Primary Care: Clinics in Office Practice, December 2014 (Vol. 41, No 4)
Nephrology
Samuel Snyder, *Editor*

THE CLINICS ARE AVAILABLE ONLINE!
Access your subscription at:
www.theclinics.com

Preface

Critical Care Nephrology

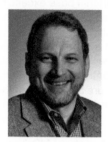

John A. Kellum, MD, FACP
Editor

It's been a decade since *Critical Care Clinics* first published an issue focusing on Critical Care Nephrology.[1] I was honored to be the guest editor, and in my preface, I emphasized the changing landscape of critical care medicine in general, and critical care nephrology in particular, arguing that the "age of empiricism" was coming to a close. Indeed, our specialty is decidedly more evidence-based today than it was ten years ago. For critical care nephrology topics such acute kidney injury (AKI),[2] renal replacement therapy,[3,4] and fluid therapy,[5,6] we now have level 1 evidence where before none existed. Admittedly, we know more about what doesn't work than what does, but this evidence base has dramatically changed the way we approach clinical practice, guideline development, and ultimately, standardization of care.[7]

Yet as I reflect on the past ten years it occurs to me that there are some disturbingly familiar themes. Through much of the decade we sought to treat or prevent AKI by augmenting renal blood flow either with drugs or with fluids. What we continue to demonstrate but never actually learn is that kidney injury isn't "fixed" by giving more fluids or renal vasodilators. Fortunately, there are some new therapies on the horizon and even some simple procedures that might be effective.[8] However, some of the most important things we can (and should) do are not very "sexy." Early antibiotics and source control for sepsis and avoiding nephrotoxins[9] would go a long way. Our reluctance to give up long-held beliefs has set us back in part because we have failed to look for alternatives.[10] Unfortunately, our reluctance to abandon old concepts is also coupled with a desire to embrace things we like. This can lead us to early adoption of treatments we should be more skeptical of (eg, early goal-directed therapy, tight glucose control) and ultimately overturn with large randomized trials.[11,12]

However, not every question we wish to answer should require or is even best answered by mega-trials. If we randomize millions of people to receive one type of chemotherapy or another, we will obscure any effectiveness signal for the very small

Crit Care Clin 31 (2015) xiii–xv
http://dx.doi.org/10.1016/j.ccc.2015.07.001
0749-0704/15/$ – see front matter © 2015 Elsevier Inc. All rights reserved.

number who have cancer. Even interventions that are given to virtually everyone (eg, fluids) might work differently in different patients. Would we seriously advocate the same intravenous fluid for a patient with watery diarrhea and serum sodium of 158 mmol/L as we would for a patient with the same amount of fluid deficit secondary to furosemide and with a serum chloride of 87 mmol/L and an arterial base excess of 10 mEq/L? Understanding human physiology and the pathobiology of disease is no less important that knowing the results of large randomized trials.

In the articles that follow, leading experts from around world synthesize data and review pathophysiology. They provide the latest insights drawn from trials, basic science, and personal experience. They do not shy away from controversy but defend their positions with evidence. They provide a glimpse into the future and review of the past. I hope you will find this collection of articles as interesting and thought-provoking as I have.

John A. Kellum, MD, FACP
Center for Critical Care Nephrology
University of Pittsburgh
604 Scaife Hall
Pittsburgh, PA 15213, USA

E-mail address:
kellumja@upmc.edu

REFERENCES

1. Kellum JA. Preface. Crit Care Clin 2005;21(2):xiii–xv.
2. Bove T, Zangrillo A, Guarracino F, et al. Effect of fenoldopam on use of renal replacement therapy among patients with acute kidney injury after cardiac surgery: a randomized clinical trial. JAMA 2014;312(21):2244–53.
3. VA/NIH Acute Renal Failure Trial Network, Palevsky PM, Zhang JH, et al. Intensity of renal support in critically ill patients with acute kidney injury. N Engl J Med 2008;359(1):7–20.
4. RENAL Replacement Therapy Study Investigators, Bellomo R, Cass A, et al. Intensity of continuous renal-replacement therapy in critically ill patients. N Engl J Med 2009;361(17):1627–38.
5. Perner A, Haase N, Guttormsen AB, et al. Hydroxyethyl starch 130/0.42 versus Ringer's acetate in severe sepsis. N Engl J Med 2012;367(2):124–34.
6. Myburgh JA, Finfer S, Bellomo R, et al. Hydroxyethyl starch or saline for fluid resuscitation in intensive care. N Engl J Med 2012;367(20):1901–11.
7. Kidney Disease: Improving Global Outcomes (KDIGO) Acute Kidney Injury Work Group. KDIGO Clinical Practice Guideline for Acute Kidney Injury. Kidney Int Suppl 2012;2:1–138.
8. Zarbock A, Schmidt C, Van Aken H, et al. Effect of remote ischemic preconditioning on kidney injury among high-risk patients undergoing cardiac surgery: a randomized clinical trial. JAMA 2015;313(21):2133–41.
9. Goldstein SL, Kirkendall E, Nguyen H, et al. Electronic health record identification of nephrotoxin exposure and associated acute kidney injury. Pediatrics 2013; 132(3):e756–67.
10. Kellum JA. Impaired renal blood flow and the "spicy food" hypothesis of acute kidney injury. Crit Care Med 2011;39(4):901–3.

11. Angus DC, Barnato AE, Bell D, et al. A systematic review and meta-analysis of early goal-directed therapy for septic shock: the ARISE, ProCESS and ProMISe Investigators. Intensive Care Med 2015. [Epub ahead of print].
12. NICE-SUGAR Study Investigators, Finfer S, Chittock DR, et al. Intensive versus conventional glucose control in critically ill patients. N Engl J Med 2009; 360(13):1283–97.

Diagnostic Criteria for Acute Kidney Injury
Present and Future

John A. Kellum, MD, FACP

KEYWORDS

- Acute kidney injury • Renal-replacement therapy • Dialysis • Clinical trials
- Biomarkers • Renal recovery • Mortality

KEY POINTS

- The criteria for acute kidney are based on changes in serum creatinine and urine output. Standardized criteria, such as KDIGO criteria, allow for uniform implementation of guidelines and reliable estimates of incidence and outcomes.
- However, acute kidney injury (AKI) remains a clinical diagnosis and clinical judgment is necessary to apply diagnostic criteria and to evaluate the changing clinical status of the patient.
- Baseline renal function is also based on clinical judgment and is best determined by prior serum creatinine measurements; when none are available estimating equations can be used with caution.
- Both serum creatinine and urine output provide independent and complementary information on renal function. Novel biomarkers can provide information on kidney damage and the latest markers can assess kidney stress.
- In the near future, function, damage, and stress may all be used to define AKI.

INTRODUCTION

Acute kidney injury (AKI) is a clinical diagnosis. Already in ancient times it was noted that the failure to pass urine was lethal if untreated and might be caused by either "an

Disclosure: This work was supported in part by R01DK070910 and R01DK083961 from the National Institute of Diabetes and Digestive and Kidney Diseases (NIDDK). The content of this article is solely the responsibility of the authors and does not necessarily represent the official views of NIDDK or National Institutes of Health.
Competing Financial Interest: J.A. Kellum has received grant support and consulting fees from Alere, Astute Medical, Bard and numerous companies developing treatments for Acute Kidney Injury.
Department of Critical Care Medicine, Center for Critical Care Nephrology, University of Pittsburgh Medical Center, University of Pittsburgh School of Medicine, 604 Scaife Hall, 3550 Terrace Street, Pittsburgh, PA 15261, USA
E-mail address: kellumja@upmc.edu

empty bladder" or an obstruction. Indeed, urinary catheters were used as early as 3000 BC. It was Galen who first established the kidneys as the source of urine and as organs that "filtered the blood."[1] Before this, it was generally believed that urine was made in the bladder from food and drink. Progress in the clinical assessment of renal function was quite limited from the time of Galen until the eighteenth century when urea was discovered. However, it would be more than a century later before increases in blood urea and serum creatinine would be used to quantify azotemia ("azote" is a very old name for nitrogen). Azotemia results from reductions in glomerular filtration rate (GFR) and together with oliguria ("small" urine) or anuria (no urine) form the cardinal features of kidney failure.

However, azotemia and oliguria represent not only disease but a normal response of the kidney to extracellular volume depletion or a decreased renal blood flow. Conversely, a "normal" urine output and GFR in the face of volume depletion could only be viewed as renal dysfunction. Thus, changes in urine output and GFR are neither necessary nor sufficient for the diagnosis of renal pathology.[2] Still, they serve as the backbone for the existing diagnostic criteria.[3]

CRITERIA FOR ACUTE KIDNEY INJURY

Little progress was made in the understanding of AKI throughout the first two millennia AD. Although the term nephritis dates back to the sixteenth century it was not really until the late nineteenth century that Bright described renal failure (Bright disease) and included acute and chronic forms.[4] A century later Bywaters and Beall described "acute renal failure" following crush injury.[5] Throughout the remainder of the twentieth century, however, acute renal failure had no widely accepted biochemical definition. As many as 60 different definitions littered the field. In 2004 the RIFLE criteria (Risk Injury Failure Loss End-stage renal disease) were put forth by the Acute Dialysis Quality Initiative.[6] RIFLE included either change in serum creatinine or urine output as criteria recognizing that AKI could be nonoliguric but at the same time creatinine may not increase as rapidly as urine output falls and it is therefore better to have both criteria available. It was not understood at the time, the degree to which urine output and creatinine criteria interact (discussed later in the section on creatinine and urine output). One shortcoming of the RIFLE criteria was its application in patients with preexisting chronic kidney disease (CKD). In patients with elevated baseline creatinines, the proportional changes required by RIFLE seemed excessive. For example, although a patient with a baseline creatinine of 1.0 mg/dL would fulfill criteria for AKI with an increase to 1.5, a patient with a baseline of 2.0 mg/dL would need to reach 3.0. Furthermore, the higher the baseline creatinine the longer the time required to reach a 50% increase. In essence it does not seem credible that a patient with a baseline of 2.6 mg/dL would need to increase to 3.9 and take 3 days to do it just to get to RIFLE-R. For this reason the AKI Network proposed a modification to RIFLE that would also classify AKI when only a small increase in creatinine (0.3 mg/dL or greater) is observed in a short period of time (48 hours or less).[7] Finally, to harmonize RIFLE, AKI Network, and pRIFLE (a modification for pediatrics), the Kidney Disease Improving Global Outcomes (KDIGO) proposed a unified version of these rules (**Table 1**).[3]

THE PURPOSE OF STANDARDIZED CRITERIA FOR ACUTE KIDNEY INJURY

If AKI is clinical diagnosis, why are standard criteria desirable? The answer to this question comes in two parts. First, even though clinical judgment is required, a framework for the clinical diagnosis is needed. In general diagnoses are not based on pure

Table 1
Criteria and staging for acute kidney injury

Stage	Serum Creatinine	Urine Output
1	1.5–1.9 times baseline OR ≥0.3 mg/dL (>26.5 μmol/L) increase	<0.5 mL/kg/h for 6–12 h
2	2.0–2.9 times baseline	<0.5 mL/kg/h for ≥12 h
3	3.0 times baseline OR Increase in serum creatinine to ≥4.0 mg/dL (353.6 μmol/L) OR Initiation of renal-replacement therapy OR In patients <18 y, decrease in eGFR to <35 mL/min per 1.73 m^2	<0.3 mL/kg/h for ≥24 h OR Anuria for ≥12 h

Minimum criteria for acute kidney injury include an increase in serum creatinine by ≥0.3 mg/dL (>26.5 μmol/L) observed within 48 hours; or an increase in serum creatinine to ≥1.5 times baseline, which is known or presumed to have occurred within the prior 7 days; or urine volume less than 0.5 mL/kg/h for 6 hours.

speculation; clinicians consider a set of diagnostic features and use these to guide their judgment. These criteria are not "cook book" but they do serve as a frame of reference so that the average patient with the disease in question fulfills the criteria put forth. Second, standardized criteria for diagnosis of AKI serve multiple purposes (**Fig. 1**) and it is neither feasible nor desirable to have a clinical adjudication for all of these. For example, in large epidemiologic studies it is not practical to examine each patient. In these studies clinicians accept diagnostic constructs as long as

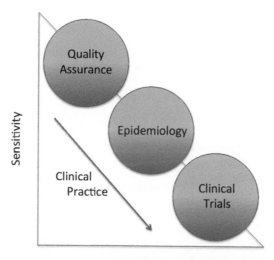

Fig. 1. Sensitivity/specificity tradeoffs for various applications of clinical definitions. For research and quality improvement, fixed thresholds are usually needed, whereas for clinical application diagnoses can be more flexible depending on the actions they elicit.

they achieve reasonable sensitivity and specificity for the disease in question. However, diagnostic criteria, just like a diagnostic test, have test characteristics and specific "cut points" are chosen to maximize sensitivity, specificity, or some degree of both. For quality improvement one might be interested in casting the widest possible net, maximizing sensitivity. If certain things can be done for all patients with "possible AKI," such as avoiding unnecessary nephrotoxic medications, clinicians would want to identify these patients. Conversely, for ascertaining outcomes in clinical trials clinicians tend to favor specificity over sensitivity.

For clinical use, the preference for maximizing sensitivity or specificity depends on the clinical actions intended to be taken. The decision to admit a patient with chest pain to the hospital is best supported by tests that are highly sensitive because the chief concern is about missing a myocardial infarction. Giving that same patient thrombolytic therapy calls for higher specificity. Importantly, however, there is another feature that exists in clinical practice that clinical studies or quality improvement projects usual do not enjoy: time. For clinical studies and for most quality improvement projects, a diagnosis is fixed. A patient either has AKI or they do not. For clinical purposes there is the luxury of provisional diagnoses. As more information becomes available clinicians can and do change their diagnoses. Thus, it may be very appropriate to use a set of diagnostic criteria that are very sensitive for initial evaluation and to require greater specificity for final diagnosis. Over time one can include the patient's clinical course and response to therapy in the assessment (**Fig. 2**).

BASELINE RENAL FUNCTION

A reference serum creatinine is used to apply the diagnostic criteria shown in **Table 1** and to stage patients. When determining the most suitable reference creatinine, the first consideration is the timing of the acute illness believed to be the cause of the AKI. For example, in a patient admitted on Friday with unstable angina who then

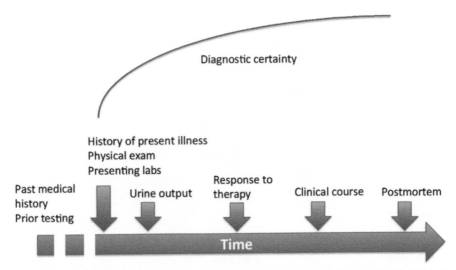

Fig. 2. Diagnostic certainty. Diagnostic certainty is usually low at the outset of a clinical evaluation but improves with time as more information and diagnostic testing results become available.

has three daily serum creatinine measures, all essentially the same, before undergoing cardiac surgery on Monday, there is a need to have a historical baseline to evaluate the serum creatinine on postoperative Day 1. In this example, the preoperative serum creatinine is a suitable reference. By contrast, consider the patient who presents with a 2-day history of fever and cough and an elevated creatinine. Let us say the creatinine continues to increase after admission. If there is an increase of at least 0.3 mg/dL over a period of 48 hours or less (any 48-hour period not only the first 48 hours), the patient meets criteria for AKI. However, assume that the patient's creatinine reaches 2.2 mg/dL. What stage is the AKI? Staging is important because the stage correlates with clinical outcomes, such as receipt of renal-replacement therapy (RRT) and mortality.[8-10] A serum creatinine might mean stage 3 AKI, for example, in a patient with a reference creatinine of 0.7 mg/dL, or it could be stage 1 in a patient with a reference creatinine of 1.4 mg/dL. Thus, the reference is extremely important. The best reference creatinine for a patient presenting with AKI is not the admission value because it is likely already abnormal (unless the patient presented only with oliguria). Therefore a baseline creatinine obtained before the current illness but still recent is ideal. Unfortunately, patients rarely have the intuition to get their creatinine checked just before developing AKI. As such one is left with deciding between various less ideal baseline values or no value at all. Various studies have shown that even an old baseline (up to 1 year prior) is better than nothing.[11,12] When multiple baseline values are available, particularly when no clear pattern is discernable, a median is probably the most representative.[11] However, even here, judgment can be important. In a patient whose last six serum creatinines (one each month for the last 6 months) have been slowly rising, the most recent creatinine is probably the best reference. Similarly, some prior baselines might have been in the setting of prior episodes of AKI and it might be possible to select a more representative value out of the series of prior values if the history is known. The best reference creatinine is the one that the clinician believes is most representative of the patient's premorbid renal function.

One of the most difficult clinical problems is the assessment of a patient with abnormal renal function and an uncertain past medical history. The problem is not dissimilar to the cardiac patient with an abnormal but nondiagnostic electrocardiogram (eg, nonspecific T-wave abnormalities) and no prior electrocardiogram on record for comparison. Importantly, a patient presenting with previously unknown kidney disease might have CKD, AKI, or both. In any case, the patient does have "something" and it is incumbent on the heath care system to determine what and to manage it appropriately. Ancillary tests, such as renal ultrasound, can be helpful to determine kidney size and examination of the urine can provide other clues. For example, a 40-year-old white woman presenting with an acute illness and a serum creatinine of 2.0 mg/dL who has normal kidney size on ultrasound and unremarkable urine sediment has AKI until proved otherwise. Conversely, a similar patient with small kidneys and albuminuria has some element of CKD; however, she may well have AKI on CKD. Obviously clinical judgment is required in these cases and what might serve as a provisional diagnosis might well change over time.[3]

If a patient presents with a clinical history compatible with AKI and an abnormal creatinine with no evidence of CKD by history or examination, the best reference creatinine may be a derived one. Because a normal creatinine may vary by more than two-fold based on demographics (especially age, race, and sex) it is not appropriate to use a single normal value for all patients. Instead, the patient's demographics can be fitted into the estimated GFR equations, such as the Modification of Diet in Renal Diseases equation using a GFR of 75 mL/min/1.73 m^2 (**Table 2**).[6] This approach has been validated in multiple studies; one shows that it tends to overestimate the

	Black Men (mg/dL [μmol/L])	Other Men (mg/dL [μmol/L])	Black Women (mg/dL [μmol/L])	Other Women (mg/dL [μmol/L])
Table 2 Estimated baseline creatinine				
Age (y)				
20–24	1.5 (133)	1.0 (88)	1.3 (115)	1.2 (106)
25–29	1.5 (133)	1.2 (106)	1.1 (97)	1.0 (88)
30–39	1.4 (124)	1.2 (106)	1.1 (97)	0.9 (80)
40–54	1.3 (115)	1.1 (97)	1.0 (88)	0.9 (80)
55–65	1.3 (115)	1.1 (97)	1.0 (88)	0.8 (71)
>65	1.2 (106)	1.0 (88)	0.9 (80)	0.8 (71)

Estimated glomerular filtration rate = 75 (mL/min per 1.73 m^2) = 186 × (serum creatinine) − 1.154 × (age) − 0.203 × (0.742 if female) × (1.210 if black) = exp(5.228 − 1.154 × ln [serum creatinine]) − 0.203 × ln(age) − (0.299 if female) + (0.192 if black).

From Bellomo R, Ronco C, Kellum JA, et al, Acute Dialysis Quality Initiative Workgroup. Acute renal failure - definition, outcome measures, animal models, fluid therapy and information technology needs: the Second International Consensus Conference of the Acute Dialysis Quality Initiative (ADQI) Group. Crit Care 2004;8:R207; with permission.

severity of AKI,[11] whereas another shows just the opposite.[12] Differences are likely the result of the frequency of undetected CKD in the population.

SERUM CREATININE AND URINE OUTPUT

Older systems to classify AKI and non–renal-specific organ failure scores, such as the Sepsis-related Organ Failure Assessment,[13] use fixed thresholds for serum creatinine (eg, 2.0 mg/dL) to classify renal "organ failure." This approach is not appropriate for AKI for two reasons. First, normal creatinine may vary by two-fold depending on age, race, and sex (see **Table 2**). Second, a fixed creatinine does not distinguish between acute and chronic abnormalities. Thus, modern methods to quantify severity of AKI are based on relative azotemia, defined by an increase in serum creatinine, or oliguria defined by a decrease in urine output (see **Table 1**). However, patients manifesting both oliguria and azotemia and those in which these impairments are persistent are more likely to have worse disease and therefore worse outcomes.[14]

Recently, using a large heterogeneous series of patients cared for over an 8-year period, we examined the associations between AKI and short- and long-term outcomes as functions of serum creatinine and urine output criteria alone and in combination.[14] Our results demonstrated that despite relatively minor differences in baseline characteristics, patients meeting both serum creatinine and urine output criteria for AKI have dramatically worse outcomes compared with patients who manifest AKI solely or predominantly by one criterion. Indeed as seen in **Table 3**, hospital mortality was less than 18% and RRT was less than 3.5% for the 11,897 (37.1%) patients manifesting AKI by only one parameter. Meanwhile, mortality reached 51.1% and RRT 55.3% for the 2200 (6.9%) patients meeting stage 3 criteria by both serum creatinine and urine output. Even stage 3 criteria in one domain with stage 1 criteria in another was associated with greater than 30% hospital mortality and greater than 10% use of RRT.[14] These results establish the absolute necessity for urine output assessment for staging of AKI. They also seem to contrast with prior work by Ralib and colleagues[15] who found that the oliguria threshold of 0.5 mL/kg/h was not predictive of survival, whereas 0.3 mL/kg/h was. These authors did not examine the effects of serum creatinine and urine output together and their sample size was only 725

Table 3
Relationship between urine output and serum creatinine criteria and clinical outcomes

KDIGO Stage		Urine Output Only				
		No AKI	Stage 1	Stage 2	Stage 3	Total
Serum Creatinine Only	**No AKI**	8179	3158	5421	440	17,198
	Dead	4.3%	5.3%	7.9%	17.7%	5.9%
	RRT	0.0%	0.0%	0.1%	1.1%	0.1%
	Stage 1	1889	1262	3485	842	7478
	Dead	8.0%	11.3%	13.0%	32.1%	13.6%
	RRT	0.3%	0.7%	0.6%	10.9%	1.7%
	Stage 2	618	476	1533	831	3458
	Dead	11.3%	23.9%	21.5%	44.2%	25.5%
	RRT	1.0%	1.3%	1.7%	21.7%	6.3%
	Stage 3	371	321	1019	2200	3911
	Dead	11.6%	38.6%	28.0%	51.1%	40.3%
	RRT	3.2%	17.8%	14.2%	55.3%	36.6%
	Total	11,057	5217	11,458	4313	32,045
	Dead	5.6%	10.5%	13.0%	42.6%	14.0%
	RRT	0.3%	1.4%	1.7%	34.6%	5.6%

Shown are the number of patients, % hospital mortality, and % RRT for patients by maximum AKI criteria (urine output, serum creatinine, or both). Colors denote similar outcome patterns.

Data from Kellum JA, Sileanu FE, Murugan R, et al. Classifying AKI by urine output versus serum creatinine level. J Am Soc Nephrol 2015. [Epub ahead of print].

patients, limiting their statistical power. Other investigators have found urine output to be a sensitive and early marker for AKI and to be associated with adverse outcomes in critically ill patients.[16] Urine output is also affected by renal tubular function as evidenced by response to a "furosemide stress test."[17] Importantly, 1-year outcomes parallel hospital outcomes for the various combinations of serum creatinine and urine output criteria. Indeed the survival curves continue to separate for much of the year following an AKI event.[14]

In addition, isolated oliguria (no creatinine criteria present) is surprisingly frequent and seems to be associated with a long-term hazard. Stage 2 and 3 AKI by urine output criteria alone are associated with decreased 1-year survival. Several studies have emphasized the importance of fluid overload in terms of its effect on clinical outcomes[18–20] and on serum creatinine measurements.[21] It is likely that most patients with oliguria are volume overloaded and it is reasonable to deduce that this represents an adverse effect on survival. It is also conceivable that volume overload masks some degree of azotemia and thus profound oliguria is not just an early indicator of AKI but may be the only indicator.

It is also clear that AKI persistence has a substantial influence on outcome. For example, we found that 4 days at stage 3 AKI results in an approximately 30% rate of death or dialysis at 1 year, whereas it requires more than a week at stage 1 to incur the same hazard.[14] Similarly, Coca and colleagues[22] demonstrated that duration of AKI based on creatinine following surgery was independently associated with subsequent outcome. Thus, risk for death or dialysis following AKI is greatest for patients that meet both serum creatinine and urine output criteria and for those in whom the abnormalities persist longer. However, even a brief episode of isolated oliguria without subsequent azotemia seems to be associated with decreased 1-year survival.

Apart from clinical use, trials of diagnostics and therapeutics for AKI are challenging for several reasons.[23–25] The selection of short-term AKI end points requires an understanding of the relationship between AKI severity and duration and long-term outcomes. In the critically ill, AKI is very common; upward of 75% of patients manifest the syndrome when defined by the full KDIGO criteria.[26] However, spontaneous resolution (or rapid response to treatment) occurs in some patients. Such patients may be less appropriate for enrollment in clinical trials of novel therapeutics. Similarly, for various clinical trial applications, it may be important to select end points that are more closely tied to clinical outcomes.

NOVEL BIOMARKERS

Over the last decade several novel biomarkers have been evaluated for their capacity to detect kidney damage and predict the development of AKI.[27] Most novel markers were developed for their capacity to detect damage and as such they can provide additional insight into AKI, complementary to functional tests, such as serum creatinine and urine output.[28] Note that the relationship between decreasing function and increasing damage is not as straightforward as might be assumed (**Fig. 3**). The characteristic pattern whereby damage proceeds loss of function (**Fig. 3**A) may be seen in some cases of AKI and affords an opportunity to detect "subclinical" AKI before function starts to fall. The problem is that other patterns also occur. For example, functional decline may start to occur alongside damage (**Fig. 3**B) or in some cases

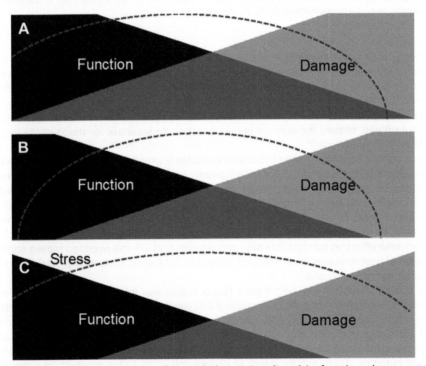

Fig. 3. Various clinical scenarios of acute kidney injury based in function, damage, and stress. The change in kidney function (eg, glomerular filtration rate) is shown in *black* and damage is shown in *gray*. (A) Classic case where damage increases and is followed by a decline in function only after some time (time shown on the x-axis). (B, C) Alternate scenarios where function may change coincidental to or even before damage. The *dashed arc* represents renal cell stress.

function may start to decline even before damage (**Fig. 3**C). This makes damage markers hard to use to forecast AKI. However, other markers might actually measure "stress" occurring at the cellular level before damage or loss of function.

In 2013 we reported the results of a prospective, observational, international investigation (Sapphire study) of tissue inhibitor of metalloproteinases-2 (TIMP-2) and insulin-like growth factor binding protein 7 (IGFBP7) in a heterogeneous group of critically ill patients.[29] In the validation phase we enrolled 744 adults without evidence of AKI. The primary end point was moderate-severe AKI (KDIGO stage 2–3)[3] within 12 hours of sample. The area under the receiver operating characteristic curve was 0.80 for [TIMP-2]•[IGFBP7] and these markers were significantly superior to all previously described markers of AKI (*P*<.002) including neutrophil gelatinase-associated lipocalin and kidney injury molecule-1, none of which achieved an area under the receiver operating characteristic curve greater than 0.72.[29] Two subsequent studies, Opal[30] and Topaz,[31] using the same end point in new cohorts confirmed the test characteristics for predicting AKI.

One of the reasons that [TIMP-2]•[IGFBP7] works for predicting AKI is that the markers relate to a cellular defense mechanism known as cell-cycle arrest. Each phase of the cell cycle has a specific function that is required for appropriate cell proliferation. Quiescent cells are normally in G_0. For cells to divide and begin the process of repair, they must enter and exit each phase of the cell cycle on schedule.[32–34] If the cell exits a phase too soon, or stays in a phase too long, the normal repair and recovery process can become maladaptive.[33] For instance, if epithelial cells remain arrested in G_1 or G_2, it favors a hypertrophic and fibrotic phenotype.[32,34] Conversely, exit from cell cycle in late G_1 leads to apoptosis.[35] Cyclins, cyclin-dependent kinases, and cyclin-dependent kinase inhibitors control each phase of the cell cycle.[33] The cell uses cell-cycle arrest as a protective mechanism to avoid cell-division when potentially damaged.[33,36] By initiating cell-cycle arrest, cells can thus avoid cell division during stress and injury, which is protective. However, if the cells do not reinitiate the cell-cycle and remain arrested at G_1 or G_2 (or possibly other phases of cell cycle), a fibrotic phenotype can ensue. By detecting cell-cycle arrest markers in the urine one may actually be detecting cell stress (depicted as the *dashed lines* in **Fig. 3**). This stress may or may not lead to damage and functional decline but it is the earliest possible point the process can be detected.

DIAGNOSTIC UNCERTAINTY AND FUTURE CLASSIFICATION SYSTEMS

No diagnostic criteria based on serum creatinine and urine output will ever be perfect. Some patients will meet these criteria and not have AKI. For example, a vegetarian with a baseline serum creatinine of 0.4 mg/dL who develops a creatinine of 0.6 after a large protein load may not have any kidney abnormality at all. A patient with short-term dehydration will experience oliguria and yet kidney injury is unlikely in absence of underlying disease or acute nephrotoxic exposures (eg, myoglobin, radiocontrast). A fairly common scenario in hospitalized patients is to see the serum creatinine fall sharply on the first hospital day. Then over the next 48 hours the creatinine rebounds to baseline value. The increase in serum creatinine over the 48 hours may reach 0.3 mg/dL and thus meet AKI criteria. AKI should not be diagnosed in a vacuum and clinical context should always be considered. Conversely, some patients with AKI may not fulfill the diagnostic criteria. A patient receiving large-volume resuscitation or massive transfusion may not achieve the changes in serum creatinine especially early on. Similarly, patients receiving large amounts of diuretics may maintain urine output at least for a time. Clinical judgment works both ways and should always be exercised in evaluating a patient with suspected AKI. Importantly, some investigators have shown that small absolute changes in serum creatinine in patients with low baseline creatinine are less significant than larger changes in the same relative magnitude in patients with high baseline levels.[37] However, our study in critically ill patients found that in those with very low baseline creatinine AKI is nevertheless associated with adverse long-term outcomes.[14]

Novel biomarkers of kidney damage or stress add information to help clinicians arrive at prompt and accurate diagnoses. In the future clinicians may well talk not just about the stage of AKI but the associated biomarker pattern. Patients with the same stage of AKI but with very different urinary [TIMP-2]•[IGFBP7] levels have different long-term outcomes (death or dialysis).[38] In the future clinicians may well speak of "stress positive/damage negative" AKI the way they currently speak of non–ST elevation myocardial infarction or "BRCA1-positive breast cancer."[26,39]

REFERENCES

1. Diamandopoulos A. Twelve centuries of nephrological writings in the Graeco-Roman world of the Eastern Mediterranean (from Hippocrates to Aetius Amidanus). Nephrol Dial Transplant 1999;14(Suppl 2):2–9.
2. Kellum JA. Acute kidney injury. Crit Care Med 2008;36:S141–5.
3. Kidney disease: improving global outcomes (KDIGO) clinical practice guideline for acute kidney injury work group (AKIWG). Kidney Int Suppl 2012;2:1–138, 1–141.
4. Eknoyan G. Emergence of the concept of acute kidney injury. Adv Chronic Kidney Dis 2008;15:308–13.
5. Bywaters EG, Beall D. Crush injuries with impairment of renal function. Br Med J 1941;1:427–32.
6. Bellomo R, Ronco C, Kellum JA, et al, Acute Dialysis Quality Initiative Workgroup. Acute renal failure - definition, outcome measures, animal models, fluid therapy and information technology needs: the Second International Consensus Conference of the Acute Dialysis Quality Initiative (ADQI) Group. Crit Care 2004;8: R204–12.
7. Mehta RL, Kellum JA, Shah SV, et al, Acute Kidney Injury Network. Acute Kidney Injury Network: report of an initiative to improve outcomes in acute kidney injury. Crit Care 2007;11:R31.
8. Hoste EAJ, Clermont G, Kersten A, et al. RIFLE criteria for acute kidney injury are associated with hospital mortality in critically ill patients: a cohort analysis. Crit Care 2006;10:R73.
9. Uchino S, Bellomo R, Goldsmith D, et al. An assessment of the RIFLE criteria for acute renal failure in hospitalized patients*. Crit Care Med 2006;34:1913–7.
10. Sileanu FE, Murugan R, Lucko N, et al. AKI in low-risk versus high-risk patients in intensive care. Clin J Am Soc Nephrol 2015;10(2):187–96. Available at: http://eutils.ncbi.nlm.nih.gov/entrez/eutils/elink.fcgi?dbfrom=pubmed&id=25424992&retmode=ref&cmd=prlinks.
11. Siew ED, Matheny ME, Ikizler TA, et al. Commonly used surrogates for baseline renal function affect the classification and prognosis of acute kidney injury. Kidney Int 2010;77:536–42.
12. Závada J, Hoste E, Cartin-Ceba R, et al. AKI6 investigators: a comparison of three methods to estimate baseline creatinine for RIFLE classification. Nephrol Dial Transplant 2010;25:3911–8.

13. Vincent JL, Moreno R, Takala J, et al. The SOFA (Sepsis-related Organ Failure Assessment) score to describe organ dysfunction/failure. On behalf of the Working Group on Sepsis-Related Problems of the European Society of Intensive Care Medicine. Intensive Care Med 1996;22:707–10.

14. Kellum JA, Sileanu FE, Murugan R, et al. Classifying AKI by urine output versus serum creatinine level. J Am Soc Nephrol 2015. [Epub ahead of print].

15. Ralib AM, Pickering JW, Shaw GM, et al. The urine output definition of acute kidney injury is too liberal. Crit Care 2013;17:R112.

16. Macedo E, Malhotra R, Bouchard J, et al. Oliguria is an early predictor of higher mortality in critically ill patients. Kidney Int 2011;80:760–7.

17. Chawla LS, Davison DL, Brasha-Mitchell E, et al. Development and standardization of a furosemide stress test to predict the severity of acute kidney injury. Crit Care 2013;17:R207.

18. Sutherland SM, Zappitelli M, Alexander SR, et al. Fluid overload and mortality in children receiving continuous renal replacement therapy: the prospective pediatric continuous renal replacement therapy registry. Am J Kidney Dis 2010;55:316–25.

19. Bouchard J, Soroko SB, Chertow GM, et al, Program to Improve Care in Acute Renal Disease (PICARD) Study Group. Fluid accumulation, survival and recovery of kidney function in critically ill patients with acute kidney injury. Kidney Int 2009;76:422–7.

20. Boyd JH, Forbes J, Nakada T-A, et al. Fluid resuscitation in septic shock: a positive fluid balance and elevated central venous pressure are associated with increased mortality. Crit Care Med 2011;39:259–65.

21. Liu KD, Thompson BT, Ancukiewicz M, et al, National Institutes of Health National Heart, Lung, and Blood Institute Acute Respiratory Distress Syndrome Network. Acute kidney injury in patients with acute lung injury: impact of fluid accumulation on classification of acute kidney injury and associated outcomes. Crit Care Med 2011;39:2665–71.

22. Coca SG, King JT, Rosenthal RA, et al. The duration of postoperative acute kidney injury is an additional parameter predicting long-term survival in diabetic veterans. Kidney Int 2010;78:926–33.

23. Palevsky PM, Molitoris BA, Okusa MD, et al. Design of clinical trials in acute kidney injury: report from an NIDDK workshop on trial methodology. Clin J Am Soc Nephrol 2012;7(5):844–50.

24. Okusa MD, Molitoris BA, Palevsky PM, et al. Design of clinical trials in acute kidney injury: a report from an NIDDK workshop–prevention trials. Clin J Am Soc Nephrol 2012;7(5):851–5.

25. Molitoris BA, Okusa MD, Palevsky PM, et al. Design of clinical trials in AKI: a report from an NIDDK workshop. Trials of patients with sepsis and in selected hospital settings. Clin J Am Soc Nephrol 2012;7(5):856–60.

26. Murugan R, Kellum JA. Acute kidney injury: what's the prognosis? Nat Rev Nephrol 2011;7:209–17.

27. Chen L, Koyner JL. Biomarkers in Acute Kidney Injury. 2015, in press.

28. Murray PT, Mehta RL, Shaw A, et al. Potential use of biomarkers in acute kidney injury: report and summary of recommendations from the 10th acute dialysis quality initiative consensus conference. Kidney Int 2014;85:513–21.

29. Kashani K, Al-Khafaji A, Ardiles T, et al. Discovery and validation of cell cycle arrest biomarkers in human acute kidney injury. Crit Care 2013;17:R25.

30. Hoste EAJ, McCullough PA, Kashani K, et al, Sapphire Investigators. Derivation and validation of cutoffs for clinical use of cell cycle arrest biomarkers. Nephrol Dial Transplant 2014;29:2054–61.

31. Bihorac A, Chawla LS, Shaw AD, et al. Validation of cell-cycle arrest biomarkers for acute kidney injury using clinical adjudication. Am J Respir Crit Care Med 2014;189:932–9.
32. Preisig PA, Franch HA. Renal epithelial cell hyperplasia and hypertrophy. Semin Nephrol 1995;15:327–40.
33. Shankland SJ. Cell cycle regulatory proteins in glomerular disease. Kidney Int 1999;56:1208–15.
34. Yang L, Besschetnova TY, Brooks CR, et al. Epithelial cell cycle arrest in G2/M mediates kidney fibrosis after injury. Nat Med 2010;16:535–43.
35. Meikrantz W, Schlegel R. Apoptosis and the cell cycle. J Cell Biochem 1995;58: 160–74.
36. Megyesi J, Safirstein RL, Price PM. Induction of p21WAF1/CIP1/SDI1 in kidney tubule cells affects the course of cisplatin-induced acute renal failure. J Clin Invest 1998;101:777–82.
37. Zeng X, McMahon GM, Brunelli SM, et al. Incidence, outcomes, and comparisons across definitions of AKI in hospitalized individuals. Clin J Am Soc Nephrol 2014; 9:12–20.
38. Koyner JL, Shaw AD, Chawla LS, et al. Tissue inhibitor metalloproteinase-2 (TIMP-2) and IGF-binding protein-7 (IGFBP7) levels are associated with adverse long-term outcomes in patients with AKI. J Am Soc Nephrol 2015;26:1747–54.
39. Kellum JA, Devarajan P. What can we expect from biomarkers for acute kidney injury? Biomark Med 2014;8:1239–45.

Biomarkers in Acute Kidney Injury

Ling-Xin Chen, MD, Jay L. Koyner, MD*

KEYWORDS

- Biomarkers • Acute kidney injury • Renal replacement therapy • Mortality

KEY POINTS

- Biomarkers of acute kidney injury (AKI) not only predict the development of AKI earlier than serum creatinine levels do but are also associated with a variety of adverse patient events, including AKI severity, need for renal replacement therapy (RRT), and inpatient mortality.
- Urinary biomarkers of AKI, including tissue injury metaloproteinase-2 (TIMP2), insulinlike growth factor binding protein-7 (IGFBP7), interleukin (IL)-18, and albumin to creatinine ratio, measured around the time of AKI have all been shown to predict long-term mortality after hospital discharge.
- Several biomarkers of AKI, including neutrophil gelatinase-associated lipocalin (NGAL), TIMP2, and IGFBP7, are available for clinical use around the world.
- The combination of functional and tubular damage biomarkers improves the discrimination of AKI over serum creatinine level alone and is strongly associated with adverse patient outcomes.

INTRODUCTION

AKI is a common syndrome, defined as the abrupt and often reversible decline in glomerular filtration, and portends increased morbidity and mortality, especially in the intensive care unit (ICU) patient population.[1] Actual rates of AKI vary depending on the definition of AKI used.[2,3] Data published from the National Hospital Discharge Survey based on the International Classification of Diseases 9 codes estimated AKI incidence to be 1.9% of all hospital discharges, which is likely a gross underestimation of the total number of AKI cases.[2,3] An international study of AKI in 15,132 critically ill patients demonstrated that AKI (defined according to the Kidney Disease: Improving Global Outcomes [KDIGO] serum creatinine criteria) developed in 32% of subjects and

Disclosures: J.L. Koyner: Consulting and research funding from Astute Medical, research funding from Satellite HealthCare, Abbott/Abbvie; L.X. Chen: Nothing to disclose.
Section of Nephrology, Department of Medicine, University of Chicago, 5841 South Maryland Avenue, Suite S-504, MC 5100, Chicago, IL 60637, USA
* Corresponding author. Section of Nephrology, University of Chicago, 5841 South Maryland Avenue, Suite S-504, MC 5100, Chicago, IL 60637.
E-mail address: jkoyner@uchicago.edu

Crit Care Clin 31 (2015) 633–648
http://dx.doi.org/10.1016/j.ccc.2015.06.002
0749-0704/15/$ – see front matter © 2015 Elsevier Inc. All rights reserved.

criticalcare.theclinics.com

carried a crude mortality rate of 27%.[4] Incident rates have been shown to vary with the definition of AKI.[4,5] However, regardless of its incidence, AKI is known to correlate with poor outcomes, including longer hospitalizations and higher mortality.[6,7] During the last decade the diagnostic criteria of AKI have been standardized, most recently with the aforementioned KDIGO criteria in 2012 (**Table 1**).[8,9] However, these guidelines are still heavily reliant on serum creatinine levels and urine output rates as determinants of AKI, which can often lag behind the actual occurrence of tubular or other intrarenal cellular injury. Serum creatinine is also limited in that its concentrations are affected by factors such as muscle mass, intravascular volume, assay interference, and drug interactions.[10,11] Thus, changes in serum creatinine levels do not accurately or consistently reflect real-time changes in renal function. Similarly, damage to the renal tubular epithelia may not be reflected in serum creatinine levels or urine output until the damage progresses to a critical threshold.

These failings of serum creatinine levels and urine output have, in concert with a call for increased investigation,[12] led to the expansion of the AKI biomarker field in the past decade.[13] Countless investigations have sought to identify markers that can facilitate the early diagnosis, differential diagnosis, and short- and long-term prognosis of AKI. Several of these biomarkers provide information regarding tubular injury, which often precedes functional changes (as determined by serum creatinine), thus not only assisting in earlier diagnosis of AKI but also potentially distinguishing a particular type of AKI. Ideally, a biomarker should be specific to kidney injury, predict the earlier onset of AKI, identify the site and/or cause of injury, and predict significant adverse outcomes. The search for the ideal kidney injury biomarker has been limited by the lack of a perfect gold standard, because using the KDIGO guidelines mentioned earlier as gold standard relies on the imperfections of serum creatinine levels.[14]

At a recent Acute Dialysis Quality Initiative (ADQI) international consensus conference, experts assessed the utilization biomarkers for the differential diagnosis, the prognosis, and management of AKI.[15] The findings and utility of biomarkers were presented in several summary statements from this conference.[16–19] One of the end products of this conference was a reconceptualization of biomarkers via the combination of functional (eg, serum creatinine) and damage biomarkers (**Table 2**). This review discusses the current state of AKI biomarkers, how they perform in the early diagnosis of AKI, what further information they yield, and how they can be used in various clinical settings.

Table 1		
KDIGO criteria for acute kidney injury		
Stage	**Serum Creatinine**	**Urine Output**
1	1.5–1.9 times baseline or $\geq$0.3 mg/dL ($\geq$26.5 µmol/L) increase	<0.5 mL/kg/h for 6–12 h
2	2.0–2.9 times baseline	<0.5 mL/kg/h for $\geq$12 h
3	3.0 times baseline or Increase in serum creatinine level to $\geq$4.0 mg/dL ($\geq$353.6 µmol/L) or Initiation of renal replacement therapy or In patients <18 y, decrease in eGFR to <35 mL/min per 1.73 m²	<0.3 mL/kg/h for $\geq$24 h or anuria for $\geq$12 h

Abbreviation: eGFR, estimated glomerular filtration rate.

From Kidney Disease: Improving Global Outcomes (KDIGO) Acute Kidney Injury Work Group. KDIGO clinical practice guideline for acute kidney injury. Kidney Int Suppl 2012;2:19; with permission.

Table 2
ADQI criteria: incorporating biomarkers into the definition of AKI

	No Damage/Biomarker Negative	Damage Present/Biomarker Positive
No functional change/ creatinine negative	No functional changes or damage	Damage without loss of function
Functional change/creatinine positive	Loss of function without damage	Damage with loss of function

Adapted from Endre ZH, Kellum JA, Di Somma S, et al. Differential diagnosis of AKI in clinical practice by functional and damage biomarkers: workgroup statements from the tenth Acute Dialysis Quality Initiative Consensus Conference. Contrib Nephrol 2013;182:32; with permission.

SUMMARY OF KEY BIOMARKERS

To date, there have been more than 30 candidate biomarkers for AKI identified and investigated.[13,20,21] **Table 3** describes the 8 most widely investigated biomarkers and their physiologic actions.

CLINICAL SETTINGS
Cardiac Surgery

Biomarkers of AKI are well studied in the population undergoing cardiac surgery because postoperative AKI is a common adverse event and is independently associated with morbidity and mortality.[22–24] A seminal paper by Mishra and colleagues[25] investigating serum and urine NGAL levels in the setting of pediatric cardiac surgery heralded the explosion of biomarker papers during the last decade. In this single-center study of 71 children, urinary NGAL level was found to be an almost perfect predictor of AKI with an area under the curve (AUC) of 0.99. The performance of urine NGAL (and other promising biomarkers) has not been duplicated; however, there have been countless studies investigating biomarkers of AKI after cardiac surgery.

This review focuses on larger multicenter biomarker investigations. In the setting of AKI associated with cardiac surgery, the authors highlight the Translational Research Investigating Biomarkers and Endpoints for Acute Kidney Injury (TRIBE-AKI) study. TRIBE-AKI is a large multicenter international prospective observational investigation of AKI biomarkers after adult and pediatric cardiac surgery. In this study of 1219 adults, several plasma and urinary biomarkers were measured at various perioperative time points. The researchers investigated a variety of AKI end points, including mild AKI, defined as a 50% increase in serum creatinine level from baseline, and severe AKI, defined as a doubling of preoperative serum creatinine level or the need for RRT. Many of the biomarkers investigated demonstrated associations with the development of postoperative mild and severe AKI. Although the TRIBE-AKI study involved an adult cohort of individuals at high risk for AKI, it was limited by a predominantly Caucasian population and a low number of severe AKI events (n = 60).

The TRIBE-AKI cohort found that, although plasma and urinary NGAL and urine IL-18 levels were diagnostic of early AKI, the effect was not significant for urine NGAL level when adjusting for factors known to contribute to AKI.[26] However, plasma and urinary NGAL and urinary IL-18 levels were all significantly associated with other clinical outcomes, such as length of hospital stay, need for dialysis, and inpatient mortality.[26] A follow-up study of this same adult cohort found that plasma NGAL (AUC [SE], 0.74 [0.04]) and urinary IL-18 (0.63 [0.05]) levels along with urinary albumin to creatinine ratio (0.67 [0.04]) were also predictive of AKI progression (defined as a worsening of Acute Kidney Injury Network [AKIN] AKI stage) when measured at the time of

Table 3
Characteristics and physiologic action for biomarkers of AKI

Category	Biomarker	Description	Physiologic Action
GFR markers	Serum cystatin C	13 kDa protein produced at a constant rate with little protein binding[20,74]	Inhibitors of cysteine proteinases cathepsin H, B, L and calpains.[20,74] Serum levels affected by diabetes, corticosteroids, hyperthyroidism, hypertriglyceridemia, hyperbilirubinemia, rheumatoid factor, inflammation[75,76]
Tubular injury markers	Urine cystatin C	13 kDa protein produced at a constant rate with little protein binding[20,74]	Freely filtered in glomerulus and degraded in proximal tubules, so usually not present in urine.[20] Urinary level may increase with albuminuria through competitive inhibition of reabsorption[77]
	Interleukin (IL)-18	IL-1 family cytokine precursor cleaved by caspase-1 to 17.2 kDa active form[78]	Induces IFN-γ and T-cell activation.[78] Urinary IL-18 found to mediate ATN in mice[79] and to be a marker of ATN in humans[62]
	Kidney injury molecule 1 or T-cell immunoglobulin and mucin domain containing protein 1 (KIM-1 or TIM-1)	40–70 kDa glycosylated transmembrane protein receptor expressed in proximal tubules, important in recognizing apoptotic cells[80,81]	Upregulated after proximal tubule ischemic injury.[80] Expressed by immune cells to activate differentiation of T helper 1, 2, and 17 cells[82] FDA approved for use in preclinical drug development
	Liver-type fatty acid-binding protein	15 kDa protein expressed in proximal tubules[83]	Binds free fatty acids and transports them to mitochondria or peroxisomes. Found to be upregulated after ischemic injury.[20,84] In mouse models found also a marker for COX-inhibitor and cisplatin-induced AKI[85,86]
	Urinary N-acetyl-β-glucosaminidase	~140 kDa proximal tubule enzyme, not renally filtered[20]	A sensitive urinary marker of loss of lysosomal integrity in proximal tubule and may reflect improvements in proximal tubular function. Inhibited by urea, industrial solvents, heavy metals.[20] Not elevated with sepsis[87]
	Neutrophil gelatinase-associated lipocalin (NGAL)	25 kDa lipocalin protein covalently bound to gelatinase from neutrophils. May exist as monomer or dimer. Expressed in lung, liver, kidney[88]	Binds to free iron and assists in response to bacterial infection.[89] Upregulated in distal nephron in response to AKI but also released from liver and neutrophils in sepsis.[90] Assay differences due to different forms of NGAL[91]

| Cell cycle arrest | Tissue inhibitor metalloproteinase-2 and insulinlike growth factor binding protein-7 (TIMP-2 and IGFBP7) | TIMP-2 is part of the TIMP family of protease inhibitors expressed ubiquitously[92] IGFBP7 is expressed in vascular endothelial cells, binds to insulin and insulinlike growth factor[93] | TIMP-2 inhibits matrix metalloproteinases, thus promoting fibrosis and blocking endothelial proliferation.[94,95] IGFBP7 inhibits endothelial angiogenesis, among other functions.[93,96] Both are markers of cell-cycle arrest and are upregulated after kidney injury[45,97] |

Abbreviations: ATN, acute tubular necrosis; COX, cyclooxygenase; FDA, US Food and Drug Administration; GFR, glomerular filtration rate; IFN, interferon.

creatinine-based diagnosis of AKI.[27] The ability of these biomarkers to identify those with the most severe forms of AKI may be useful in the future for studies of AKI therapies, allowing targeting of those who are least likely to recover spontaneously and those at the highest risk for the most adverse patient outcomes.[27]

Both urinary and serum cystatin C have been studied in the TRIBE-AKI cardiac surgery population; it was found that preoperative serum cystatin C levels predicted postoperative AKI better than serum creatinine-based glomerular filtration rate (GFR) estimations, indicating superiority of serum cystatin C as an index of baseline GFR.[28] Preoperative urinary albumin and plasma brain natriuretic peptide levels were found to be associated with postoperative AKI and other clinical outcomes such as the need for postoperative dialysis and length of ICU stay and hospitalization.[29,30] However, not every biomarker measured in the TRIBE AKI cohort was successful in predicting postoperative AKI; when measured within the first postoperative hour, urinary cystatin C level was not associated with the postoperative AKI in either the adult or pediatric TRIBE-AKI cohorts.[31] In the TRIBE-AKI pediatric cohort, serum cystatin C levels independently predicted longer duration of mechanical ventilation and longer length of ICU stay.[32] However, in the adult population, postoperative serum cystatin C level was not as sensitive as postoperative serum creatinine level in identifying AKI cases.[33] The TRIBE-AKI group also assessed the performance of other biomarkers, including kidney injury molecule (KIM)-1 and liver-type fatty acid-binding protein (L-FABP), both of which performed modestly in their ability to predict early postoperative AKI, but neither was able to predict AKI progression. Finally, in an attempt to combine data from the different biomarkers, the TRIBE-AKI group demonstrated that the combination of 3 biomarkers in the early postoperative period (urinary KIM-1, urinary IL-18, and plasma NGAL) yielded the highest AUC of 0.78 for the prediction of AKI, thus suggesting that a panel of biomarkers may provide more information than each biomarker taken individually.[34]

The TRIBE-AKI group has published on the association of these same perioperative biomarkers of AKI with long-term, post-hospital, all-cause mortality (median follow-up [interquartile range], 3.0 years [2.2–3.6]).[31] As expected, long-term mortality was higher in those with AKI (80 deaths per 1000 person-years) than in those with no postoperative AKI (40 deaths per 1000 years). In addition, in those with and without AKI, the highest tertile of peak postoperative urinary biomarker concentration was associated with increased mortality. The hazard ratios for those with AKI ranged from 2.0 to 3.2 (for IL-18, urine albumin creatinine ratio (ACR), and KIM-1), whereas the association was attenuated in those without AKI, with hazard ratios 1.2 to 1.8 (KIM-1 and IL-18).[31] Although it was not formally compared in the analyses, the urinary biomarker-associated mortality risk was strikingly similar between those in the highest biomarker tertile without AKI (elevated biomarkers of injury but no change in glomerular function) and those in the lowest biomarker tertile with AKI (no change in biomarkers of injury but change in glomerular function/serum creatinine level) (see **Table 2**). Although there are differences between these biomarker positive/creatinine negative and biomarker negative/creatinine positive cohorts, they appear to be similar on some levels, and these subgroups require further investigation.

Critical Illness and Sepsis

Sepsis accounts for almost half of AKI cases in the critically ill, and about 30% of these are community acquired.[13,35] In the setting of sepsis, ICU admission, or critical illness, several biomarkers have demonstrated an association with AKI and other adverse patient outcomes. The first large-scale head-to-head comparison of biomarkers of AKI in the critically ill was the EARLY-Acute Renal Failure (ARF) trial, which included

528 critically ill patients across 2 regional ICUs in New Zealand.[36] The EARLY-ARF trial originally set out to study erythropoietin as an intervention for AKI therapy and relied on urinary levels of γ-glutamyl transpeptidase (GGT) and alkaline phosphatase (AP) to guide patient enrollment.[37] Although the trial result showed no effect from early erythropoietin in AKI outcomes, the samples collected from the study led to a series of secondary analyses of AKI biomarkers, including GGT, AP, NGAL, cystatin C, KIM-1, and IL-18. Unfortunately, none of these were found to have an AUC more than 0.7, for the prediction of early AKI. Urinary cystatin C, NGAL, IL-18, and KIM-1 all performed similarly in AKI identification at study entry (AUCs between 0.62 and 0.67). Urinary NGAL levels predicted RRT within 7 days, the best with an AUC of 0.79 (0.65–0.94), whereas the other biomarkers performed slightly worse (AUCs 0.62–0.73). Urinary cystatin C, NGAL, and IL-18 performed similarly in prediction of death within 7 days (AUC, 0.66–0.68).[36] When the cohort was stratified by baseline estimated GFR (eGFR) and the timing of biomarker measurement, biomarker performance for the prediction of early AKI improved significantly in all the biomarkers studied, with IL-18 levels measured at 12 to 36 hours after kidney insult reaching an AUC of 0.94 (0.80–1) for those with eGFR less than 60 mL/min.[36] Others have demonstrated a similar benefit to stratifying biomarkers by preexisting chronic kidney disease (CKD) status and timing after injury.[38,39] Thus, biomarker usage and future tests of a biomarker's predictive ability should potentially consider not only the patient's baseline eGFR but also perhaps the timing after injury.[39]

In a large single-center case-control study of 380 critically ill patients across various ICUs (130 of who had AKI defined as AKIN stage 1), Siew and colleagues[40] demonstrated that urinary cystatin C, NGAL, and L-FABP yielded AUCs less than 0.60 for prediction of AKI. This same group also found that urinary IL-18 was not useful in the prediction of AKI in the ICU setting.[41] In both studies, these biomarkers had some predictive value for outcomes such as death or dialysis. In prediction of death or acute dialysis within 28 days, urine NGAL had an odds ratio (OR) of 1.53 (95% confidence interval [CI], 1.07–2.19) and IL-18 had an OR of 1.86 (95% CI, 1.31–2.64).[41] Other smaller trials have also found mixed predictive ability in these biomarkers.[42,43] Given that NGAL, IL-18, and KIM-1 are inflammatory markers the levels of which may be increased in sepsis, regardless of the presence or absence of AKI, their use for AKI diagnosis is perhaps limited in the setting of sepsis. When patients without sepsis in the ICU were studied, the levels of NGAL and KIM-1 were found to increase 1 day before the increase of serum creatinine levels in AKI.[44]

Urinary markers TIMP-2 and IGFBP7 have been found to be highly predictive of AKI in the ICU population.[45] The SAPPHIRE study included a 3-center discovery cohort of 522 critically ill patients who suffered AKI from multiple causes (sepsis, shock, major surgery, and trauma) as well as a prospective observational international validation cohort of 728 critically ill subjects.[45] In the validation arm, patients were selected to be at high risk for AKI due to the presence of cardiovascular or respiratory dysfunction (as measured by sequential organ failure assessment (SOFA) score) at the time of ICU admission with a primary end point being the progression to KDIGO stages 2 or 3 within the first 12 postenrollment hours.[45] When compared with other biomarkers, including NGAL, KIM-1, and IL-18, TIMP-2*IGFBP7 demonstrated better prediction of stage 2–3 AKI with a C-statistic (95% CI) of 0.8 (0.75–0.84).[45] These markers have been subsequently validated in follow-up studies; they have been approved for clinical use to predict stage 2 or 3 AKI within the first 12 to 24 hours of ICU admission in the United States.[46,47]

The strength of TIMP-2*IGFBP7 largely lies within its extremely high negative predictive value (NPV) at low values (eg, 0.3 [ng/mL]^2/1000 NPV [95% CI, 97

(96–99)]).[46] Thus, critically ill patients with low TIMP-2*IGFBP7 levels are at low risk for the development of severe AKI even in the setting of elevated clinical suspicion. At higher values, TIMP-2*IGFBP7 remains useful, but the interpretation of values 0.3 to 2.0 (ng/mL)^2/1000 is more reliant on clinical suspicion for AKI. At these higher values, the NPV remains between 85% and 93%, with the positive predictive value (PPV) ranging from 30% to 65%.[46,47] TIMP-2*IGFBP7 has been recently approved for clinical use, but there has not been much published about the day-to-day clinical use of the assay outside of the aforementioned discovery and validation studies.[45–47] The publication of several investigations of these biomarkers over the next several years will foster new knowledge on the utility of these markers in the day to day care of critically ill patients at risk for severe AKI. In the interim, Kellum and Chawla[48] have proposed a potential clinical approach for the use of this new test in the specific setting of individuals undergoing cardiac surgery.

The 9-month outcomes data from the validation arm of the SAPPHIRE trial showed that patients with AKI whose levels of TIMP-2*IGFBP7 greater than 2.0 at the time of study enrollment (roughly 6–12 hours after ICU admission) had a hazard ratio of 2.16 (95% CI, 1.32–3.53) for the composite incidence of all-cause mortality or RRT compared with those without elevation of TIMP-2*IGFBP7 levels (<0.3) .[49] In this adjusted analysis, the 692-subject cohort was stratified by AKI status (defined as any KDIGO stage AKI within the first 72 hours of ICU stay) to account for the interaction between the biomarkers and AKI. This association between TIMP-2*IGFBP7 and the 9-month incidence of the composite end point was specific to AKI whereby there was a stepwise increase in death or dialysis in those with AKI based on their admission TIMP-2*IGFBP7 concentration but no increased risk for those without AKI, regardless of TIMP-2*IGFBP7 concentration.[49] These results, taken in concert with aforementioned data from the TRIBE-AKI long-term follow-up, are promising for the future of biomarkers in the prediction of poor post-hospitalization clinical outcomes,[31,50] although further investigation is needed to examine the utility of biomarkers in predicting end points such as the development of post-AKI CKD or renal recovery.

Although these studies represent some of the largest biomarker studies in the critically ill, several smaller studies have used biomarkers for a variety of novel purposes. In a post hoc analysis of the Genetic and Inflammatory Markers of Sepsis study cohort (a multicenter prospective study of 1836 patients admitted with community-acquired pneumonia), Srisawat and colleagues[51] identified 189 patients who achieved RIFLE-F AKI (Risk, Injury, Failure, Loss of kidney function, and End Stage Renal Disease which is a diagnostic criteria for AKI - where F stand for the level of failure) during hospitalization and compared plasma NGAL levels between those who did and did not recover (defined as either being alive off RRT or having persistent RIFLE-F at hospital discharge). They found that using plasma NGAL levels measured on the first day of RIFLE-F AKI, pedicted failure of renal recovery with an AUC of 0.74 (95% CI, 0.66–0.81). Biomarkers may be useful predictors of short and long-term mortality when measured at the time of RRT initiation, as demonstrated by Lin and colleagues[50] in a single-center study of 101 critically ill patients who developed AKI requiring RRT. Levels of IL-18 and cystatin C collected on the first day of RRT were independent predictors of hospital mortality, with IL-18 levels also predicting 6-month mortality.[50] Finally, in the setting of critical illness, investigators have begun to investigate the combination of functional and structural biomarkers of renal function to predict adverse patient outcomes, as described by the ADQI consensus conference.[16] A prospective single-center study of mechanically ventilated patients in the ICU combined biomarkers of glomerular filtration and tubular damage measured at ICU admission for prediction of dialysis. Of the

106 subjects, 50 required dialysis within 10 days of ICU admission. They found that the combination of serum cystatin C ($\geq$1.4 mg/L) and urine NGAL ($\geq$106.7 ng/mL) concentrations was the best predictor for RRT initiation (AUC 0.8, positive predictive value of 0.67, and NPV 0.87).[52]

Emergency Department

AKI biomarkers have also been investigated at the time of emergency room presentation. In a single-center prospective cohort study of 635 patients presenting to the emergency room, of which only 30 developed RIFLE-R criteria AKI that did not reverse in 3 days, Nickolas and colleagues[53] found that urinary NGAL levels yielded an AUC of 0.94 (0.881–1.000) for AKI prediction. The NGAL level was also highly predictive of clinical outcomes, including inpatient nephrology consultation, need for RRT, and admission to the ICU. However, serum creatinine also performed well in AKI prediction, with an AUC of 0.92 (0.86–0.98). This study specifically defined AKI separately from prerenal azotemia, which was defined as any AKI that resolved within 3 days of treatment or was accompanied by fractional excretion of sodium (FENa) of less than 1%.[53] This approach highlights the possibility of biomarkers as markers specific to irreversible renal injury or renal injury that has progressed to the point of tubular damage. A follow-up international multicenter prospective study of 1635 unselected patients presenting to the emergency department (ED) who were subsequently admitted to the hospital also sought to examine biomarkers in a discriminatory role between prerenal azotemia, intrinsic AKI, and stable CKD.[54] Of the biomarkers studied (urinary levels of NGAL, KIM-1, IL-18, L-FABP, and cystatin C), none performed better than serum creatinine in the diagnosis of intrinsic AKI, although urinary NGAL did have the highest AUC among biomarkers at 0.81 (0.76–0.86). The AUC of NGAL also increased in parallel with RIFLE severity class and, when combined with serum creatinine, improved prediction for in-hospital dialysis or mortality.[54]

Perhaps most impressive in this study was the examination combining biomarkers of function and damage to improve patient risk assessment. In this cohort of 1635 subjects, a cutoff of 104 ng/mL for urine NGAL and 1.4 mg/dL for creatinine meant that 5.3% of those who were NGAL positive/creatinine negative received RRT or experienced inpatient mortality. This result was not statistically different from the 5.1% of those who were NGAL negative/creatinine positive who experienced the same composite end point but was significantly higher than those who were NGAL negative/creatinine negative (see **Table 2**).[54] The investigators demonstrated a similar finding for KIM-1 (cutoff, 2.82 ng/mL) and creatinine (cutoff, 1.4 mg/dL), with KIM-1-positive/creatinine-negative subjects being at increased risk for the same composite end point. Thus, even in the setting of the ED there is utility in combining functional and structural biomarkers of kidney function, with those who are biomarker positive/creatinine positive being at highest risk for all of the adverse patient outcomes.[54,55]

Others have investigated biomarkers in patients in the ED for their ability to differentiate between prerenal azotemia and intrinsic AKI. In a single-center observational cohort of 616 patients presenting to the ED, Soto and colleagues[56] examined the predictive ability of plasma NGAL for intrinsic AKI, as defined by RIFLE or AKIN criteria that did not resolve by 3 days after admission. Plasma NGAL levels had the highest AUC (95% CI) for prediction of AKI at time 12 hours after presentation (0.85 [0.81–0.90]) and had an AUC of 0.73 (0.68–0.79) for distinguishing between prerenal azotemia and intrinsic AKI.[56] This same group investigated the performance of serum and urine cystatin C, which did not perform as well as NGAL for the prediction of AKI or the discrimination between prerenal and intrinsic AKI.[57] Plasma NGAL was separately studied in a secondary analysis of a multicenter prospective observational cohort of

661 patients in the ED with suspected sepsis (systemic inflammatory response syndrome criteria or serum lactate concentration >2.5 mmol/L).[58] AKI was defined as a greater than 0.5 mg/dL increase in serum creatinine level within 72 hours or need for RRT and occurred in 24 (3.6%) patients. Plasma NGAL level had an AUC of 0.82 (95% CI, 0.76–0.88) for prediction of AKI, as compared with serum creatinine level, which had an AUC of 0.73 (95% CI, 0.63–0.84). Although this study did not discriminate between prerenal azotemia and intrinsic AKI, it examined the predictive ability of NGAL for all-cause in-hospital mortality, AUC 0.75 (0.68–0.82) as compared with the AUC of serum creatinine level of 0.65 (0.57–0.73).[58]

The above-mentioned studies have important limitations in that different NGAL assays and cutoffs were used across studies for their different desired outcomes. These studies also used different patient selection criteria, and none of them included a component of urine microscopy or physician assessment, both of which have been shown to improve patient risk stratification in the ED.[59,60] These issues need to be further studied and validated in larger multicenter ED studies.

DISCRIMINATORY FUNCTION

As discussed earlier, an important function of an ideal biomarker is to discriminate between different types of renal injury, especially prerenal azotemia and intrinsic renal damage, because this distinction is difficult to define using creatinine levels and urine output. Although the limited literature on biomarkers and the differential diagnosis of AKI in the ED was discussed earlier,[53,54,56] this discriminatory function has been investigated in other clinical settings. Early studies demonstrated that urinary IL-18 and KIM-1 levels can distinguish between acute tubular necrosis (ATN) and other renal processes, including CKD and prerenal azotemia.[61–63] However, secondary analysis of the EARLY-ARF study (n = 529) demonstrated that several biomarkers (IL-18, cystatin C, NGAL, and KIM-1) also increased in prerenal AKI, which was defined as AKI with FENa less than 1% and recovery within 48 hours of treatment.[64] In this study, only urine cystatin C and IL-18 exhibited a significant stepwise increase in concentration in those with no AKI to those with prerenal AKI to those with AKI that lasted longer than 48 hours. Similarly, in a study of critically ill patients with AKI, Doi and colleagues[65] showed elevations in urinary L-FABP, NGAL, IL-18, and albumin concentrations in patients in the ICU with prerenal AKI, compared with those with no AKI. These findings are in line with the ongoing controversy of whether separation of prerenal azotemia and ATN is a valid diagnostic approach because it is becoming increasingly recognized that prerenal azotemia and ATN occur along the spectrum of AKI.[61,66,67] Further complicating the issue is lack of a true gold standard for diagnosis of prerenal azotemia, which is why the authors favor the aforementioned paradigm advocated by the ADQI consensus conference (see **Table 2**).[16]

This ADQI approach was used by Basu and colleagues[68] who used urinary NGAL as a marker of tubular injury and plasma cystatin C as a marker of functional damage. In their single-center retrospective study of 345 pediatric patients undergoing cardiopulmonary bypass, patients were grouped into 1 of 4 groups according to the urine NGAL (cutoff 200 ng/mg creatinine) and serum cystatin C (cutoff, 0.8 mg/L) concentrations and they compared the performance of these biomarkers for the prediction of persistent AKI (defined as AKI lasting more than 48 hours). They found that the dual-positive NGAL+/cystatin C+ composite was a better predictor of persistent AKI than serum creatinine and that the NGAL+/cystatin C− composite also trended toward better prediction of persistent AKI than serum creatinine. In the NGAL−/cystatin C+ group, all had reversible AKI (recovery within 48 hours).[68] Thus, in yet another study, the combination of a glomerular function and tubular injury biomarker improved diagnostic precision over serum creatinine alone.

One final example of the benefit of combining functional and structural biomarkers in predicting adverse patient outcomes in the setting of AKI is the furosemide stress test (FST). Koyner and colleagues demonstrated that in those with early AKI (AKIN stage 1 or 2), the 2-hour urine output following a standardized one-time intravenous dose of furosemide (1.0 mg/kg in furosemide-naive patients and 1.5 mg/kg in those with prior exposure) was highly predictive of adverse patient outcomes.[69] Urine output of less than 100 mL/h in the first 2 hours following furosemide administration was associated with a sensitivity and specificity of 87% and 84% for the progression to stage 3 AKI (AUC 0.87). In these 77 patients with early AKI and the absence of hypovolemia, the urine output following the FST was also associated with an increased risk of the need for RRT and inpatient mortality. In a post hoc analysis, when FST results were analyzed in those with elevated AKI biomarkers (NGAL >150 ng/mL [n = 44] or TIMP-2*IGFBP7 >0.3 [n = 32]), the ability to predict these same adverse events was even better.[69] Thus, combining biomarkers of injury with a functional marker of nephron integrity in the setting of early AKI allows for the rapid identification of patients at the highest risk for the most adverse outcomes, and this may be useful as nephrologist and intensivists move forward into clinical trials to treat AKI.[70]

SUMMARY

During the last decade, AKI biomarkers have gone from being at the top of a clinical nephrologist's wish list to a clinical reality. Recent data demonstrate that biomarkers can determine which patients are at risk for the future development of not only AKI (as measured by serum creatinine and urine output) but also other adverse events, such as the need for RRT and inpatient and long-term postdischarge mortality. With several different biomarkers being clinically available around the world, one can begin to use them to test the efficacy of potential AKI interventions. The EARLY-ARF trial was the first trial to use biomarkers to select patients for an AKI intervention.[37] Others have used biomarkers as part of an interventional trial to trigger the early initiation of RRT.[71,72] In the future, biomarkers will be used to select patients at the highest risk for the most adverse outcomes to prioritize enrollment for interventional trials. This is not to say that our current panel of biomarkers are perfect, they are not; nephrologists and intensivists still desperately need tools to better understand the pathophysiology and epidemiology of AKI, renal recovery, and the links between AKI and the development of CKD.[73] As the investigation of biomarkers continues and expands from the emergency room, ICU, and post cardiac surgery to include more specific clinical settings such as organ transplant or cardiorenal syndromes, it is expected that the use of biomarkers will result in changes in clinical outcomes, giving clinicians more powerful tools to make important clinical decisions.

REFERENCES

1. Bagshaw SM, Mortis G, Doig CJ, et al. One-year mortality in critically ill patients by severity of kidney dysfunction: a population-based assessment. Am J Kidney Dis 2006;48:402–9.
2. Liangos O, Wald R, O'Bell JW, et al. Epidemiology and outcomes of acute renal failure in hospitalized patients: a national survey. Clin J Am Soc Nephrol 2006;1: 43–51.
3. Palevsky PM. Epidemiology of acute renal failure: the tip of the iceberg. Clin J Am Soc Nephrol 2006;1:6–7.

4. Srisawat N, Sileanu FE, Murugan R, et al. Variation in risk and mortality of acute kidney injury in critically ill patients: a multicenter study. Am J Nephrol 2015;41: 81–8.

5. Uchino S, Kellum JA, Bellomo R, et al. Acute renal failure in critically ill patients: a multinational, multicenter study. JAMA 2005;294:813–8.

6. Chertow GM, Burdick E, Honour M. Acute kidney injury, mortality, length of stay, and costs in hospitalized patients. J Am Soc Nephrol 2005;16:3365–70.

7. Hoste EA, Clermont G, Kersten A. RIFLE criteria for acute kidney injury are associated with hospital mortality in critically ill patients: a cohort analysis. Crit Care 2006;10:R73.

8. Kidney Disease: Improving Global Outcomes (KDIGO) Acute Kidney Injury Work Group. KDIGO clinical practice guideline for acute kidney injury. Kidney Int Suppl 2012;2:1–138.

9. Singbartl K, Kellum JA. AKI in the ICU: definition, epidemiology, risk stratification, and outcomes. Kidney Int 2012;81(9):819–25.

10. Baum N, Dichoso CC, Carlton CE Jr. Blood urea nitrogen and serum creatinine: physiology and interpretations. Urology 1975;5:583–8.

11. Ducharme MP, Smythe M, Strohs G. Drug-induced alterations in serum creatinine concentrations. Ann Pharmacother 1993;27:622–33.

12. American Society of Nephrology. The American Society of Nephrology renal research report. J Am Soc Nephrol 2005;16:1886–903.

13. Koyner JL, Parikh CR. Clinical utility of biomarkers of AKI in cardiac surgery and critical illness. Clin J Am Soc Nephrol 2013;8:1034–42.

14. Waikar SS, Betensky RA, Emerson SC, et al. Imperfect gold standards for kidney injury biomarker evaluation. J Am Soc Nephrol 2012;23:13–21.

15. Murray PT, Mehta RL, Shaw A, et al. Potential use of biomarkers in acute kidney injury: report and summary of recommendations from the 10th Acute Dialysis Quality Initiative consensus conference. Kidney Int 2014;85:513–21.

16. Endre ZH, Kellum JA, Di Somma S, et al. Differential diagnosis of AKI in clinical practice by functional and damage biomarkers: workgroup statements from the tenth Acute Dialysis Quality Initiative Consensus Conference. Contrib Nephrol 2013;182:30–44.

17. Okusa MD, Jaber BL, Doran P, et al. Physiological biomarkers of acute kidney injury: a conceptual approach to improving outcomes. Contrib Nephrol 2013; 182:65–81.

18. Cruz DN, Bagshaw SM, Maisel A, et al. Use of biomarkers to assess prognosis and guide management of patients with acute kidney injury. Contrib Nephrol 2013;182:45–64.

19. McCullough PA, Shaw AD, Haase M, et al. Diagnosis of acute kidney injury using functional and injury biomarkers: workgroup statements from the tenth Acute Dialysis Quality Initiative Consensus Conference. Contrib Nephrol 2013;182: 13–29.

20. Charlton JR, Portilla D, Okusa MD. A basic science view of acute kidney injury biomarkers. Nephrol Dial Transplant 2014;29(7):1301–11.

21. Vanmassenhove J, Vanholder R, Nagler E, et al. Urinary and serum biomarkers for the diagnosis of acute kidney injury: an in-depth review of the literature. Nephrol Dial Transplant 2013;28:254–73.

22. Hansen MK, Gammelager H, Mikkelsen MM, et al. Post-operative acute kidney injury and five-year risk of death, myocardial infarction, and stroke among elective cardiac surgical patients: a cohort study. Crit Care 2013;17:R292.

23. Hansen MK, Gammelager H, Jacobsen CJ, et al. Acute kidney injury and long-term risk of cardiovascular events after cardiac surgery: a population-based cohort study. J Cardiothorac Vasc Anesth 2015;29(3):617–25.

24. Chertow G, Levy E, Hammermeister K, et al. Independent association between acute renal failure and mortality following cardiac surgery. Am J Med 1998;104: 343–8.

25. Mishra J, Dent C, Tarabishi R, et al. Neutrophil gelatinase-associated lipocalin (NGAL) as a biomarker for acute renal injury after cardiac surgery. Lancet 2005;365:1231–8.

26. Parikh CR, Coca SG, Thiessen-Philbrook H, et al. Postoperative biomarkers predict acute kidney injury and poor outcomes after adult cardiac surgery. J Am Soc Nephrol 2011;22:1748–57.

27. Koyner JL, Garg AX, Coca SG, et al. Biomarkers predict progression of acute kidney injury after cardiac surgery. J Am Soc Nephrol 2012;23:905–14.

28. Shlipak MG, Coca SG, Wang Z, et al. Presurgical serum cystatin C and risk of acute kidney injury after cardiac surgery. Am J Kidney Dis 2011;58:366–73.

29. Coca SG, Jammalamadaka D, Sint K, et al. Pre-operative proteinuria predicts acute kidney injury in patients undergoing cardiac surgery. J Thorac Cardiovasc Surg 2012;143:495–502.

30. Patel UD, Storti S, Lorenzoni V, et al. Pre-operative serum brain natriuretic peptide and risk of acute kidney injury after cardiac surgery. Circulation 2012;125:1347–55.

31. Coca SG, Garg AX, Thiessen-Philbrook H, et al. Urinary biomarkers of AKI and mortality 3 years after cardiac surgery. J Am Soc Nephrol 2014;25(5):1063–71.

32. Zappitelli M, Krawczeski CD, Devarajan P, et al. Early postoperative serum cystatin C predicts severe acute kidney injury following pediatric cardiac surgery. Kidney Int 2011;80:655–62.

33. Spahillari A, Parikh CR, Sint K, et al. Serum cystatin C– versus creatinine-based definitions of acute kidney injury following cardiac surgery: a prospective cohort study. Am J Kidney Dis 2012;60:922–9.

34. Parikh CR, Thiessen-Philbrook H, Garg AX, et al. Performance of kidney injury molecule-1 and liver fatty acid-binding protein and combined biomarkers of AKI after cardiac surgery. Clin J Am Soc Nephrol 2013;8:1079–88.

35. Bagshaw SM, Uchino S, Bellomo R, et al. Septic acute kidney injury in critically ill patients: clinical characteristics and outcomes. Clin J Am Soc Nephrol 2007;2: 431–9.

36. Endre ZH, Pickering JW, Walker RJ, et al. Improved performance of urinary bio-markers of acute kidney injury in the critically ill by stratification for injury duration and baseline renal function. Kidney Int 2011;79:1119–30.

37. Endre ZH, Walker RJ, Pickering JW, et al. Early intervention with erythropoietin does not affect the outcome of acute kidney injury (the EARLYARF trial). Kidney Int 2010;77:1020–30.

38. McIlroy DR, Wagener G, Lee HT. Neutrophil gelatinase-associated lipocalin and acute kidney injury after cardiac surgery: the effect of baseline renal function on diagnostic performance. Clin J Am Soc Nephrol 2010;5:211–9.

39. Koyner JL, Vaidya VS, Bennett MR, et al. Urinary biomarkers in the clinical prognosis and early detection of acute kidney injury. Clin J Am Soc Nephrol 2010;5: 2154–65.

40. Siew ED, Ware LB, Bian A, et al. Distinct injury markers for the early detection and prognosis of incident acute kidney injury in critically ill adults with preserved kidney function. Kidney Int 2013;84:786–94.

41. Siew ED, Ikizler TA, Gebretsadik T, et al. Elevated urinary IL-18 levels at the time of ICU admission predict adverse clinical outcomes. Clin J Am Soc Nephrol 2010; 5:1497–505.

42. Martensson J, Bell M, Oldner A. Neutrophil gelatinase-associated lipocalin in adult septic patients with and without acute kidney injury. Intensive Care Med 2010;36:1333–40.

43. Tu Y, Wang H, Sun R, et al. Urinary netrin-1 and KIM-1 as early biomarkers for septic acute kidney injury. Ren Fail 2014;36:1559–63.

44. de Geus HR, Fortrie G, Betjes MG, et al. Time of injury affects urinary biomarker predictive values for acute kidney injury in critically ill, non-septic patients. BMC Nephrol 2013;14:273.

45. Kashani K, Al-Khafaji A, Ardiles T, et al. Discovery and validation of cell cycle arrest biomarkers in human acute kidney injury. Crit Care 2013;17:R25.

46. Hoste EA, McCullough PA, Kashani K, et al. Derivation and validation of cutoffs for clinical use of cell cycle arrest biomarkers. Nephrol Dial Transplant 2014;29: 2054–61.

47. Bihorac A, Chawla LS, Shaw AD, et al. Validation of cell-cycle arrest biomarkers for acute kidney injury using clinical adjudication. Am J Respir Crit Care Med 2014;189:932–9.

48. Kellum JA, Chawla LS. Cell-cycle arrest and acute kidney injury: the light and the dark sides. Nephrol Dial Transplant 2015. [Epub ahead of print].

49. Koyner JL, Shaw AD, Chawla LS, et al. Tissue inhibitor metalloproteinase-2 (TIMP-2) IGF-binding protein-7 (IGFBP7) levels are associated with adverse long-term outcomes in patients with AKI. J Am Soc Nephrol 2015;26:1747–54.

50. Lin CY, Chang CH, Fan PC, et al. Serum interleukin-18 at commencement of renal replacement therapy predicts short-term prognosis in critically ill patients with acute kidney injury. PLoS One 2013;8:e66028.

51. Srisawat N, Murugan R, Lee M, et al. Plasma neutrophil gelatinase-associated lipocalin predicts recovery from acute kidney injury following community-acquired pneumonia. Kidney Int 2011;80:545–52.

52. Pipili C, Ioannidou S, Tripodaki ES, et al. Prediction of the renal replacement therapy requirement in mechanically ventilated critically ill patients by combining biomarkers for glomerular filtration and tubular damage. J Crit Care 2014;29: 692.e7–13.

53. Nickolas TL, O'Rourke MJ, Yang J, et al. Sensitivity and specificity of a single emergency department measurement of urinary neutrophil gelatinase-associated lipocalin for diagnosing acute kidney injury. Ann Intern Med 2008; 148:810–9.

54. Nickolas TL, Schmidt-Ott KM, Canetta P, et al. Diagnostic and prognostic stratification in the emergency department using urinary biomarkers of nephron damage: a multicenter prospective cohort study. J Am Coll Cardiol 2012;59:246–55.

55. Haase M, Devarajan P, Haase-Fielitz A, et al. The outcome of neutrophil gelatinase-associated lipocalin-positive subclinical acute kidney injury a multicenter pooled analysis of prospective studies. J Am Coll Cardiol 2011;57:1752–61.

56. Soto K, Papoila AL, Coelho S, et al. Plasma NGAL for the diagnosis of AKI in patients admitted from the emergency department setting. Clin J Am Soc Nephrol 2013;8:2053–63.

57. Soto K, Coelho S, Rodrigues B, et al. Cystatin C as a marker of acute kidney injury in the emergency department. Clin J Am Soc Nephrol 2010;5:1745–54.

58. Shapiro NI, Trzeciak S, Hollander JE, et al. The diagnostic accuracy of plasma neutrophil gelatinase-associated lipocalin in the prediction of acute kidney injury

in emergency department patients with suspected sepsis. Ann Emerg Med 2010; 56:52–9.

59. Schinstock CA, Semret MH, Wagner SJ, et al. Urinalysis is more specific and urinary neutrophil gelatinase-associated lipocalin is more sensitive for early detection of acute kidney injury. Nephrol Dial Transplant 2013;28:1175–85.

60. Somma Di, Magrini L, De Berardinis BS, et al. Additive value of blood neutrophil gelatinase-associated lipocalin to clinical judgement in acute kidney injury diagnosis and mortality prediction in patients hospitalized from the emergency department. Crit Care 2013;17:R29.

61. Parikh CR, Han G. Variation in performance of kidney injury biomarkers due to cause of acute kidney injury. Am J Kidney Dis 2013;62:1023–6.

62. Parikh CR, Jani A, Melnikov VY, et al. Urinary interleukin-18 is a marker of human acute tubular necrosis. Am J Kidney Dis 2004;43:405–14.

63. Han WK, Bailly V, Abichandani R, et al. Kidney injury molecule-1 (KIM-1): a novel biomarker for human renal proximal tubule injury. Kidney Int 2002;62:237–44.

64. Nejat M, Pickering JW, Devarajan P, et al. Some biomarkers of acute kidney injury are increased in pre-renal acute injury. Kidney Int 2012;81(12):1254–62.

65. Doi K, Katagiri D, Negishi K, et al. Mild elevation of urinary biomarkers in prerenal acute kidney injury. Kidney Int 2012;82:1114–20.

66. Belcher JM, Parikh CR. Is it time to evolve past the prerenal azotemia versus acute tubular necrosis classification? Clin J Am Soc Nephrol 2011;6:2332–4.

67. Bellomo R, Bagshaw S, Langenberg C, et al. Pre-renal azotemia: a flawed paradigm in critically ill septic patients? Contrib Nephrol 2007;156:1–9.

68. Basu RK, Wong HR, Krawczeski CD, et al. Combining functional and tubular damage biomarkers improves diagnostic precision for acute kidney injury after cardiac surgery. J Am Coll Cardiol 2014;64:2753–62.

69. Koyner JL, Davison DL, Brasha-Mitchell E, et al. Furosemide stress test and biomarkers for the prediction of AKI severity. J Am Soc Nephrol 2015. [Epub ahead of print].

70. Faubel S, Chawla LS, Chertow GM, et al. Ongoing clinical trials in AKI. Clin J Am Soc Nephrol 2012;7:861–73.

71. Smith OM, Wald R, Adhikari NK, et al. Standard versus accelerated initiation of renal replacement therapy in acute kidney injury (STARRT-AKI): study protocol for a randomized controlled trial. Trials 2013;14:320.

72. Srisawat N, Tiranathanagul K, Susantitaphong P, et al. The effect of early intervention with renal replacement therapy guiding by plasma neutrophil gelatinase associated lipocalin and the outcome of acute kidney injury (the EARLYRRT trial): a randomized controlled trial. J Am Soc Nephrol 2014;25:7A [Abstract TH-OR029].

73. Chawla LS, Eggers PW, Star RA, et al. Acute kidney injury and chronic kidney disease as interconnected syndromes. N Engl J Med 2014;371:58–66.

74. Zhang Z, Lu B, Sheng X, et al. Cystatin C in prediction of acute kidney injury: a systemic review and meta-analysis. Am J Kidney Dis 2011;58:356–65.

75. Herget-Rosenthal S, Bökenkamp A, Hofmann W. How to estimate GFR-serum creatinine, serum cystatin C or equations? Clin Biochem 2007;40:153–61.

76. Séronie-Vivien S, Delanaye P, Piéroni L, et al. Cystatin C: current position and future prospects. Clin Chem Lab Med 2008;46(12):1664–86.

77. Nejat M, Hill JV, Pickering JW, et al. Albuminuria increases cystatin C excretion: implications for urinary biomarkers. Nephrol Dial Transplant 2012;27:iii96–103.

78. Dinarello CA, Novick D, Kim S, et al. Interleukin-18 and IL-18 binding protein. Front Immunol 2013;4:289.

79. Melnikov VY, Faubel S, Siegmund B, et al. Neutrophil-independent mechanisms of caspase-1– and IL-18–mediated ischemic acute tubular necrosis in mice. J Clin Invest 2002;110:1083–91.

80. Ichimura T, Bonventre JV, Bailly V, et al. Kidney injury molecule-1 (KIM-1), a putative epithelial cell adhesion molecule containing a novel immunoglobulin domain, is up-regulated in renal cells after injury. J Biol Chem 1998;273:4135–42.

81. Bonventre JV. Kidney injury molecule-1: a translational journey. Trans Am Clin Climatol Assoc 2014;125:293–9.

82. Ichimura T, Brooks CR, Bonventre JV. Kim-1/Tim-1 and immune cells: shifting sands. Kidney Int 2012;81:809–11.

83. Maatman RG, van de Westerlo EM, van Kuppevelt TH, et al. Molecular identification of the liver- and the heart-type fatty acid-binding proteins in human and rat kidney. Use of the reverse transcriptase polymerase chain reaction. Biochem J 1992;288:285–90.

84. Yamamoto T, Noiri E, Ono Y, et al. Renal L-type fatty acid–binding protein in acute ischemic injury. J Am Soc Nephrol 2007;18:2894–902.

85. Tanaka T, Noiri E, Yamamoto T, et al. Urinary human L-FABP is a potential biomarker to predict COX-inhibitor-induced renal injury. Nephron Exp Nephrol 2008;108:e19–26.

86. Negishi K, Noiri E, Sugaya T, et al. A role of liver fatty acid-binding protein in cisplatin-induced acute renal failure. Kidney Int 2007;72:348–58.

87. Yamashita T, Doi K, Hamasaki Y, et al. Evaluation of urinary tissue inhibitor of metalloproteinase-2 in acute kidney injury: a prospective observational study. Crit Care 2014;18(6):716.

88. Kjeldsen L, Johnsen AH, Sengelov H, et al. Isolation and primary structure of NGAL, a novel protein associated with human neutrophil gelatinase. J Biol Chem 1993;268:10425–32.

89. Haase-Fielitz A, Haase M, Devarajan P. Neutrophil gelatinase-associated lipocalin as a biomarker of acute kidney injury: a critical evaluation of current status. Ann Clin Biochem 2014;51:335–51.

90. Singer E, Markó L, Paragas N, et al. Neutrophil gelatinase-associated lipocalin: pathophysiology and clinical applications. Acta Physiol (Oxf) 2013;207:663–72.

91. Martensson J, Bellomo R. The rise and fall of NGAL in acute kidney injury. Blood Purif 2014;37:304–10.

92. Chang C, Werb Z. The many faces of metalloproteases: cell growth, invasion, angiogenesis and metastasis. Trends Cell Biol 2001;11:S37–43.

93. Tamura K, Hashimoto K, Suzuki K, et al. Insulin-like growth factor binding protein-7 (IGFBP7) blocks vascular endothelial cell growth factor (VEGF)-induced angiogenesis in human vascular endothelial cells. Eur J Pharmacol 2009;610:61–7.

94. Mazanowska O, Zabińska M, Kościelska-Kasprzak K, et al. Increased plasma matrix metalloproteinase-2 (MMP-2), tissue inhibitor of proteinase-1 (TIMP-1), TIMP-2, and urine MMP-2 concentrations correlate with proteinuria in renal transplant recipients. Transplant Proc 2014;46:2636–9.

95. Seo DW, Li H, Qu CK, et al. Shp-1 mediates the antiproliferative activity of tissue inhibitor of metalloproteinase-2 in human microvascular endothelial cells. J Biol Chem 2006;281:3711–21.

96. Hwa V, Oh Y, Rosenfeld RG. The insulin-like growth factor-binding protein (IGFBP) superfamily. Endocr Rev 1999;20:761–87.

97. Meersch M, Schmidt C, Van Aken H, et al. Urinary TIMP-2 and IGFBP7 as early biomarkers of acute kidney injury and renal recovery following cardiac surgery. PLoS One 2014;9:e93460.

Sepsis-Induced Acute Kidney Injury

Johan Mårtensson, MD, PhD, DESA[a,b], Rinaldo Bellomo, MD, FRACP, FCICM[a,c],*

KEYWORDS

- Sepsis • Acute kidney injury • Inflammation • Renal replacement therapy

KEY POINTS

- Acute kidney injury (AKI) is a common and potentially fatal complication of sepsis.
- Sepsis-induced immune cells seems to release reactive oxygen and nitrogen species, which can damage tubular cells directly.
- Nephrons seem to adapt to sepsis-induced renal stress by conserving energy, removing dysfunctional cells, decreasing the glomerular filtration rate, and possibly recruiting shunt pathways, which attenuate their contact with toxin-rich blood.
- It is likely that progression of septic AKI can, in part, be prevented by avoiding hypotension, fluid overload, and venous congestion.
- Future therapeutic options for septic AKI may include antiinflammatory drugs targeting molecular mechanisms involved in the pathogenesis of septic AKI, and/or blood purification techniques.

INTRODUCTION

Severe sepsis is the trigger for the development of approximately 50% of cases of acute kidney injury (AKI) among critically ill patients.[1] Even in patients with less severe infections, the incidence of AKI is as high as 16% to 25%.[2] Sepsis-induced AKI is associated with mortality rates of up to 50% to 60%, depending on severity.[3] Septic AKI is characterized by a rapid and often profound decline in the kidneys' ability to filter blood and eliminate nitrogen waste products, usually evolving over hours to days after the onset of sepsis.[4] Limited understanding of pathophysiologic mechanisms has precluded the development of effective therapies for sepsis-induced AKI. However,

Conflicts of Interest: None declared.

[a] Department of Intensive Care, Austin Hospital, 145 Studley Road, Heidelberg, Victoria 3084, Australia; [b] Department of Physiology and Pharmacology, Section of Anaesthesia and Intensive Care Medicine, Karolinska Institutet, 171 77 Stockholm, Sweden; [c] Department of Epidemiology and Preventive Medicine, Australian and New Zealand Intensive Care Research Centre, School of Preventive Medicine and Public Health, Monash University, 99 Commercial Road, Melbourne, Victoria 3004, Australia

* Corresponding author. Department of Epidemiology and Preventive Medicine, Australian and New Zealand Intensive Care Research Centre, Monash University, Melbourne, Australia.

E-mail addresses: rinaldo.bellomo@monash.edu; rinaldo.bellomo@austin.org.au

Crit Care Clin 31 (2015) 649–660
http://dx.doi.org/10.1016/j.ccc.2015.06.003
criticalcare.theclinics.com
0749-0704/15/$ – see front matter © 2015 Elsevier Inc. All rights reserved.

early infectious source control and supportive care, with vasopressors, intravenous fluids and renal replacement therapy (RRT) seem to be logical and are likely to impact favorably outcomes among patients with septic AKI. This review summarizes our current understanding of the pathogenesis of sepsis-induced AKI. Moreover, because changes in glomerular hemodynamics are thought to play a major role in septic AKI, they are given special attention in this article. Management of septic AKI with special reference to systemic blood pressures, fluid management, vasopressor therapy, red blood cell (RBC) transfusion and RRT is also discussed. Finally, we highlight some potential future pharmacologic therapies for septic AKI.

THE KIDNEYS' RESPONSE TO SEPSIS
Cellular Adaptation

The innate immune response to infections triggers adaptive mechanisms affecting the kidneys' tubular, vascular and glomerular functions. Invading pathogens release molecules, for example, lipopolysaccharide, lipoteichoic acid, or DNA, known as pathogen-associated molecular patterns (PAMPs), into the blood. Additionally, cellular injury and disruption release intracellular contents, the so-called damage-associated molecular patterns (DAMPs). PAMPs and DAMPs are recognized by pattern recognition receptors, such as Toll-like receptors, on immune cells.[5] In response to this activation, immune cells release cytokines, chemokines and reactive oxygen (ROS) and nitrogen (RNS) species (**Fig. 1**). Such release of ROS and RNS

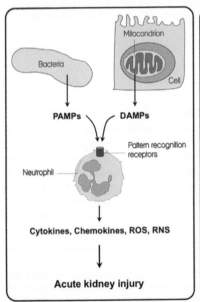
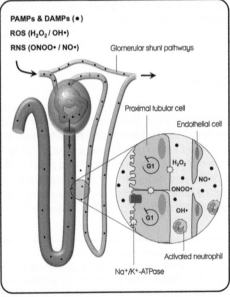

Fig. 1. Pathophysiology of septic acute kidney injury. The systemic inflammatory response is triggered by PAMPs from invading microorganisms and by DAMPs from damaged cells. Activated neutrophils release inflammatory mediators, ROS and RNS, which cause kidney tubular cell stress and injury. Tubules adapt to cellular stress by conserving energy through G1 cell-cycle arrest. Mislocation of Na⁺/K⁺-adenosine triphosphatase prevents energy-consuming NaCl reuptake. Recruitment of glomerular shunt pathways may protect the tubules from further harm by shunting toxin-rich blood away from the kidneys. DAMPs, damage-associated molecular patterns; PAMPs, pathogen-associated molecular patterns; RNS, reactive nitrogen species; ROS, reactive oxygen species.

cause additional direct cell injury via oxidative degradation of intracellular lipids, proteins, and DNA.[6]

Because the kidneys receive a major portion of cardiac output (approximately one-fifth) and filter large plasma volumes every hour, the tubules in septic patients are logically likely to be continuously exposed to DAMPs, PAMPs, ROS, and RNS, either through blood or via its filtrate in the tubular lumen. Logically, this toxic milieu poses a threat to the nephrons and cellular stress or injury could be expected. However, despite the common complete loss of kidney function in sepsis, histologic evidence of cell injury is remarkably scarce.[7–9] These observations suggest that important adaptive mechanisms may be at work, which, at least partly, can protect the kidneys until the septic state has resolved.

Cytoprotective mechanisms include the ability to reduce energy demands and use, restrict formation of ROS, remove dysfunctional organelles, and regulate cell death. For example, stressed tubular cells are able to enter cell-cycle arrest, which stops normal cell division and conserves energy until the injurious stimuli have abated.[10] Energy consumption is further decreased because sodium chloride reabsorption, the most energy-consuming process along the nephron, is decreased owing to decreased glomerular filtration rate (GFR) and redistribution of Na^+/K^+-adenosine triphosphatase from basal to apical or lateral cell segments (see **Fig. 1**).[11]

Formation of ROS is catalyzed by free iron. Excessive release of free iron and generation of ROS seem to be involved in cardiac surgery-associated AKI and may contribute to septic AKI.[12] The upregulation of iron scavengers by tubular cells, such as neutrophil-gelatinase associated lipocalin and hepcidin may limit extracellular iron-induced injury in these patients.[13] The increased levels of neutrophil-gelatinase associated lipocalin and hepcidin seen in septic AKI patients suggest that disturbed iron homeostasis might be an important mechanism in sepsis-induced AKI as well.[14–16]

DAMPs and PAMPs can, by binding to pattern recognition receptors, trigger intracellular molecular pathways, ultimately leading to regulated tubular cell death (ie, necroptosis and/or apoptosis).[17] Although the purpose of such cell death would be to defend the organism against intracellular invaders (eg, microbes), the release of DAMPs from necroptotic cells might create a vicious circle, which might support and even amplify the systemic inflammatory response.

GLOMERULAR HEMODYNAMICS IN SEPTIC ACUTE KIDNEY INJURY

A decreased GFR is the major functional event of septic AKI. Low GFR can be regarded as a protective mechanism against further insults. Decreased GFR means less filtration of toxins such as DAMPs and PAMPs, which limits further tubular cell toxin exposure and stress. Decreased GFR also means lower energy consumption, because less sodium chloride is filtered and needs to be reabsorbed. GFR is ultimately determined by the net filtration pressure (NFP), which can be expressed by the following equation:

$$NFP = P_C - P_B - \pi_C$$

where P_C is the hydrostatic pressure in the glomerular capillaries, P_B is the hydrostatic pressure in Bowman's space, and π_C is the oncotic pressure in the glomerular capillaries (**Fig. 2**).

Mean arterial pressure (MAP) and the relative tone in the afferent and the efferent arterioles determine P_C. Autoregulatory mechanisms allow P_C to be maintained across a wide MAP range. Below this autoregulatory range, for example, during septic shock, the P_C, NFP, and GFR decrease with blood pressure. Decreased GFR can logically be

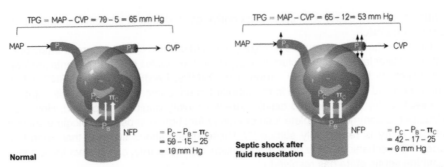

Fig. 2. Normal glomerular hemodynamics (*left column*) and theoretic changes associated with septic shock after fluid resuscitation leading to abolished NFP and GFR (*right column*). CVP, central venous pressure; GFR, glomerular filtration rate; MAP, mean arterial pressure; NFP, net filtration pressure; P_a, afferent arteriolar pressure; P_e, efferent arteriolar pressure; P_C, glomerular capillary pressure; P_B, pressure within Bowman's space; π_C, capillary oncotic pressure; TPG, transrenal pressure gradient.

the consequence of decreased MAP, increased afferent arteriolar tone, decreased efferent arteriolar tone, or a combination of these 3 alterations.

Despite normal or increased global renal blood flow during septic AKI,[18] GFR sometimes ceases completely. Predominant efferent arteriolar vasodilatation causing a decrease in P_C and hence NFP is a possible mechanism behind this phenomenon (see **Fig. 2**). In fact, less pronounced vasodilatation in the afferent arteriole could be explained physiologically. As a consequence of impaired reabsorption of sodium chloride by injured tubules, as discussed elsewhere in this article, increased salt delivery to the 'salt-detecting' macula densa cells in the distal part of the nephron, which triggers constriction of the afferent arteriole, may blunt the sepsis-induced afferent vasodilatation. Additionally, activation of the renal sympathetic nervous system during sepsis may further counteract afferent vasodilatation and contribute to decreased GFR and oliguria.[19] Finally, infusion of efferent arteriolar vasoconstrictors, such as angiotensin II and vasopressin, during experimental hyperdynamic sepsis improve MAP, GFR, and urine output despite reduced global RBF.[20,21] This observation further supports the role of prevailing efferent arteriolar relaxation in septic AKI.

The presence of vascular pathways bypassing the glomerular capillaries (glomerular shunt pathways) provides another potential explanation to the loss of GFR in sepsis.[22,23] Recruitment of such shunt pathways may be an important defense mechanism blunting the kidneys' exposure to PAMPs, DAMPs, ROS, and RNS.

Elevated central venous pressure (CVP) with renal venous congestion and renal interstitial edema may contribute to the onset and maintenance of sepsis-induced kidney dysfunction.[24] Owing to the noncompliant renal capsule, intrarenal pressure increases exponentially with renal volume.[25] Reduced transrenal pressure gradient (TPG = MAP − CVP) causing reduced RBF as well as increased intratubular pressure (P_B) counteracting NFP are potential consequences of renal venous congestion (see **Fig. 2**).

MANAGEMENT OF PATIENTS WITH SEPTIC ACUTE KIDNEY INJURY
Systemic Blood Pressure

Arterial hypotension frequently complicates severe infections and is likely to contribute to the development and progression of AKI (**Table 1**).[26] The optimal blood pressure target needed to prevent kidney damage and/or delay mortality in individual patients remains to be determined. However, in a recent multicenter, randomized

Table 1
Therapeutic targets in patients with or at risk of septic acute kidney injury, physiology, and current evidence

Targets	Physiologic Renal Effects	Clinical Renal Effects
MAP 80–85 vs 65–70 mm Hg	Higher MAP increases renal perfusion pressure and blood flow	SEPSISPAM trial: lower need for RRT with higher blood pressure target in patients with chronic hypertension[27]
CVP >12 mm Hg	Renal perfusion pressure (MAP – CVP) decreases when CVP increases. Elevated CVP increase intratubular pressure, which counteracts GFR	Elevated CVP (>12 mm Hg) is associated with the development or progression of AKI in observational studies[26,38]
Protocol-based EGDT[28]	NA	ARISE and ProCESS trials: no effect on mortality or RRT requirement compared with "usual care"[31,32]
Hemoglobin 90 vs 70 g/L	Increased oxygen delivery to kidney tubular cells	TRISS trial: no effect on dialysis-free survival with a target hemoglobin of 90 g/L compared with a target of 70 g/L[47]
Vasopressin	Increase MAP; maintain GFR by mainly contracting the efferent arteriole	VASST: no effect on mortality; Prevented AKI progression and need for RRT in post hoc analysis[39,40]
RRT	NA	Observational data; better renal recovery with continuous than with intermittent RRT; should be initiated when fluid balance cannot be managed with diuretics alone[48,54]

Abbreviations: AKI, acute kidney injury; CVP, central venous pressure; EGDT, early goal-directed therapy; GFR, glomerular filtration rate; MAP, mean arterial pressure; NA, not applicable; RRT, renal replacement therapy; VASST, Vasopressin and Septic Shock Trial.

controlled trial (RCT), the SEPSISPAM trial, 776 patients with septic shock were resuscitated to a MAP of either 80 to 85 mm Hg or 65 to 70 mm Hg[27] using higher dose norepinephrine infusion. This trial found no significant difference in 90-day mortality between the high-target and the low-target group. Moreover, the occurrence of worsening kidney function and the need for RRT was similar in the 2 groups. Blood pressure deficits (decrease in blood pressure relative to the patient's premorbid value) may still be important in situations with impaired renal autoregulation, such as in patients with chronic kidney disease and arterial hypertension, and in the elderly. The importance of individualized blood pressure targets was highlighted in a secondary analysis of patients with chronic hypertension in the SEPSISPAM trial. In this subpopulation, a target MAP of 65 to 70 mm Hg increased the need for RRT compared with a MAP of 80 to 85 mm Hg.[27] Finally, an important and logical corollary of the findings of SEPSISPAM is that norepinephrine infusion at higher doses is safe from a renal point of view, not contraindicated in septic patients with AKI, and possibly beneficial to GFR preservation in selected patients.

Fluid Management and Central Venous Pressure

The mainstay of treatment of septic shock is to give intravenous fluids, vasopressors and inotropes guided by physiologic endpoints.[28] Although such early goal-directed therapy is recommended in the Surviving Sepsis Campaign guidelines,[29] its benefits are open to challenge.[30] In fact, in 2 recent large multicenter RCTs, early goal-directed therapy did not reduce mortality or prevent RRT requirements in patients with early septic shock.[31,32] Moreover, fluid resuscitation fails to revert hemodynamic instability in a significant proportion of critically ill patients.[33] When fluid therapy does improve physiologic parameters, the effect is transient and repeated fluid boluses are required to maintain the effect.[34] In both cases, unnecessary and repeated fluid administration leads to gradual fluid accumulation over days. Observational studies suggest that fluid accumulation is associated with development and progression of AKI[35,36] and increased mortality in AKI patients.[37] This association is particularly strong when CVP is allowed to increase beyond 12 mm Hg,[26,38] supporting the role of venous congestion in the pathogenesis of AKI.

Vasopressor Therapy

In contrast with fluid resuscitation, vasopressors can restore blood pressure reliably in most septic patients. Optimal timing and choice of vasopressor therapy is, however, uncertain. In the Vasopressin and Septic Shock Trial (VASST), administration of low-dose vasopressin (0.01–0.03 U/min) instead of norepinephrine did not decrease mortality in patients with septic shock.[39] However, a secondary analysis of the VASST showed attenuated progression of AKI and decreased need for RRT in vasopressin-treated patients.[40] Furthermore, terlipressin, a vasopressin analog with greater selectivity for the vasopressin 1 receptor, prevented worsening renal function compared with placebo in patients with the hepatorenal syndrome,[41] a condition that shares many pathophysiologic features with sepsis-induced AKI. Benefits, if any, of terlipressin in septic shock patients need to be confirmed in future RCTs.

Red Blood Cell Transfusion

Septic AKI patients treated with RRT are particularly prone to anemia and hence to receive RBC transfusions. First, the frequent blood sampling needed to monitor electrolyte balance during RRT contributes to low hemoglobin levels.[42] Second, both filter clotting and increased bleeding risk owing to circuit anticoagulation are recognized complications during RRT.[43] Third, AKI is associated with disturbed red cell production owing to an altered response to erythropoietin.[44] Additionally, many AKI patients have chronic kidney disease with associated chronic anemia. Finally, fluid overload is common in AKI and might dilute hemoglobin.

In the Surviving Sepsis Campaign guidelines, a restrictive RBC transfusion strategy, targeting a hemoglobin of 70 g/L, is recommended[29] and results from observational studies show that RBC transfusion in response to the anemia of critical illness is associated with increased morbidity and mortality.[45,46] A recent RCT therefore explored the safety of targeting a hemoglobin level of 70 g/L compared with 90 g/L in 998 patients with septic shock, of which 12% were treated with RRT at baseline.[47] No differences in mortality, ischemic events, or further RRT requirements were found. Thus, a hemoglobin target just above 70 g/L seems to be safe and appropriate.

Renal Replacement Therapy

Continuous RRT (CRRT) rather than intermittent RRT or extended daily hemofiltration is preferred in AKI patients with severe sepsis.[48,49] Although differences in survival are absent when comparing these modalities, the rate of renal recovery is better with CRRT, probably owing to the lower rate of hypotensive episodes and better fluid homeostasis achieved with CRRT.[48,50] In contrast, optimal timing of CRRT initiation relative to the onset and severity of septic AKI as well as the optimal intensity of such therapy remains uncertain. In a secondary analysis of the Randomized Evaluation of Normal versus Augmented Level (RENAL) replacement therapy study, where 50% of patients had severe sepsis,[51] the time between a doubling of serum creatinine and CRRT start had no impact on mortality.[52] In addition, early CRRT, initiated before conventional criteria were met, failed to improve outcomes in patients with severe sepsis.[53] In contrast, others suggest that CRRT initiation before fluid overload has evolved improves survival.[54]

A CRRT intensity of 20 to 25 mL/kg per hour is recommended for critically ill AKI patients.[55] Based on large RCTs, higher intensities do not offer additional survival benefit in general patients in the intensive care unit.[51,56] Yet, high-volume hemofiltration (65–70 mL/kg/h) has been suggested in patients with septic shock. Although high-volume hemofiltration decreased vasopressor requirements in 1 study,[57] no effect on survival was demonstrated.[58]

FUTURE THERAPIES

The molecular mechanisms involved in the sepsis-induced inflammatory response are potential targets for future therapies (**Table 2**). Alkaline phosphatase obtunds the

Table 2
Future therapies

Therapy	Mechanism	Evidence
Recombinant human soluble thrombomodulin	Reduce thrombin mediated clotting. Enhance protein C activation. Inactivate high-mobility group protein B1.	Phase 2b clinical trial in patients with sepsis and disseminated intravascular coagulation: Trend toward lower 28-day mortality. (Vincent 2013 2070–2079).
Acetylsalicylic acid	Induce synthesis of antiinflammatory molecules (lipoxins, resolvins, protectins).	Associated with reduced ICU mortality in observational studies.[62,63] Protected against endotoxin-induced AKI in animal model.[64]
Alkaline phosphatase	Endogenous enzyme. Detoxify endotoxins through dephosphorylation. iNOS inhibitor.	Phase 2a clinical trial: Improved creatinine clearance. Trend toward reduced RRT requirements. Decreased ICU duration of stay.[60]
Anti-histone antibody	Block cytotoxic extracellular histones released during sepsis.	Prevented death and AKI in experimental sepsis.[67]
Polymyxin B hemoperfusion	Polymyxin B adsorbed to a polystyrene fiber in a hemoperfusion device has the ability to bind and neutralize lipopolysaccharide. Inactivates circulating proapoptotic factors.	EUPHAS trial: Improved hemodynamics, lung function, SOFA score and survival at 28 d in patients with intraabdominal sepsis.[68]

Abbreviations: AKI, acute kidney injury; ICU, intensive care unit; iNOS, inducible nitrous oxide; RRT, renal replacement therapy.

inflammatory response by detoxifying endotoxin, and by attenuating RNS production.[59] Intravenous injection of alkaline phosphatase in patients with early septic AKI significantly improved creatinine clearance with a trend toward a reduced need for RRT.[60] No large RCT has yet explored its efficacy in septic humans.

Activated platelets trigger several proinflammatory pathways involved in sepsis-induced organ damage.[61] Acetylsalicylic acid (aspirin) interferes with several of these pathways by stimulating the synthesis of antiinflammatory molecules such as lipoxins, resolvins, and protectins. Observational data suggest that aspirin treatment before[62] or during[63] intensive care unit admission is associated independently with lower mortality. Moreover, animal studies confirm an aspirin-induced resolvin-mediated attenuation of AKI during endotoxemia.[64]

Like other DAMPs, histones (nuclear gene-regulating proteins) are released by necroptotic cells, activate the immune system and promote sepsis-induced organ injury.[65] Activated protein C, which degrades extracellular histones, was a previously approved therapy for sepsis but was removed from the market owing to lack of efficacy in a large RCT.[66] Antihistone antibodies were recently shown to prevent death and AKI in a septic mouse model.[67] Their role as therapeutic agents in human septic AKI is yet to be determined.

Removal (adsorption) of circulating endotoxin by polymyxin B hemoperfusion in patients with severe abdominal sepsis improved hemodynamics, organ function, and survival significantly in a recent, small RCT.[68] An ongoing phase 3 trial, including 650 patients with septic shock and elevated endotoxin levels, will provide more robust evidence on the potential benefits of polymyxin B hemoperfusion on clinical outcomes.[69]

SUMMARY

Sepsis-induced systemic inflammation triggers protective mechanisms within the nephron, affecting tubular and glomerular functions. Depending on the severity of this inflammatory response, a varying degree of kidney impairment can be expected, from a small decrease in GFR to complete shutdown and permanent dysfunction. At present, no specific therapy for septic AKI exists. Although novel drugs and blood purification techniques for sepsis-induced AKI are being tested, supportive care to prevent further kidney insults, such as those induced by hypotension, renal edema, and renal venous congestion, is likely to allow kidney structure and function to more easily recover once the septic state has resolved.

REFERENCES

1. Uchino S, Kellum JA, Bellomo R, et al. Acute renal failure in critically ill patients: a multinational, multicenter study. JAMA 2005;294(7):813–8.
2. Murugan R, Karajala-Subramanyam V, Lee M, et al. Acute kidney injury in non-severe pneumonia is associated with an increased immune response and lower survival. Kidney Int 2010;77(6):527–35.
3. Bagshaw SM, Uchino S, Bellomo R, et al. Septic acute kidney injury in critically ill patients: clinical characteristics and outcomes. Clin J Am Soc Nephrol 2007;2(3):431–9.
4. Hoste EA, Lameire NH, Vanholder RC, et al. Acute renal failure in patients with sepsis in a surgical ICU: predictive factors, incidence, comorbidity, and outcome. J Am Soc Nephrol 2003;14(4):1022–30.
5. Zhang Q, Raoof M, Chen Y, et al. Circulating mitochondrial DAMPs cause inflammatory responses to injury. Nature 2010;464(7285):104–7.

6. Bosmann M, Ward PA. The inflammatory response in sepsis. Trends Immunol 2013;34(3):129–36.
7. Brun C, Munck O. Lesions of the kidney in acute renal failure following shock. Lancet 1957;272(6969):603–7.
8. Lerolle N, Nochy D, Guerot E, et al. Histopathology of septic shock induced acute kidney injury: apoptosis and leukocytic infiltration. Intensive Care Med 2010; 36(3):471–8.
9. Langenberg C, Bagshaw SM, May CN, et al. The histopathology of septic acute kidney injury: a systematic review. Crit Care 2008;12(2):R38.
10. Yang QH, Liu DW, Long Y, et al. Acute renal failure during sepsis: potential role of cell cycle regulation. J Infect 2009;58(6):459–64.
11. Zuk A, Bonventre JV, Brown D, et al. Polarity, integrin, and extracellular matrix dynamics in the postischemic rat kidney. Am J Physiol 1998;275(3 Pt 1):C711–731.
12. Martines AM, Masereeuw R, Tjalsma H, et al. Iron metabolism in the pathogenesis of iron-induced kidney injury. Nat Rev Nephrol 2013;9(7):385–98.
13. Haase M, Bellomo R, Haase-Fielitz A. Novel biomarkers, oxidative stress, and the role of labile iron toxicity in cardiopulmonary bypass-associated acute kidney injury. J Am Coll Cardiol 2010;55(19):2024–33.
14. Martensson J, Bell M, Oldner A, et al. Neutrophil gelatinase-associated lipocalin in adult septic patients with and without acute kidney injury. Intensive Care Med 2010;36(8):1333–40.
15. Martensson J, Bell M, Xu S, et al. Association of plasma neutrophil gelatinase-associated lipocalin (NGAL) with sepsis and acute kidney dysfunction. Biomarkers 2013;18(4):349–56.
16. Martensson J, Glassford NJ, Jones S, et al. Urinary neutrophil gelatinase-associated lipocalin to hepcidin ratio as a biomarker of acute kidney injury in intensive care unit patients. Minerva Anestesiol 2014. [Epub ahead of print].
17. Linkermann A, Green DR. Necroptosis. N Engl J Med 2014;370(5):455–65.
18. Langenberg C, Wan L, Egi M, et al. Renal blood flow in experimental septic acute renal failure. Kidney Int 2006;69(11):1996–2002.
19. Calzavacca P, May CN, Bellomo R. Glomerular haemodynamics, the renal sympathetic nervous system and sepsis-induced acute kidney injury. Nephrol Dial Transplant 2014;29(12):2178–84.
20. Wan L, Langenberg C, Bellomo R, et al. Angiotensin II in experimental hyperdynamic sepsis. Crit Care 2009;13(6):R190.
21. Ishikawa K, Wan L, Calzavacca P, et al. The effects of terlipressin on regional hemodynamics and kidney function in experimental hyperdynamic sepsis. PLoS One 2012;7(2):e29693.
22. Ljungqvist A. Ultrastructural demonstration of a connection between afferent and efferent juxtamedullary glomerular arterioles. Kidney Int 1975;8(4):239–44.
23. Casellas D, Mimran A. Shunting in renal microvasculature of the rat: a scanning electron microscopic study of corrosion casts. Anat Rec 1981;201(2):237–48.
24. Prowle JR, Kirwan CJ, Bellomo R. Fluid management for the prevention and attenuation of acute kidney injury. Nat Rev Nephrol 2014;10(1):37–47.
25. Cruces P, Salas C, Lillo P, et al. The renal compartment: a hydraulic view. Intensive Care Med Exp 2014;2:26.
26. Legrand M, Dupuis C, Simon C, et al. Association between systemic hemodynamics and septic acute kidney injury in critically ill patients: a retrospective observational study. Crit Care 2013;17(6):R278.
27. Asfar P, Meziani F, Hamel JF, et al. High versus low blood-pressure target in patients with septic shock. N Engl J Med 2014;370(17):1583–93.

28. Rivers E, Nguyen B, Havstad S, et al. Early goal-directed therapy in the treatment of severe sepsis and septic shock. N Engl J Med 2001;345(19):1368–77.
29. Dellinger RP, Levy MM, Rhodes A, et al. Surviving sepsis campaign: international guidelines for management of severe sepsis and septic shock: 2012. Crit Care Med 2013;41(2):580–637.
30. Maitland K, Kiguli S, Opoka RO, et al. Mortality after fluid bolus in African children with severe infection. N Engl J Med 2011;364(26):2483–95.
31. Yealy DM, Kellum JA, Huang DT, et al. A randomized trial of protocol-based care for early septic shock. N Engl J Med 2014;370(18):1683–93.
32. Peake SL, Delaney A, Bailey M, et al. Goal-directed resuscitation for patients with early septic shock. N. Engl. J Med 2014;371(16):1496–506.
33. Bihari S, Prakash S, Bersten AD. Post resuscitation fluid boluses in severe sepsis or septic shock: prevalence and efficacy (price study). Shock 2013;40(1):28–34.
34. Glassford NJ, Eastwood GM, Bellomo R. Physiological changes after fluid bolus therapy in sepsis: a systematic review of contemporary data. Crit Care 2014;18:696.
35. Payen D, de Pont AC, Sakr Y, et al. A positive fluid balance is associated with a worse outcome in patients with acute renal failure. Crit Care 2008;12(3):R74.
36. Grams ME, Estrella MM, Coresh J, et al. Fluid balance, diuretic use, and mortality in acute kidney injury. Clin J Am Soc Nephrol 2011;6(5):966–73.
37. Bouchard J, Soroko SB, Chertow GM, et al. Fluid accumulation, survival and recovery of kidney function in critically ill patients with acute kidney injury. Kidney Int 2009;76(4):422–7.
38. Boyd JH, Forbes J, Nakada TA, et al. Fluid resuscitation in septic shock: a positive fluid balance and elevated central venous pressure are associated with increased mortality. Crit Care Med 2011;39(2):259–65.
39. Russell JA, Walley KR, Singer J, et al. Vasopressin versus norepinephrine infusion in patients with septic shock. N Engl J Med 2008;358(9):877–87.
40. Gordon AC, Russell JA, Walley KR, et al. The effects of vasopressin on acute kidney injury in septic shock. Intensive Care Med 2010;36(1):83–91.
41. Sanyal AJ, Boyer T, Garcia-Tsao G, et al. A randomized, prospective, double-blind, placebo-controlled trial of terlipressin for type 1 hepatorenal syndrome. Gastroenterology 2008;134(5):1360–8.
42. Chant C, Wilson G, Friedrich JO. Anemia, transfusion, and phlebotomy practices in critically ill patients with prolonged ICU length of stay: a cohort study. Crit Care 2006;10(5):R140.
43. Maynar Moliner J, Honore PM, Sanchez-Izquierdo Riera JA, et al. Handling continuous renal replacement therapy-related adverse effects in intensive care unit patients: the daily trauma concept. Blood Purif 2012;34(2):177–85.
44. von Ahsen N, Muller C, Serke S, et al. Important role of nondiagnostic blood loss and blunted erythropoietic response in the anemia of medical intensive care patients. Crit Care Med 1999;27(12):2630–9.
45. Marik PE, Corwin HL. Efficacy of red blood cell transfusion in the critically ill: a systematic review of the literature. Crit Care Med 2008;36(9):2667–74.
46. Rohde JM, Dimcheff DE, Blumberg N, et al. Health care-associated infection after red blood cell transfusion: a systematic review and meta-analysis. JAMA 2014; 311(13):1317–26.
47. Holst LB, Haase N, Wetterslev J, et al. Lower versus higher hemoglobin threshold for transfusion in septic shock. N Engl J Med 2014;371(15):1381–91.
48. Wald R, Shariff SZ, Adhikari NK, et al. The association between renal replacement therapy modality and long-term outcomes among critically ill adults with acute kidney injury: a retrospective cohort study. Crit Care Med 2014;42(4):868–77.

49. Sun Z, Ye H, Shen X, et al. Continuous venovenous hemofiltration versus extended daily hemofiltration in patients with septic acute kidney injury: a retrospective cohort study. Crit Care 2014;18(2):R70.
50. Schneider AG, Bellomo R, Bagshaw SM, et al. Choice of renal replacement therapy modality and dialysis dependence after acute kidney injury: a systematic review and meta-analysis. Intensive Care Med 2013;39(6):987–97.
51. Bellomo R, Cass A, Cole L, et al. Intensity of continuous renal-replacement therapy in critically ill patients. N Engl J Med 2009;361(17):1627–38.
52. Jun M, Bellomo R, Cass A, et al. Timing of renal replacement therapy and patient outcomes in the randomized evaluation of normal versus augmented level of replacement therapy study. Crit Care Med 2014;42(8):1756–65.
53. Payen D, Mateo J, Cavaillon JM, et al. Impact of continuous venovenous hemofiltration on organ failure during the early phase of severe sepsis: a randomized controlled trial. Crit Care Med 2009;37(3):803–10.
54. Vaara ST, Korhonen AM, Kaukonen KM, et al. Fluid overload is associated with an increased risk for 90-day mortality in critically ill patients with renal replacement therapy: data from the prospective FINNAKI study. Crit Care 2012;16(5):R197.
55. Lameire N, Kellum JA. Contrast-induced acute kidney injury and renal support for acute kidney injury: a KDIGO summary (Part 2). Crit Care 2013;17(1):205.
56. Palevsky PM, Zhang JH, O'Connor TZ, et al. Intensity of renal support in critically ill patients with acute kidney injury. N Engl J Med 2008;359(1):7–20.
57. Boussekey N, Chiche A, Faure K, et al. A pilot randomized study comparing high and low volume hemofiltration on vasopressor use in septic shock. Intensive Care Med 2008;34(9):1646–53.
58. Joannes-Boyau O, Honore PM, Perez P, et al. High-volume versus standard-volume haemofiltration for septic shock patients with acute kidney injury (IVOIRE study): a multicentre randomized controlled trial. Intensive Care Med 2013;39(9):1535–46.
59. Peters E, van Elsas A, Heemskerk S, et al. Alkaline phosphatase as a treatment of sepsis-associated acute kidney injury. J Pharmacol Exp Ther 2013;344(1):2–7.
60. Pickkers P, Heemskerk S, Schouten J, et al. Alkaline phosphatase for treatment of sepsis-induced acute kidney injury: a prospective randomized double-blind placebo-controlled trial. Crit Care 2012;16(1):R14.
61. Akinosoglou K, Alexopoulos D. Use of antiplatelet agents in sepsis: a glimpse into the future. Thromb Res 2014;133(2):131–8.
62. Winning J, Neumann J, Kohl M, et al. Antiplatelet drugs and outcome in mixed admissions to an intensive care unit. Crit Care Med 2010;38(1):32–7.
63. Eisen DP. Manifold beneficial effects of acetyl salicylic acid and nonsteroidal anti-inflammatory drugs on sepsis. Intensive Care Med 2012;38(8):1249–57.
64. Chen J, Shetty S, Zhang P, et al. Aspirin-triggered resolvin D1 down-regulates inflammatory responses and protects against endotoxin-induced acute kidney injury. Toxicol Appl Pharmacol 2014;277(2):118–23.
65. Allam R, Kumar SV, Darisipudi MN, et al. Extracellular histones in tissue injury and inflammation. J Mol Med 2014;92(5):465–72.
66. Ranieri VM, Thompson BT, Barie PS, et al. Drotrecogin alfa (activated) in adults with septic shock. N Engl J Med 2012;366(22):2055–64.
67. Xu J, Zhang X, Pelayo R, et al. Extracellular histones are major mediators of death in sepsis. Nat Med 2009;15(11):1318–21.

68. Cruz DN, Antonelli M, Fumagalli R, et al. Early use of polymyxin B hemoperfusion in abdominal septic shock: the EUPHAS randomized controlled trial. JAMA 2009; 301(23):2445–52.
69. Klein DJ, Foster D, Schorr CA, et al. The EUPHRATES trial (Evaluating the Use of Polymyxin B Hemoperfusion in a Randomized controlled trial of Adults Treated for Endotoxemia and Septic shock): study protocol for a randomized controlled trial. Trials 2014;15:218.

Thrombocytopenia-Associated Multiple Organ Failure and Acute Kidney Injury

CrossMark

Trung C. Nguyen, MD[a],*, Miguel A. Cruz, PhD[b],
Joseph A. Carcillo, MD[c]

KEYWORDS

- TAMOF • AKI • TTP • HUS • DIC • ADAMTS-13 • VWF • Platelet

KEY POINTS

- Thrombocytopenia-associated multiple organ failure (TAMOF) is a clinical phenotype that encompasses a spectrum of syndromes associated with disseminated microvascular thromboses, such as thrombotic thrombocytopenic purpura (TTP), hemolytic uremic syndrome (HUS), and disseminated intravascular coagulation.
- Acute kidney injury (AKI) is a common finding in patients with TAMOF, especially those with TTP and HUS.
- Patients with TAMOF with genetic predisposition leading to dysregulation of the complement pathway and/or Von Willebrand factor/platelet-mediated microvascular thrombosis may be more at risk to develop AKI.
- There are sufficient preliminary data to support the design of randomized controlled trials to evaluate the role of therapeutic plasma exchange in patients with TAMOF.

INTRODUCTION

Thrombocytopenia-associated multiple organ failure (TAMOF) is a clinical phenotype that encompasses a spectrum of syndromes associated with disseminated microvascular thromboses, such as the thrombotic microangiopathies (TMAs) thrombotic

Disclosures: Drs Nguyen and Cruz received grant support from the National Institute of General Medical Sciences (NIGMS) (NIH R01 GM112806). Dr Carcillo received grant support from NIGMS (NIH R01 GM109618).
[a] Section of Critical Care Medicine, Department of Pediatrics, Baylor College of Medicine/Texas Children's Hospital, Center for Translational Research on Inflammatory Diseases (CTRID), Michael DeBakey VA Medical Center, Houston, TX 77030, USA; [b] Department of Medicine, Baylor College of Medicine, Center for Translational Research on Inflammatory Diseases (CTRID), Michael DeBakey VA Medical Center, Houston, TX 77030, USA; [c] Department of Critical Care Medicine and Pediatrics, University of Pittsburgh School of Medicine, Pittsburgh, PA 15261, USA
* Corresponding author.
E-mail address: tcnguyen@texaschildrenshospital.org

Crit Care Clin 31 (2015) 661–674
http://dx.doi.org/10.1016/j.ccc.2015.06.004
0749-0704/15/$ – see front matter © 2015 Elsevier Inc. All rights reserved.

thrombocytopenic purpura/hemolytic uremic syndromes (TTP/HUS) and dissemi-nated intravascular coagulation (DIC). TAMOF is characterized by new-onset throm-bocytopenia with progression to multiple organ failure (MOF) in critically ill patients. The decrease in platelet counts reflects their involvement in causing disseminated microvascular thromboses, which lead to organ ischemia and dysfunction. Autopsy studies from patients who died with TAMOF reveal widespread microvascular throm-boses in all organs.[1–4] With the current management strategy, mortalities from TAMOF remain high, ranging from 5% to 80%.[5–13]

The past decade has brought significant advances in our knowledge of the patho-physiologic processes of TTP, HUS, and DIC. Von Willebrand factor (VWF) and ADAMTS-13 (also known as VWF-cleaving protease) play a central role in TTP.[14,15] Shiga toxins and the complement pathway are vital in the development of HUS.[15,16] Tissue factor is the major protease that drives the pathology of DIC.[17]

Acute kidney injury (AKI) is a common feature in patients with TAMOF with incidences as high as 58% in TTP, 100% in HUS, and 42% in DIC.[18–20] Because of the progress made in the field, we have better insight into the development of AKI in patients with TAMOF and, it is hoped, better innovative approaches to reverse their pathologic consequences.

THROMBOTIC THROMBOCYTOPENIA PURPURA

In 1924 Dr Moschowitz[21] was the first to describe a case of TTP in a girl who suddenly died with petechiae, paralysis, and coma. Autopsy findings revealed that she had disseminated occlusions of her terminal arterioles and capillaries with hyaline thrombi. For decades, the diagnosis of TTP remained a clinical diagnosis with the classic clin-ical pentad of thrombocytopenia, hemolytic anemia, fever, and neurologic and renal involvement. In 1982 Dr Moake and colleagues[22] identified ultralarge VWF (ULVWF) as the "powerful poison which had both agglutinative and hemolytic properties"[22] that caused disseminated microvascular thromboses in TTP. Not until 1998 did Dr Tsai and Lian[23] and Dr Lammle, from 2 different laboratories, simultaneously report that ADAMTS-13 (also known as VWF-cleaving protease) deficiency was the underly-ing pathophysiologic process in TTP.[24] With ADAMTS-13 deficiency, the ULVWF and large plasma VWF remained uncleaved and maintain their prothrombotic properties in the blood.

TTP is divided into 2 categories: congenital and acquired. In both categories, the ADAMTS-13 activity level is less than 10%. In congenital TTP, more than 80 mutations of the *ADAMTS13* gene have been identified.[25,26] In acquired TTP, ADAMTS-13 inhib-itors, such as immunoglobulin G (IgG) autoantibodies to ADAMTS-13 have been reported.[23,24] Autopsies in patients who have died with TTP reveal characteristic VWF/platelet-rich microthrombi in all organs.[1,2,4,27]

Von Willebrand Factor and ADAMTS-13 in Thrombotic Thrombocytopenic Purpura

VWF is the largest multimeric glycoprotein in plasma with a molecular weight ranging from 500 to 20,000 kDa.[28] VWF mediates platelet adhesion to sites of vascular damage by binding to the platelet receptor glycoprotein Ib-IX-V (GP Ib-IX-V) complex and to exposed subendothelial collagen. VWF is synthesized by endothelial cells and megakaryocytes as monomers with subsequent dimerization and multimerization in the endoplasmic reticulum and Golgi apparatus, respectively. After synthesis, VWF is secreted by either the constitutive pathway of lower molecular mass (~500 kDa) di-mers or the inducible pathway of larger VWF and ULVWF.[28,29] The inducible pathway is induced by inflammation.[30–32] VWF adhesiveness is associated with its larger size.

Thus, ULVWF is extremely large and hyperadhesive. ULVWF can spontaneously aggregate platelets by forming high-strength bonds with the platelet receptor GP Ib-IX-V complex.[33] This ULVWF is rapidly and partially cleaved by ADAMTS-13 before being released into the plasma. Consequently, plasma VWF binds and aggregates platelets only in the presence of modulators, such as ristocetin, or *at high shear stress*.[34,35] Deficiency of ULVWF proteolysis results in the accumulation of ULVWF in plasma and on endothelial surfaces as observed in patients with TTP.

ADAMTS-13 is a member of the ADAMTS family of proteases (*A Disintegrin And Metalloproteinase with ThromboSpondin motifs*).[25] The *ADAMTS13* gene encodes a protein with 1427 amino acids, and its mRNA is detected in hepatic stellate cells, endothelial cells, platelets, and glomeruli podocytes.[25,36–39] ADAMTS-13 cleaves VWF at a single peptide bond Tyr842-Met843 in the VWF A2 domain. This cleavage reduces the ULVWF, which spontaneously aggregates platelets, to smaller plasma forms that bind to platelets only with modulators or high fluid shear stress. The cleaved VWF is no longer prothrombotic but maintains hemostatic functions.

Thrombotic Thrombocytopenic Purpura and Acute Kidney Injury

Before the widespread measurement of ADAMTS-13 in patients with TMAs, AKI and neurologic injury were used to discriminate between the TMAs, HUS, and TTP. Severe AKI was sufficient to diagnosis HUS, and severe neurologic injury was sufficient to diagnosis TTP in patients with TMA. This simple clinical differentiation may have led to the underestimation of the incidence of TTP or AKI-associated TTP. Furthermore, old definitions of kidney injury were more restrictive, which might have led to the underdiagnosis of AKI. Thus, with the current use of the ADAMTS-13 assay and a new standardized AKI definition, investigators are now reporting that AKI is much more prevalent in patients with TTP, with up to 58.7% of patients presenting with AKI compared with approximately 20.0% in older studies.[20,40,41]

In a retrospective study, Zafrani and colleagues[20] reported that by using the Kidney Disease–Improving Global Outcomes 2012 guidelines, 54 (58.7%) out of 92 patients with TTP (ADAMTS-13 <10%) presented with AKI, including 46.3% of patients with stage 3 AKI. Renal replacement therapy was required in 25.9% of patients. Mild or moderate chronic renal disease occurred in 42.6% of the patients with AKI. These investigators also found that patients with TTP-induced AKI had lower serum levels of C3 compared with patients with TTP without AKI. C3 deposition in the kidney was observed in all 4 of their patients who underwent kidney biopsy and 3 of whom had low serum C3 levels. These findings suggested that the alternative complement pathway is activated in TTP-induced patients with AKI. In another study, investigators reported 2 sisters who presented with congenital TTP with one presenting with severe renal failure and the other presenting with exclusive neurologic injury. Both had heterozygous mutations of the *ADAMTS13* gene. However, the sister who developed renal failure also had a heterozygous mutation in factor H of the complement gene.[42] These two studies suggest that patients with TTP-induced AKI may have a genetic disposition to complement pathway hyperactivation.

Manea and colleagues[39] revealed that glomeruli podocytes synthesized and secreted ADAMTS-13 into the glomerular circulation. They described 2 patients with congenital TTP-induced AKI with *ADAMTS13* mutations that impaired the secretion of synthesized ADAMTS-13. They proposed that ADAMTS-13 in the glomeruli protected VWF/platelet-rich microthrombi formation in the *high-shear glomerular circulation*. Thus, a defect in ADAMTS-13 secretion could explain a subset of patients with TTP who are predisposed to develop AKI.

Acquired TTP can be a manifestation of autoimmune diseases, such as systemic lupus erythematosus.[41,43,44] These autoimmune diseases with their associated glomerulopathies and interstitial nephropathies can rapidly worsen the already fragile renal function during an acute TTP episode and manifest as TTP-induced AKI.

Managing Thrombotic Thrombocytopenic Purpura

The clinical pentad of TTP (thrombocytopenia, hemolytic anemia, fever, neurologic, and renal injuries) will trigger the clinicians to work up TMA. ADAMTS-13, VWF, and complement assays should be sent. Elevated lactate dehydrogenase and the presence of schistocytes would suggest the pathophysiologic process of TMA. The confirmatory diagnosis of TTP will be made with ADAMTS-13 activity less than 10%, the presence of ULVWF, and clinical signs/symptoms of TTP. The therapeutic strategies for TTP are (1) replenish ADAMTS-13 activity, (2) remove ADAMTS-13 inhibitors, and (3) remove ULVWF. Transfusion with fresh frozen plasma (FFP), which contains ADAMTS-13, addresses the first strategy. The second strategy is addressed by steroids and/or rituximab (anti-CD20 on B-lymphocytes), which can be given to reduce the synthesis of IgG inhibitory autoantibodies to ADAMTS-13.[45] The third strategy is addressed by therapeutic plasma exchange, which is now the standard therapy for newly diagnosed TTP. It has decreased TTP mortality from 100% down to less than 20%.[7,9]

The recognition that AKI is prevalent in TTP is important. TTP and HUS need to be differentiated by molecular diagnosis because they have potentially different management strategies. Plasma therapies including therapeutic plasma exchange (TPE) are best for TTP, whereas TPE is not recommended for infection-induced HUS. If uncontrolled complement pathway activation is involved as reported in some patients with TTP-induced AKI earlier, anti-C5 monoclonal antibody eculizumab may also have a role. A multidisciplinary approach is warranted including early involvement from hematology, transfusion medicine, nephrology, and immunology.

HEMOLYTIC UREMIC SYNDROME

The clinical triad of HUS is thrombocytopenia, hemolytic anemia, and AKI. Most cases require only supportive care and do not progress into MOF. However, cases with brain injuries, such as coma, seizures, and stroke, are more likely to develop TAMOF and are associated with higher mortality.[11] HUS is divided into 2 major clinical phenotypes: infection-induced HUS and atypical HUS with complement dysregulation. Autopsies in patients who have died with HUS reveal disseminated fibrin-rich microthrombi in most cases, but a subset of patients do have VWF/platelet-rich microthrombi.[1,27] These HUS autopsies reveal that the kidneys are markedly involved compared with other organs, contrasting with TTP and DIC whereby all organs are involved.[1]

Infection-induced HUS accounts for 90% of all HUS cases; most cases (~85%) are caused by Shiga toxin-producing *Escherichia coli* (STEC) and several other bacteria, including *Streptococcus pneumonia*.[13,46] HUS develops in 6% to 15% of the infected patients 2 to 10 days after bloody diarrhea.[46] STEC-HUS has commonly been affecting children until the recent 2011 outbreak in Germany that affected mostly adults.[10] Mortality for STEC-HUS ranges from 5% to 9%.[11]

Atypical HUS accounts for approximately 10% of all HUS cases.[13] The complement pathway genetic mutations account for 50% to 60%, and thrombomodulin mutations account for 5% of atypical HUS cases. Mortality is approximately 25% for all atypical HUS but is 50% to 80% for the familial form of atypical HUS.[12,13]

Shiga Toxins and Complement Pathway in Hemolytic Uremic Syndrome

Shiga toxins produced by enterohemorrhagic *Escherichia coli* bind to the glycosphin-golipid surface receptor globotriaosyl ceramide expressed on the renal microvascular endothelium. The toxins are then internalized leading to protein synthesis inhibition and cell death.[47] In addition, Shiga toxins can cause a prothrombotic state in a host by activating monocytes to release inflammatory cytokines,[48] activating platelets,[49] increasing tissue factor activity on glomerular endothelial cells,[50] inhibiting ADAMTS-13, stimulating ULVWF release from glomerular endothelial cells,[51] and activating the complement alternative pathway.[52] Recently, investigators proposed a link between the ULVWF and the alternative complement pathway in HUS. They showed that the endothelial cells can synthesize the alternative complement components that are assembled and activated on the endothelial cells-secreted ULVWF.[53] The activated complement complex on ULVWF could then cause local endothelial damage.

The complement system is essential for immune surveillance and homeostasis.[54] The complement genetic mutations associated with atypical HUS allow for the tightly regulated complement pathway to become unregulated and hyperactive after an inflammatory trigger. This process leads to inflammation and, if severe, will lead to uncontrolled systemic inflammation, disseminated microvascular thromboses, and MOF. More than 120 complement genetic mutations have been linked to atypical HUS.[16] Autoantibodies to factor H, a regulatory complement protein, can also cause HUS.[55]

Hemolytic Uremic Syndrome and Acute Kidney Injury

Shiga toxins directly bind to the renal microvascular endothelium, as described earlier, to cause renal damage. All STEC-HUS manifest some renal impairment. About 30% to 40% of cases require renal support therapy for an average of 10 days, and 25% of cases have long-term renal sequelae.[11,56] Complement regulatory factors are expressed on or bound to the endothelium. These regulatory factors protect the endothelium from complement-induced damage. In atypical HUS, the genetic mutations to these complement regulatory factors lead to uncontrolled complement activation and endothelial damage. Certain vascular beds are at increased risk for hyperactive complement activation. In particular, the glomerular capillary bed has a fenestrated endothelium, which continually exposes the subendothelial matrix to circulating proteins and peptides and, thus, is very vulnerable to complement attack. Overall, atypical HUS has worse morbidities and mortality than STEC-HUS. The severity depends on the underlying complement abnormality. Up to 70% of patients with complement mutations die or progress to end-stage renal disease.[13]

Managing Hemolytic Uremic Syndrome

Complement pathway interrogation and a genetic workup should be initiated in patients with the clinical triad of HUS. ADAMTS-13 and VWF assays should be sent to rule out TTP. For most STEC-HUS, supportive care is the current recommendation. The American Society for Apheresis (ASFA) gives a category I recommendation ("apheresis [i.e. TPE] is accepted as a first line therapy")[7] for atypical HUS caused by autoantibody to factor H. ASFA gives TPE a category II recommendation ("apheresis is accepted as a second-line therapy"[7]) for atypical HUS caused by complement factor gene mutation. Currently, TPE is not recommended for STEC-HUS (category IV recommendation). Direct complement inhibition with monoclonal antibody eculizumab should be considered for atypical HUS.[57,58]

Diarrhea/infection-associated HUS with brain injuries and/or rapid progression into TAMOF poses a significant therapeutic strategy dilemma for intensivists. These patients may have a mixture of pathologic mechanisms involving Shiga toxins, VWF, ADAMTS-13, platelets, complements, fibrin, and endothelium. Until clinicians have the ability to rapidly tease out the exact pathologic mechanism, there is a biological plausibility for the benefit of TPE with the aim of restoring the homeostatic milieu of the plasma. More recent case series have highlighted the benefit of TPE in severe diarrhea/infection-associated HUS.[59,60] Eculizumab also has recently been suggested to be beneficial in STEC-HUS.[19,61]

DISSEMINATED INTRAVASCULAR COAGULATION

The consensus definition of DIC by the Scientific Subcommittee on DIC of the International Society of Thrombosis and Hemostasis is "an acquired syndrome characterized by the intravascular activation of coagulation with loss of localization arising from different causes. It can originate from and cause damage to the microvasculature, which if sufficiently severe, can produce organ dysfunction."[62] Conditions that can trigger DIC include sepsis, cancer, trauma/burns, obstetric complications, toxin exposure, and vascular abnormalities. DIC can occur in 39% of patients with severe sepsis, with a mortality of up to 50%.[5,6] Clinically, the patients present with shock caused by poor perfusion of the organs and petechiae and purpura on the skin. Autopsies in patients who have died with DIC reveal fibrin-rich microthrombi in small and midsize vessels in all organs.[2,4,27]

Tissue Factor in Disseminated Intravascular Coagulation

Tissue factor plays a key role in the initiation and propagation of DIC. The tissue factor is expressed from 2 major sources: the vessel wall and hematopoietic cells. When the vascular wall is injured, the extravascular tissue factor is exposed. Monocytes will express and release the tissue factor after stimulated by inflammatory cytokines or endotoxins during systemic inflammation, such as infection.[17,63,64] After expression, the tissue factor complexes with factor VIIa. This complex then activates factors IX and X, eventually leading to thrombin generation. As the tissue factor propagates thrombin formation, the endogenous anticoagulants in the body, such as antithrombin III, protein C, and tissue factor pathway inhibitor, are all found to be impaired during DIC. Decreased synthesis, increased consumption and degradation, and the development of inhibitors all contribute to the depletion of anticoagulants activities.[65] Finally, the body's natural fibrinolytic system that is responsible for the breakdown of clots during a prothrombotic state is also impaired. Plasminogen-activator inhibitor type-1, a potent inhibitor of the fibrinolytic pathway, is pathologically elevated in DIC and MOF.[66–68]

Disseminated Intravascular Coagulation and Acute Kidney Injury

The overall incidence of AKI is lower in DIC (up to 48%) than TTP or HUS.[18] Unlike TTP and HUS in which the kidneys are specifically at risk for injury, the DIC pathologic mechanism does not specifically target the kidneys compared with other organs. Of note, Ono and colleagues[69] found that 28% of patients with sepsis-induced DIC had evidence of AKI. In particular, those patients with ADAMTS-13 activity less than 20% had a significantly higher incidence of AKI compared with those with ADAMTS-13 activity greater than 20% (41% vs 15% respectively). In additions, these patients' plasma contained granulocyte elastase, a protease released by activated granulocytes during sepsis that can proteolyze ADAMTS-13 into inactive fragments. This study suggests that patients with DIC with low ADAMTS-13 activity may be prone to AKI because of the risk of the high-shear-dependent platelet/VWF-mediated thrombosis in the glomerular circulation.

Managing Disseminated Intravascular Coagulation

In 2013, the Scientific Subcommittee on DIC of the International Society of Thrombosis and Haemostasis published a guideline combining the recommendations from the British, Japanese, and Italian DIC treatment guidelines.[70] In summary, this subcommittee recommends the following: (1) There is no gold standard for the diagnosis of DIC, and no single test is capable of diagnosing DIC. (2) The key in DIC treatment is treating the underlying condition. (3) The transfusions of platelets, FFP, fibrinogen, and prothrombin complex concentrate is recommended in actively bleeding patients with low platelet counts, prolonged prothrombin time/activated partial thromboplastin time, hypofibrinogenemia, or contraindicated FFP-transfusion, respectively. (4) Therapeutic doses of low-molecular-weight heparin (LMWH) should be considered if thrombosis predominates. (5) Prophylaxis for venous thromboembolism with prophylactic doses of unfractionated heparin or LMWH is recommended in nonbleeding patients. (6) The administration of antithrombin III, recombinant thrombomodulin, or activated protein C may be considered. (7) Generally, antifibrinolytic agents should not be used. (8) Patients with severe bleeding characterized by a marked hyperfibrinolytic state, such as leukemia and trauma, could be treated with antifibrinolytic agents.

THROMBOCYTOPENIA-ASSOCIATED MULTIPLE ORGAN FAILURE

In the intensive care unit (ICU), overt DIC has been observed in 40% of patients with new-onset thrombocytopenia.[71–73] TTP and HUS are rare diagnoses in the ICU. The mechanism of the other 60% of patients with new-onset thrombocytopenia in the ICU is of great interest because new-onset thrombocytopenia has been associated with significantly higher mortality.[73–75] Investigators studying MOF have observed that pediatric patients with TAMOF defined as platelet counts less than 100,000/mm^3 and at least 2 failing organs have clinical, biomarkers, and histologic evidences of a thrombotic microangiopathic process.[76] Only 46% of these patients with TAMOF have evidence of an activated fibrin-mediated pathway as in DIC with prolonged prothrombin time. None of these patients with TAMOF have classic TTP, but 89% of the patients have evidence of increased VWF-mediated thrombosis similar to TTP pathophysiology. The mean ADAMTS-13 activity level is 39%, which is abnormally low but not less than 10% as in patients with classic TTP. ULVWF is observed in 53% of these patients. Histopathologic findings in these patients with TAMOF reveal VWF/platelet-rich and fibrin-rich microthrombi in the brain, lungs, and kidneys. Of note, all of these pediatric patients with TAMOF have concurrent sepsis. These investigators suggest that more than half of critically ill children with TAMOF have an acquired ADAMTS-13 deficiency leading to a thrombotic microangiopathic process.

Other investigators have reported that acquired ADAMTS-13 deficiency associated with systemic inflammation has higher morbidity and mortality.[69,77–80] Many molecules associated with systemic inflammation or activated coagulation can inhibit ADAMTS-13. Interleukin 6 can inhibit ADAMTS-13 from cleaving ULVWF.[30] Plasma-free hemoglobin, which is released during hemolysis, can inhibit ADAMTS-13.[81,82] Plasmin and thrombin, products of activated coagulation and inflammation, can proteolyze and inactivate ADAMTS-13.[83] Released by activated neutrophils during systemic inflammation, granulocyte elastase and reactive oxygen species that oxidize VWF can inhibit ADAMTS-13-mediated cleavage.[69,84] VWF proteolytic fragments seem to provide a negative feedback loop by inhibiting ADAMTS-13.[85]

Neutralizing IgG autoantibodies to ADAMTS-13 are the first described inhibitors of ADAMTS-13.[23,24]

Thrombocytopenia-Associated Multiple Organ Failure and Acute Kidney Injury

In patients with TAMOF but who do not have overt DIC, TTP, or HUS, evidences suggest that these patients have a thrombotic microangiopathic process that leads to disseminated microvascular thromboses. Similar to the incidence of TTP-induced AKI, a large US multicenter pediatric TAMOF registry and a pediatric Turkish TAMOF network reported that 56.8% and 47.6% of patients with TAMOF, respectively, have AKI requiring renal replacement therapy.[86,87] These studies suggest that platelet/VWF-mediated thrombosis might be the underlying pathophysiologic process.

Managing Thrombocytopenia-Associated Multiple Organ Failure (Not Overt Disseminated Intravascular Coagulation, Thrombotic Thrombocytopenic Purpura, and Hemolytic Uremic Syndrome)

Mounting evidence suggests that a nonspecific plasma therapeutic strategy, such as TPE, may have a role in reversing MOF and improving outcomes in patients with TAMOF. Of note, all of these patients with TAMOF have concurrent sepsis as a diagnosis.[76,86–88] Currently, the ASFA gives a category III recommendation ("Optimum role of apheresis therapy is not established. Decision making should be individualized"[7]) for TPE in sepsis with MOF. A randomized controlled trial for TPE in TAMOF is warranted.

Currently, there is no monotherapy for DIC and TTP. Various agents have been tried without success, such as heparin, antithrombin III, recombinant tissue factor pathway inhibitor, recombinant activated protein C, protein C concentrate, and recombinant soluble thrombomodulin.[89–96] Eculizumab, an anti-C5 monoclonal antibody, is a promising drug for atypical HUS and possibly for STEC-HUS with MOF.[19,57,58,61,97]

Investigators continue to search for effective therapeutic strategies for a TAMOF clinical phenotype. A phase I recombinant ADAMTS-13 for congenital TTP is ongoing (ClinicalTrials.gov; NCT02216084). An anti-VWF nanobody trial for acquired TTP has been completed and preliminarily reported at the American Society of Hematology meeting in 2014 "Caplacizumab improved standard of care of patients affected with acquired TTP by a more rapid achievement of platelet normalization and lower number of exacerbations with manageable side effects and bleeding episodes" (ClinicalTrials.gov; NCT01151423). N-acetylcysteine has been shown to reduce the size of VWF in human plasma and mice.[98] Recently, N-acetylcysteine was used successfully to treat a case of refractory TTP.[99] The authors have recently reported using a recombinant VWF A2 polypeptide that inhibits platelet-fibrin (estropipate [Ogen]) interaction to reduce disseminated microvascular thromboses and mortality in an endotoxemia-induced DIC murine model.[100]

Armed with a better understanding of the mechanisms of a TAMOF clinical phenotype, innovative therapeutic strategies are being tried to improve the high morbidity and mortality associated with TAMOF.

REFERENCES

1. Hosler GA, Cusumano AM, Hutchins GM. Thrombotic thrombocytopenic purpura and hemolytic uremic syndrome are distinct pathologic entities. A review of 56 autopsy cases. Arch Pathol Lab Med 2003;127(7):834–9.

2. Burke AP, Mont E, Kolodgie F, et al. Thrombotic thrombocytopenic purpura causing rapid unexpected death: value of CD61 immunohistochemical staining in diagnosis. Cardiovasc Pathol 2005;14(3):150–5.
3. Kojima M, Shimamura K, Mori N, et al. A histological study on microthrombi in autopsy cases of DIC. Bibl Haematol 1983;(49):95–106.
4. Asada Y, Sumiyoshi A, Hayashi T, et al. Immunohistochemistry of vascular lesion in thrombotic thrombocytopenic purpura, with special reference to factor VIII related antigen. Thromb Res 1985;38(5):469–79.
5. Dhainaut JF, Yan SB, Joyce DE, et al. Treatment effects of drotrecogin alfa (activated) in patients with severe sepsis with or without overt disseminated intravascular coagulation. J Thromb Haemost 2004;2(11):1924–33.
6. Khemani RG, Bart RD, Alonzo TA, et al. Disseminated intravascular coagulation score is associated with mortality for children with shock. Intensive Care Med 2009;35(2):327–33.
7. Szczepiorkowski ZM, Winters JL, Bandarenko N, et al. Guidelines on the use of therapeutic apheresis in clinical practice–evidence-based approach from the Apheresis Applications Committee of the American Society for Apheresis. J Clin Apheresis 2010;25(3):83–177.
8. Bell WR, Braine HG, Ness PM, et al. Improved survival in thrombotic thrombocytopenic purpura-hemolytic uremic syndrome. Clinical experience in 108 patients. N Engl J Med 1991;325(6):398–403.
9. Rock GA, Shumak KH, Buskard NA, et al. Comparison of plasma exchange with plasma infusion in the treatment of thrombotic thrombocytopenic purpura. Canadian Apheresis Study Group. N Engl J Med 1991;325(6):393–7.
10. Frank C, Werber D, Cramer JP, et al. Epidemic profile of Shiga-toxin-producing Escherichia coli O104:H4 outbreak in Germany. N Engl J Med 2011;365(19):1771–80.
11. Garg AX, Suri RS, Barrowman N, et al. Long-term renal prognosis of diarrhea-associated hemolytic uremic syndrome: a systematic review, meta-analysis, and meta-regression. JAMA 2003;290(10):1360–70.
12. Kaplan BS, Meyers KE, Schulman SL. The pathogenesis and treatment of hemolytic uremic syndrome. J Am Soc Nephrol 1998;9(6):1126–33.
13. Noris M, Remuzzi G. Atypical hemolytic-uremic syndrome. N Engl J Med 2009;361(17):1676–87.
14. Moake JL. Thrombotic microangiopathies. N Engl J Med 2002;347(8):589–600.
15. George JN, Nester CM. Syndromes of thrombotic microangiopathy. N Engl J Med 2014;371(7):654–66.
16. Noris M, Mescia F, Remuzzi G. STEC-HUS, atypical HUS and TTP are all diseases of complement activation. Nat Rev Nephrol 2012;8(11):622–33.
17. Levi M, van der Poll T. Disseminated intravascular coagulation: a review for the internist. Intern Emerg Med 2013;8(1):23–32.
18. In JW, Kim JE, Jeong JS, et al. Diagnostic and prognostic significance of neutrophil gelatinase-associated lipocalin in disseminated intravascular coagulation. Clin Chim Acta 2014;430:145–9.
19. Trachtman H, Austin C, Lewinski M, et al. Renal and neurological involvement in typical Shiga toxin-associated HUS. Nat Rev Nephrol 2012;8(11):658–69.
20. Zafrani L, Mariotte E, Darmon M, et al. Acute renal failure is prevalent in patients with thrombotic thrombocytopenic purpura associated with low plasma ADAMTS13 activity. J Thromb Haemost 2015;13(3):380–9.
21. Moschcowitz E. A hitherto undescribed disease. Proceedings of New York Pathological Society 1924;(24):21–4.

22. Moake JL, Rudy CK, Troll JH, et al. Unusually large plasma factor VIII: von Willebrand factor multimers in chronic relapsing thrombotic thrombocytopenic purpura. N Engl J Med 1982;307(23):1432–5.

23. Tsai HM, Lian EC. Antibodies to von Willebrand factor-cleaving protease in acute thrombotic thrombocytopenic purpura. N Engl J Med 1998;339(22):1585–94.

24. Furlan M, Robles R, Galbusera M, et al. von Willebrand factor-cleaving protease in thrombotic thrombocytopenic purpura and the hemolytic-uremic syndrome. N Engl J Med 1998;339(22):1578–84.

25. Levy GG, Nichols WC, Lian EC, et al. Mutations in a member of the ADAMTS gene family cause thrombotic thrombocytopenic purpura. Nature 2001; 413(6855):488–94.

26. Zhou Z, Nguyen TC, Guchhait P, et al. Von Willebrand factor, ADAMTS-13, and thrombotic thrombocytopenic purpura. Semin Thromb Hemost 2010;36(1): 71–81.

27. Tsai HM, Chandler WL, Sarode R, et al. von Willebrand factor and von Willebrand factor-cleaving metalloprotease activity in Escherichia coli O157:H7-associated hemolytic uremic syndrome. Pediatr Res 2001;49(5):653–9.

28. Sadler JE. Biochemistry and genetics of von Willebrand factor. Annu Rev Biochem 1998;67:395–424.

29. Tsai HM, Nagel RL, Hatcher VB, et al. The high molecular weight form of endothelial cell von Willebrand factor is released by the regulated pathway. Br J Haematol 1991;79(2):239–45.

30. Bernardo A, Ball C, Nolasco L, et al. Effects of inflammatory cytokines on the release and cleavage of the endothelial cell-derived ultralarge von Willebrand factor multimers under flow. Blood 2004;104(1):100–6.

31. Sporn LA, Marder VJ, Wagner DD. Inducible secretion of large, biologically potent von Willebrand factor multimers. Cell 1986;46(2):185–90.

32. Wagner DD. Cell biology of von Willebrand factor. Annu Rev Cell Biol 1990;6: 217–46.

33. Moake JL, Turner NA, Stathopoulos NA, et al. Involvement of large plasma von Willebrand factor (vWF) multimers and unusually large vWF forms derived from endothelial cells in shear stress-induced platelet aggregation. J Clin Invest 1986;78(6):1456–61.

34. Arya M, Anvari B, Romo GM, et al. Ultralarge multimers of von Willebrand factor form spontaneous high-strength bonds with the platelet glycoprotein Ib-IX complex: studies using optical tweezers. Blood 2002;99(11):3971–7.

35. Chow TW, Turner NA, Chintagumpala M, et al. Increased von Willebrand factor binding to platelets in single episode and recurrent types of thrombotic thrombocytopenic purpura. Am J Hematol 1998;57(4):293–302.

36. Liu L, Choi H, Bernardo A, et al. Platelet-derived VWF-cleaving metalloprotease ADAMTS-13. J Thromb Haemost 2005;3(11):2536–44.

37. Turner N, Nolasco L, Tao Z, et al. Human endothelial cells synthesize and release ADAMTS-13. J Thromb Haemost 2006;4(6):1396–404.

38. Zhou W, Inada M, Lee TP, et al. ADAMTS13 is expressed in hepatic stellate cells. Lab Invest 2005;85(6):780–8.

39. Manea M, Kristoffersson A, Schneppenheim R, et al. Podocytes express ADAMTS13 in normal renal cortex and in patients with thrombotic thrombocytopenic purpura. Br J Haematol 2007;138(5):651–62.

40. Vesely SK, George JN, Lammle B, et al. ADAMTS13 activity in thrombotic thrombocytopenic purpura-hemolytic uremic syndrome: relation to presenting

features and clinical outcomes in a prospective cohort of 142 patients. Blood 2003;102(1):60–8.

41. Coppo P, Bengoufa D, Veyradier A, et al. Severe ADAMTS13 deficiency in adult idiopathic thrombotic microangiopathies defines a subset of patients character-ized by various autoimmune manifestations, lower platelet count, and mild renal involvement. Medicine 2004;83(4):233–44.

42. Noris M, Bucchioni S, Galbusera M, et al. Complement factor H mutation in fa-milial thrombotic thrombocytopenic purpura with ADAMTS13 deficiency and renal involvement. J Am Soc Nephrol 2005;16(5):1177–83.

43. Yamada R, Nozawa K, Yoshimine T, et al. A case of thrombotic thrombocyto-penia purpura associated with systemic lupus erythematosus: diagnostic utility of ADAMTS-13 activity. Autoimmune Dis 2011;2011:483642.

44. Yamashita H, Takahashi Y, Kaneko H, et al. Thrombotic thrombocytopenic pur-pura with an autoantibody to ADAMTS13 complicating Sjogren's syndrome: two cases and a literature review. Mod Rheumatol 2013;23(2):365–73.

45. Moake J. Thrombotic microangiopathies: multimers, metalloprotease, and beyond. Clin Transl Sci 2009;2(5):366–73.

46. Tarr PI, Gordon CA, Chandler WL. Shiga-toxin-producing Escherichia coli and haemolytic uraemic syndrome. Lancet 2005;365(9464):1073–86.

47. Johannes L, Romer W. Shiga toxins–from cell biology to biomedical applica-tions. Nat Rev Microbiol 2010;8(2):105–16.

48. van Setten PA, Monnens LA, Verstraten RG, et al. Effects of verocytotoxin-1 on nonadherent human monocytes: binding characteristics, protein synthesis, and induction of cytokine release. Blood 1996;88(1):174–83.

49. Karpman D, Papadopoulou D, Nilsson K, et al. Platelet activation by Shiga toxin and circulatory factors as a pathogenetic mechanism in the hemolytic uremic syndrome. Blood 2001;97(10):3100–8.

50. Nestoridi E, Tsukurov O, Kushak RI, et al. Shiga toxin enhances functional tissue factor on human glomerular endothelial cells: implications for the pathophysio-logy of hemolytic uremic syndrome. J Thromb Haemost 2005;3(4):752–62.

51. Nolasco LH, Turner NA, Bernardo A, et al. Hemolytic uremic syndrome-associated Shiga toxins promote endothelial-cell secretion and impair ADAMTS13 cleavage of unusually large von Willebrand factor multimers. Blood 2005;106(13):4199–209.

52. Morigi M, Galbusera M, Gastoldi S, et al. Alternative pathway activation of com-plement by Shiga toxin promotes exuberant C3a formation that triggers micro-vascular thrombosis. J Immunol 2011;187(1):172–80.

53. Turner NA, Moake J. Assembly and activation of alternative complement com-ponents on endothelial cell-anchored ultra-large von Willebrand factor links complement and hemostasis-thrombosis. PLoS One 2013;8(3):e59372.

54. Ricklin D, Hajishengallis G, Yang K, et al. Complement: a key system for immune surveillance and homeostasis. Nat Immunol 2010;11(9):785–97.

55. Dragon-Durey MA, Loirat C, Cloarec S, et al. Anti-Factor H autoantibodies asso-ciated with atypical hemolytic uremic syndrome. J Am Soc Nephrol 2005;16(2):555–63.

56. Noris M, Remuzzi G. Hemolytic uremic syndrome. J Am Soc Nephrol 2005;16(4):1035–50.

57. Legendre CM, Licht C, Muus P, et al. Terminal complement inhibitor eculizumab in atypical hemolytic-uremic syndrome. N Engl J Med 2013;368(23):2169–81.

58. Zuber J, Fakhouri F, Roumenina LT, et al. Use of eculizumab for atypical haemo-lytic uraemic syndrome and C3 glomerulopathies. Nat Rev Nephrol 2012;8(11):643–57.

59. Colic E, Dieperink H, Titlestad K, et al. Management of an acute outbreak of diarrhoea-associated haemolytic uraemic syndrome with early plasma exchange in adults from southern Denmark: an observational study. Lancet 2011; 378(9796):1089–93.

60. Kielstein JT, Beutel G, Fleig S, et al. Best supportive care and therapeutic plasma exchange with or without eculizumab in Shiga-toxin-producing E. coli O104:H4 induced haemolytic-uraemic syndrome: an analysis of the German STEC-HUS registry. Nephrol Dial Transplant 2012;27(10):3807–15.

61. Lapeyraque AL, Malina M, Fremeaux-Bacchi V, et al. Eculizumab in severe Shiga-toxin-associated HUS. N Engl J Med 2011;364(26):2561–3.

62. Taylor FB Jr, Toh CH, Hoots WK, et al. Towards definition, clinical and laboratory criteria, and a scoring system for disseminated intravascular coagulation. Thromb Haemost 2001;86(5):1327–30.

63. Conkling PR, Greenberg CS, Weinberg JB. Tumor necrosis factor induces tissue factor-like activity in human leukemia cell line U937 and peripheral blood monocytes. Blood 1988;72(1):128–33.

64. van der Poll T, Levi M, Hack CE, et al. Elimination of interleukin 6 attenuates coagulation activation in experimental endotoxemia in chimpanzees. J Exp Med 1994;179(4):1253–9.

65. Levi M, de Jonge E, van der Poll T. Rationale for restoration of physiological anti-coagulant pathways in patients with sepsis and disseminated intravascular coagulation. Crit Care Med 2001;29(7 Suppl):S90–4.

66. Madach K, Aladzsity I, Szilagyi A, et al. 4G/5G polymorphism of PAI-1 gene is associated with multiple organ dysfunction and septic shock in pneumonia induced severe sepsis: prospective, observational, genetic study. Crit Care 2010;14(2):R79.

67. Green J, Doughty L, Kaplan SS, et al. The tissue factor and plasminogen activator inhibitor type-1 response in pediatric sepsis-induced multiple organ failure. Thromb Haemost 2002;87(2):218–23.

68. Madoiwa S, Nunomiya S, Ono T, et al. Plasminogen activator inhibitor 1 promotes a poor prognosis in sepsis-induced disseminated intravascular coagulation. Int J Hematol 2006;84(5):398–405.

69. Ono T, Mimuro J, Madoiwa S, et al. Severe secondary deficiency of von Willebrand factor-cleaving protease (ADAMTS13) in patients with sepsis-induced disseminated intravascular coagulation: its correlation with development of renal failure. Blood 2006;107(2):528–34.

70. Wada H, Thachil J, Di Nisio M, et al. Guidance for diagnosis and treatment of DIC from harmonization of the recommendations from three guidelines. J Thromb Haemost 2013;11:761–7.

71. Corrigan JJ Jr. Thrombocytopenia: a laboratory sign of septicemia in infants and children. J Pediatr 1974;85(2):219–21.

72. Stephan F, Hollande J, Richard O, et al. Thrombocytopenia in a surgical ICU. Chest 1999;115(5):1363–70.

73. Vanderschueren S, De Weerdt A, Malbrain M, et al. Thrombocytopenia and prognosis in intensive care. Crit Care Med 2000;28(6):1871–6.

74. Akca S, Haji-Michael P, de Mendonca A, et al. Time course of platelet counts in critically ill patients. Crit Care Med 2002;30(4):753–6.

75. Moreau D, Timsit JF, Vesin A, et al. Platelet count decline: an early prognostic marker in critically ill patients with prolonged ICU stays. Chest 2007;131(6):1735–41.

76. Nguyen TC, Han YY, Kiss JE, et al. Intensive plasma exchange increases a disintegrin and metalloprotease with thrombospondin motifs-13 activity and

reverses organ dysfunction in children with thrombocytopenia-associated multiple organ failure. Crit Care Med 2008;36(10):2878–87.

77. Bockmeyer CL, Claus RA, Budde U, et al. Inflammation-associated ADAMTS13 deficiency promotes formation of ultra-large von Willebrand factor. Haematologica 2008;93(1):137–40.

78. Martin K, Borgel D, Lerolle N, et al. Decreased ADAMTS-13 (A disintegrin-like and metalloprotease with thrombospondin type 1 repeats) is associated with a poor prognosis in sepsis-induced organ failure. Crit Care Med 2007;35(10):2375–82.

79. Ohshiro M, Kuroda J, Kobayashi Y, et al. ADAMTS-13 activity can predict the outcome of disseminated intravascular coagulation in hematologic malignancies treated with recombinant human soluble thrombomodulin. Am J Hematol 2012;87(1):116–9.

80. Nguyen TC, Liu A, Liu L, et al. Acquired ADAMTS-13 deficiency in pediatric patients with severe sepsis. Haematologica 2007;92(1):121–4.

81. Studt JD, Hovinga JA, Antoine G, et al. Fatal congenital thrombotic thrombocytopenic purpura with apparent ADAMTS13 inhibitor: in vitro inhibition of ADAMTS13 activity by hemoglobin. Blood 2005;105(2):542–4.

82. Zhou Z, Han H, Cruz MA, et al. Haemoglobin blocks von Willebrand factor proteolysis by ADAMTS-13: a mechanism associated with sickle cell disease. Thromb Haemost 2009;101(6):1070–7.

83. Crawley JT, Lam JK, Rance JB, et al. Proteolytic inactivation of ADAMTS13 by thrombin and plasmin. Blood 2005;105(3):1085–93.

84. Chen J, Fu X, Wang Y, et al. Oxidative modification of von Willebrand factor by neutrophil oxidants inhibits its cleavage by ADAMTS13. Blood 2010;115(3): 706–12.

85. Nguyen TC, Balll C, Cruz MA, et al. A negative feedback mechanism of regulating VWF proteolysis by ADAMTS-13. J Thromb Haemost 2011; 9(Suppl 2):206.

86. Fortenberry JD, Knezevic A, Nguyen TC, et al. Outcome in children on ECMO with TAMOF receiving plasma exchange: results from the prospective pediatric TAMOF network study. Crit Care Med 2012;40(12):A520.

87. Sevketoglu E, Yildizdas D, Horoz OO, et al. Use of therapeutic plasma exchange in children with thrombocytopenia-associated multiple organ failure in the Turkish thrombocytopenia-associated multiple organ failure network. Pediatr Crit Care Med 2014;15(8):e354–9.

88. Ruth A, McCracken C, Hall M, et al. Advanced technologies in pediatric severe sepsis: findings from the PHIS database. Crit Care Med 2013;41(12):A1102.

89. Aoki N, Matsuda T, Saito H, et al. A comparative double-blind randomized trial of activated protein C and unfractionated heparin in the treatment of disseminated intravascular coagulation. Int J Hematol 2002;75(5):540–7.

90. Jaimes F, De La Rosa G, Morales C, et al. Unfractioned heparin for treatment of sepsis: a randomized clinical trial (The HETRASE Study). Crit Care Med 2009; 37(4):1185–96.

91. Warren BL, Eid A, Singer P, et al. Caring for the critically ill patient. High-dose antithrombin III in severe sepsis: a randomized controlled trial. JAMA 2001; 286(15):1869–78.

92. Abraham E, Reinhart K, Opal S, et al. Efficacy and safety of tifacogin (recombinant tissue factor pathway inhibitor) in severe sepsis: a randomized controlled trial. JAMA 2003;290(2):238–47.

93. Bernard GR, Vincent JL, Laterre PF, et al. Efficacy and safety of recombinant human activated protein C for severe sepsis. N Engl J Med 2001;344(10):699–709.

94. Ranieri VM, Thompson BT, Barie PS, et al. Drotrecogin alfa (activated) in adults with septic shock. N Engl J Med 2012;366(22):2055–64.

95. de Kleijn ED, de Groot R, Hack CE, et al. Activation of protein C following infusion of protein C concentrate in children with severe meningococcal sepsis and purpura fulminans: a randomized, double-blinded, placebo-controlled, dose-finding study. Crit Care Med 2003;31(6):1839–47.

96. Saito H, Maruyama I, Shimazaki S, et al. Efficacy and safety of recombinant human soluble thrombomodulin (ART-123) in disseminated intravascular coagulation: results of a phase III, randomized, double-blind clinical trial. J Thromb Haemost 2007;5(1):31–41.

97. Nurnberger J, Philipp T, Witzke O, et al. Eculizumab for atypical hemolytic-uremic syndrome. N Engl J Med 2009;360(5):542–4.

98. Chen J, Reheman A, Gushiken FC, et al. N-acetylcysteine reduces the size and activity of von Willebrand factor in human plasma and mice. J Clin Invest 2011; 121(2):593–603.

99. Li GW, Rambally S, Kamboj J, et al. Treatment of refractory thrombotic thrombocytopenic purpura with N-acetylcysteine: a case report. Transfusion 2014;54(5): 1221–4.

100. Nguyen TC, Gushiken F, Correa JI, et al. A recombinant fragment of von Willebrand factor reduces fibrin-rich microthrombi formation in mice with endotoxemia. Thromb Res 2015;135(5):1025–30.

Drug-Induced Acute Kidney Injury

A Focus on Risk Assessment for Prevention

Sandra L. Kane-Gill, PharmD, MS[a,b,*], Stuart L. Goldstein, MD[c]

KEYWORDS

- Drug-induced acute kidney injury
- Drug-related side effects and adverse drug reactions • Acute kidney injury
- Risk factors • Risk assessment • Prevention

KEY POINTS

- Modifiable drug-specific exposures for nephrotoxicity are the duration of nephrotoxin treatment, cumulative or total daily dose of nephrotoxin, and pharmacokinetic and pharmacodynamic drug interactions.
- Acute kidney injury (AKI) detection strategies may mitigate further kidney injury, but they do little to prevent harm and have not used systematic creatinine surveillance for AKI in at-risk patients.
- The advent and wide dissemination of hospital-based electronic health records has led to automated AKI alerting systems that need to be optimized for the prevention of drug-induced AKI.
- Once a suspected drug cause has been identified then evaluation includes temporal sequence, objective evidence, prior knowledge to support the nephrotoxin as a culprit and ruling out non-drug related causes.

EPIDEMIOLOGY OF DRUG-INDUCED ACUTE KIDNEY INJURY

Critically ill patients receive twice the number of drugs as compared with non–critically ill patients, increasing the risk of developing significantly more adverse drug events, such as acute kidney injury (AKI).[1,2] Approximately 20% of the drugs prescribed in

Funding Sources: None.
Conflict of Interest: None.
[a] Department of Pharmacy and Therapeutics, University of Pittsburgh School of Pharmacy, 918 Salk Hall, 3501 Terrace Street, Pittsburgh, PA 15261, USA; [b] Center for Critical Care Nephology, University of Pittsburgh Medical Center, University of Pittsburgh School of Medicine, 3550 Terrace Street, Pittsburgh, PA 15261, USA; [c] Center for Acute Care Nephrology, Department of Pediatrics, Cincinnati Children's Hospital Medical Center, University of Cincinnati College of Medicine, 3333 Burnet Avenue, MLC 7022, Cincinnati, OH 45229, USA
* Corresponding author. University of Pittsburgh School of Pharmacy, 918 Salk Hall, 3501 Terrace Street, Pittsburgh, PA 15261.
E-mail address: SLK54@pitt.edu

Crit Care Clin 31 (2015) 675–684
http://dx.doi.org/10.1016/j.ccc.2015.06.005
0749-0704/15/$ – see front matter © 2015 Elsevier Inc. All rights reserved.

the intensive care unit (ICU) are considered nephrotoxic.[3] Drugs are the third to fifth leading cause of AKI in this setting following sepsis and hypotension.[4–7] AKI occurs in 20% to 30% of critically ill patients, with drugs contributing to about 1 in 4 episodes of AKI. The rate of drug-induced AKI is similar in hospitalized pediatric patients at 16%.[8] Drug-induced nephrotoxicity is higher in the elderly at a rate of up to 66%.[9] According to a meta-analysis of risk factors for AKI in critically ill patients, there is a 53% greater odds of developing AKI for every nephrotoxic drug received (odds ratio 1.53; confidence interval 1.09–2.14).[10]

The negative consequences attributable to drug-induced AKI are severe. An evaluation of AKI in 5 US academic hospitals indicates that the in-hospital mortality rate from nephrotoxic causes is approximately 25%, ranging from 18% to 50% varying by institution. The rate of dialysis dependence following AKI from nephrotoxic causes is about 20%.[11] The patient outcomes for AKI from nephrotoxins are similar to AKI of other causes.[11] Over the past decade, the association between AKI and chronic kidney disease (CKD) has been repeatedly demonstrated in children and adults,[12–16] yet the studies in these reviews looked at all-cause AKI and did not separate out drug-induced AKI as an independent entity. Menon and colleagues[8] followed children from a single-center electronic health record (EHR)–driven AKI surveillance study. Although none of the patients had signs of CKD before nephrotoxic medication exposure, 70% of the children had at least one sign of chronic kidney injury (decreased estimated glomerular filtration rate, hyperfiltration, proteinuria, and/or hypertension) when assessed at follow-up. Thus, it is critical that patients who develop AKI after a nephrotoxic insult be followed longitudinally for signs of CKD.[13]

The fact that many nephrotoxic drugs are mainstays of the therapeutic advancements and improved outcomes observed in hospitalized patients has likely led to a perspective that drug-induced AKI is a necessary evil of modern medical management. Clearly, antimicrobials, antivirals, chemotherapeutics, and solid organ transplant antirejection medications represent essential medication classes, all of which can be associated with AKI. A little more discretion can be given to the prescribing of nonessential nephrotoxins, such as nonsteroidal antiinflammatories. Drug-induced nephrotoxicity is more apt to occur in those patients with risk factors. The purpose of this article is to review the risk factors, risk-assessment strategies, prevention, and management of drug-induced AKI with *emphasis on risk assessment*. The authors do not discuss the mechanisms of drug-induced AKI, as this has been well covered by others.[17–20]

RISK FACTORS FOR DRUG-INDUCED ACUTE KIDNEY INJURY

There are several susceptibilities and exposures that may contribute to AKI development as discussed in the Kidney Disease: Improving Global Outcomes (KDIGO) guidelines.[10,21] Also a recent systematic review highlighted the risk factors for AKI in critically ill patients.[9] The susceptibilities and exposures for AKI are listed in **Table 1**. Although these risks are for AKI, one assumes that they may apply to drug-induced AKI, although no specific comparison between risk factors of drug-induced AKI and AKI from other causes has been conducted.

Risk factors for consideration specific to drug-induced AKI include drug combinations, such as the "triple whammy" including nonsteroidal antiinflammatories, angiotensin-converting enzymes, and diuretics.[22–24] Dual drug combinations that have been proposed as a cause of additional risk for AKI when administered simultaneously are cisplatin plus gentamicin, simvastatin plus cyclosporine, vancomycin plus ceftazidime, and gentamicin plus cephalothin. A combination of drugs presents

Table 1	
Susceptibilities and exposures for developing AKI	
Description of Risk Factors	**Risk Factors in Critically Ill Patients**
Susceptibilities	Age, black race, female sex, history of diabetes mellitus, history of hypertension, history of AKI, dehydration, higher baseline serum creatinine
Exposures	Nephrotoxin administration, radiocontrast agents, trauma, burn, circulatory shock, sepsis, high-risk surgery, severity of disease, hypotension, fluid overload
Drug-specific exposures	Duration of nephrotoxin treatment, cumulative or total daily dose of nephrotoxin treatment, elevated drug concentrations, pharmacokinetic and pharmacodynamics drug interactions

Data from Cartin-Ceba R, Kashiouris M, Plataki M, et al. Risk factors for development of acute kidney injury in critically ill patients: a systematic review and meta-analysis of observational studies. Crit Care Res Pract 2012;2012:691013; and Kidney Disease: Improving Global Outcomes (KDIGO) Acute Kidney Injury Work Group. KDIGO clinical practice guideline for acute kidney injury. Kidney Int 2012;2(suppl 1):1–138.

additional risk caused by pharmacokinetic and pharmacodynamic drug interactions.[25] A pharmacokinetic interaction is the administration of a participant drug that alters the absorption, distribution, metabolism, and/or elimination of the object drug; in this case, the object drug is the nephrotoxin. The pharmacokinetic interactions will result in greater potential for nephrotoxicity. A pharmacodynamic interaction is the administration of 2 nephrotoxic drugs simultaneously having an additive or possibly synergistic effect. The cumulative dose and duration of treatment with a nephrotoxin enhances the risk of developing AKI. Lastly, for consideration is the individual drug nephrotoxic potential because some drugs are more nephrotoxic than others (ie, piperacillin/tazobactam, vancomycin, and amphotericin) and drug-specific nephrotoxic potential may be influenced by other patient characteristics, such as increased age.[18,20,26–28]

An example of a risk-factor assessment for drug-induced nephrotoxicity is the recent evaluation of vancomycin; this retrospective observational study revealed a prevalence of 21% for vancomycin-induced AKI in critically ill patients. The risk factors for vancomycin-associated AKI per logistic regression analysis were higher median trough concentrations, longer duration of therapy, simultaneous use of vasoactive drugs, and administration of vancomycin via intermittent infusions.[29] This evaluation was limited by the lack of a concomitant drug administration assessment to determine the contribution of drug combinations in the development of AKI. Also, susceptibilities and exposures for AKI should have been considered in more detail.

RISK ASSESSMENT FOR DRUG-INDUCED ACUTE KIDNEY INJURY

Risk assessment for drug-induced AKI has predominantly been reactive in looking for AKI in patients who have been exposed to nephrotoxic medications. The advent and wide dissemination of hospital-based EHRs has led to automated AKI alerting systems, usually based on an increase in serum creatinine.[30] EHR-based safety tools include kidney injury triggers, such as the Institute for Healthcare Improvement's Global Trigger Tool,[31] a recent tool using Acute Kidney Injury Network definition,[32] or dosing tools to improve compliance with dose adjustment of renally cleared medications after AKI has occurred.[33,34] In some studies, EHR-based AKI detection expedites time to interventions and yields a higher percentage of patients returning to baseline kidney function.[35,36] Matheny and colleagues[37] used retrospective EHR data to develop a risk stratification model to predict hospital-acquired AKI that needs to be tested for AKI prevention.

Although AKI detection strategies may mitigate further kidney injury after AKI has already occurred, they do little to prevent initial harm and have generally not used systematic creatinine surveillance for AKI in at-risk patients. Thus, many cases may go undetected because drug-induced AKI is usually nonoliguric in nature.[20] A recent pediatric single-center quality-improvement initiative used prospective screening of hospitalized children at risk for drug-induced AKI to drive systematic serum creatinine surveillance.[38] Epidemiologic data demonstrated non–critically ill children exposed to 3 or more nephrotoxic drugs simultaneously or an intravenous aminoglycoside for more than 3 days are at an increased risk of AKI.[39,40] Kirkendall and colleagues[41] developed an EHR-based trigger to alert clinical pharmacists on rounds when a patient was at increased risk, thus allowing for daily creatinine monitoring. The advantage to this automated risk identification system is that it has a dedicated person committed to an action after the alert, which is outside the workflow of prescribing or order verification. In the first year of the project, 25% of exposed patients developed AKI, which was higher than reported by administrative coding or less systematic screening.[42,43] Furthermore, this reliable detection led to AKI mitigation strategies to decrease the number of days of AKI.[37] Although these outcomes need to be validated in multiple different centers, including adult care environments, development of risk-assessment tools to foster systematic surveillance or nephrotoxic medication avoidance represents a modifiable risk factor for AKI.

In addition, patients with CKD may be at greater risk for drug-induced AKI as a result of their decreased renal reserve. The added risk baseline renal dysfunction has been studied most often in adult patients receiving intravenous contrast administration, but drug-induced AKI from other nephrotoxic medications is also increased from CKD.[43] The recent KDIGO guidelines identify other factors that increase the susceptibility to AKI, including advanced age, anemia, black race, cancer, diabetes, female sex, other chronic disease, and volume contraction.[21] Of these risk factors, only volume contraction is modifiable and, therefore, should be corrected before administration of a nephrotoxic medication. The exposures of risk for AKI described in the KDIGO guidelines are potentially modifiable or at least if treated quickly and accurately with the goal of reducing the duration of exposure that could reduce the risk for AKI.[44]

Further considerations for building an effective risk-assessment alerting system are to include risk factors combined with known nephrotoxins in the knowledge/rule logic for the alert allowing for early detection before an increase in serum creatinine. This idea is similar to the work of Goldstein (described earlier) with the addition of risk factors.[41] Another element to consider for an effective system is the provision of active alerts that require a response or provide specific recommendations to a specific individual rather than a passive, simply informational alert. A parallel group randomized controlled trial that assigned patients to medical teams receiving electronic AKI alerts and teams that did not receive such an alert failed to show a difference in patient outcomes between groups.[45] Perhaps the reason for the ineffective alert was the passive advice provided to the clinician receiving the alert, being simply a link to the KDIGO guidelines. A highly performing risk-assessment alerting system will require adjustments and evaluation to maximize benefits.

A necessary step at every institution is the optimal reporting of adverse drug reactions per institutional policies and procedures. A dedicated risk management team is needed to evaluate adverse drug reactions, in this case drug-induced AKI, so that causes of events (ie, medication errors) can be identified. Evaluating reported events provides an opportunity to identify patterns or problems in institutions and promote prevention efforts for future events with systematic changes using these data.[46] This dedicated team is especially important for those who are not fortunate to have resources for automated or manual surveillance of patients at risk for AKI.

PREVENTION OF DRUG-INDUCED ACUTE KIDNEY INJURY

Prevention is the best approach to averting harm associated with nephrotoxins. This most efficient approach to evaluating risk factors, as mentioned in the risk-assessment section (earlier), will require either manual or electronic surveillance. Early detection of patients at risk for AKI requires clinicians to shift their approach away from waiting for an increase in serum creatinine, as this biomarker lags by 24 to 48 hours behind initial kidney injury.[47] Once high-risk patients are identified, then diligent monitoring of urine output and serum creatinine is necessary. Also, attempts to manage potentially modifiable risk factors should be made, including the avoidance of nephrotoxic drugs when possible.[21,44] As the duration of AKI increases, the outcomes worsen, so prevention of AKI occurrence and prevention of AKI progression is key.[48]

Based on recent findings, we may become more focused on tracking other biomarkers that increase before serum creatinine. Kidney injury molecule 1 (KIM-1), N-acetyl-β-D-glucosaminidase (NAG), and neutrophil gelatinase-associated lipocalin demonstrated potential in the early detection of aminoglycoside-induced AKI with significant increases in neonates with AKI. However, KIM-1 was the only urinary biomarker that upheld its significance in the multivariate regression analysis.[49] The recently marketed urinary test for tissue inhibitor of metalloproteinase-2 (TIMP-2) and insulin-like growth factor binding protein-7 (IGFBP-7) biomarkers allow for identifying critically ill patients at risk for AKI at least 12 hours before an increase in serum creatinine. The value of these biomarkers for the prevention of drug-induced AKI is still under investigation.

Using therapies as prevention strategies for AKI has been attempted for recombinant human insulinlike growth factor I, atrial natriuretic peptide, N-acetylcysteine (noncontrast induced), fenoldopam, dopamine, and others with no success.[21,50] Data from animal models seem promising but have not translated well in human studies.[50] One example of this is the use of pentoxifylline for drug-induced nephrotoxicity, specifically nephrotoxicity caused by cyclosporine. Pentoxifylline demonstrated positive results in animal studies, but there is still inconclusive evidence to show a benefit in humans.[51] There are several barriers to successful pharmacologic prevention or treatment of AKI, including patient and comorbid factors, complexity of AKI, and AKI being a multisystem disease.[50]

The most promising approaches for the prevention of contrast-induced AKI are the use of preemptive hydration and N-acetylcysteine. Often the limitations associated with the studies surrounding which intravenous (IV) fluid to use and the use of oral versus IV N-acetylcysteine is highlighted to illustrate the need for further clarity in this area.[52,53] The current KDIGO guidelines recommend the use of IV volume expansion with either isotonic sodium chloride or sodium bicarbonate rather than no IV fluid expansion in patients at risk for contrast-induced AKI.[21] Also, oral N-acetylcysteine is recommended in conjunction with IV isotonic crystalloid administration in patients at risk for contrast-induced AKI per KDIGO; but it is not recommended by the American College of Cardiology/American Heart Association/Society of Cardiovascular Angiography and Interventions' guideline.[54] In an attempt to address this controversy, there is an ongoing randomized, double-blind, multicenter trial evaluating IV isotonic sodium bicarbonate versus IV isotonic sodium chloride and oral N-acetylcysteine (NAC) versus placebo called Prevention of Serious Adverse Events following Angiography (PRESERVE).[53]

MANAGEMENT OF DRUG-INDUCED ACUTE KIDNEY INJURY

One of the largest challenges in the management of drug-induced AKI is the identification of a drug-related cause. When trying to identify drug causes, we should review the patients' entire medication list, including over-the-counter drugs and herbal products. An evaluation of suspected drugs includes consideration of the temporal sequence between the event and drug administration, objective evidence including drug concentrations when appropriate, prior knowledge of the event to support the nephrotoxin as a culprit, and ruling out the other non–drug-related causes. There are adverse drug reaction causality instruments that can aid in this evaluation. Some popular examples of instruments are the Naranjo criteria, Kramer, and Jones—and all of which perform comparatively, although their reliability in the ICU has been questioned.[55,56] Often we are left with a strong hunch of causality and manage the situation with the removal of the suspected offending agent, known as a dechallenge, and then observe the patients' response for a definitive diagnosis.

Further management of drug-induced AKI, in its early stage, according to the KDIGO guidelines, includes discontinuing all nephrotoxic agents when possible, ensuring adequate volume status, monitoring serum creatinine, monitoring urine output, hemodynamic monitoring, and avoiding hyperglycemia.[21] Despite the goal of avoiding drugs that should be used cautiously or avoided in patients with kidney injury, 42% of hospitalized patients are initiated on nephrotoxins in general medicine units, although the magnitude of inappropriate prescribing in critically ill patients is unclear.[57] Also of note, up to 67% of drugs that are cleared renally are not dose adjusted appropriately based on kidney function.[58] So, overall there is an opportunity for improving the prescribing of nephrotoxins and managing renally cleared drugs in the presence of AKI.

FUTURE DIRECTIONS

Although the prevalence and impact of drug-induced AKI presents a serious health care burden, drug-induced AKI risk assessment remains generally relegated to broad demographic criteria; treatment consists of hydration and nephrotoxic medication avoidance. Recent efforts have commenced in 2 areas to personalize risk stratification and AKI detection: (1) assessment of genetic predisposition to specific nephrotoxic medications and (2) use of novel damage urinary biomarkers to identify AKI before the increase in the functional AKI marker, serum creatinine. The Drug Induced Renal Injury Consortium (DIRECT, NCT02159209) is a multicenter international pediatric and adult prospective observational collaborative study designed to determine the genetic risk factors for drug-induced AKI.[59] A blood sample for DNA is obtained for any patient with documented KDIGO stage II AKI exposed to up to 3 nephrotoxic medications before AKI development. DIRECT will perform a genome-wide association study to examine the association of common genetic variants with the development of drug-induced AKI. For assessing the association between a common single nucleotide and the risk of drug-induced AKI, association tests will be undertaken to compare genotype frequencies between cases and controls. It is hoped that results from the DIRECT study will identify patients who are at very high risk for AKI from a specific drug, or class of drugs, allowing medical teams to find suitable alternatives or lower doses, when appropriate.

The limitations of serum creatinine as a real-time AKI marker have been well documented in the literature, resulting in a concerted effort to find novel markers of kidney damage that detect AKI earlier and predict AKI severity.[60] Currently, published evaluation of the ability of these new markers to detect drug-induced AKI has been limited to drug exposure in animal studies; but several human studies are ongoing in the oncology and cystic fibrosis populations. Given that these biomarkers can identify both acute and chronic kidney damage in different nephron segments, the authors speculate that novel urinary biomarker assessment for AKI risk and AKI development will become the standard of care once validated.

SUMMARY

Drug-induced AKI is becoming recognized as a significant sequelae of care for hospitalized patients. Recent work to identify drug-induced AKI risk factors and develop systematic nephrotoxic medication exposure and AKI detection alerts and the association with the development of CKD has highlighted the enormous magnitude of the harm. It is hoped that current translational efforts to identify genetic polymorphisms that increase risk, or provide protection, to drug-induced AKI will allow us to modify practice and reduce unnecessary harm in the future.

REFERENCES

1. Cullen DJ, Sweitzer BJ, Bates DW, et al. Preventable adverse drug events in hospitalized patients: a comparative study of intensive care and general care units. Crit Care Med 1997;25:1289–97.
2. Kane-Gill SL, Kirisci L, Verrico MM, et al. Analysis of risk factors for adverse drug events in critically ill patients. Crit Care Med 2012;40:823–8.
3. Taber SS, Mueller BA. Drug-associated renal dysfunction. Crit Care Clin 2006;22: 357–74.
4. Brivet FG, Kleinknecht DJ, Loirat P, et al. Acute renal failure in intensive care units - causes, outcome, and prognostic factors of hospital mortality; a prospective, multicenter study. French Study Group on Acute Renal Failure. Crit Care Med 1996;24: 192–8.
5. Mehta RL, Pascual MT, Soroko S, et al. Spectrum of acute renal failure in the intensive care unit: the PICARD experience. Kidney Int 2004;66:1613–21.
6. Uchino S, Kellum JA, Bellomo R, et al. Acute renal failure in critically ill patients: a multinational, multicenter study. JAMA 2005;294:813–8.
7. Uchino S. The epidemiology of acute renal failure in the world. Curr Opin Crit Care 2006;12:538–43.
8. Menon S, Kirkendall ES, Nguyen H, et al. Acute kidney injury associated with high nephrotoxic medication exposure leads to chronic kidney disease after 6 months. J Pediatr 2014;165:522–7.e2.
9. Kohli HS, Bhaskaran MC, Muthukumar T, et al. Treatment-related acute renal failure in the elderly: a hospital-based prospective study. Nephrol Dial Transplant 2000;15:212–7.
10. Cartin-Ceba R, Kashiouris M, Plataki M, et al. Risk factors for development of acute kidney injury in critically ill patients: a systematic review and meta-analysis of observational studies. Crit Care Res Pract 2012;2012:691013 [article ID 691013].
11. Mehta RL, Pascual MT, Soroko S, et al. Spectrum of acute kidney failure in the intensive care unit: the PICARD experience. Kidney Int 2004;66:1613–21.

12. Goldstein SL, Devarajan P. Acute kidney injury in childhood: should we be worried about progression to CKD? Pediatr Nephrol 2011;26:509–22.
13. Goldstein SL, Jaber BL, Faubel S, et al, Acute Kidney Injury Advisory Group of American Society of Nephrol. Aki transition of care: a potential opportunity to detect and prevent CKD. Clin J Am Soc Nephrol 2013;8:476–83.
14. Chawla LS, Amdur RL, Amodeo S, et al. The severity of acute kidney injury predicts progression to chronic kidney disease. Kidney Int 2011;79(12):1361–9.
15. Hsu CY. Yes, AKI truly leads to CKD. J Am Soc Nephrol 2012;23:967–9.
16. Chawla LS, Eggers PW, Star RA, et al. Acute kidney injury and chronic kidney disease as interconnected syndromes. N Engl J Med 2014;371:58–66.
17. Parzella MA, Makowitz GS. Drug-induced acute interstitial nephritis. Nat Rev Nephrol 2010;6:461–70.
18. Bentley ML, Corwin HL, Dasta J. Drug-induced acute kidney injury in the critically ill adult: recognition and prevention strategies. Crit Care Med 2010;38(6 Suppl): S169–74.
19. Nolin TD, Himmelfarb J. Mechanisms of drug-induced nephrotoxicity. Handb Exp Pharmacol 2010;196:111–30.
20. Schetz M, Dasta J, Goldstein S, et al. Drug-induced acute kidney injury. Curr Opin Crit Care 2005;11:555–65.
21. Kidney Disease: Improving Global Outcomes (KDIGO) Acute Kidney Injury Work Group. KDIGO clinical practice guideline for acute kidney injury. Kidney Int 2012;2(suppl 1):1–138.
22. Loboz KK, Shienfield GM. Drug combinations and impaired renal function- the 'triple whammy'. Br J Clin Pharmacol 2004;59:239–43.
23. Fournier JP, Sommet A, Durrieu G, et al. Drug interactions between antihypertensive drugs and non-steroidal anti-inflammatory agents: a descriptive study using the French pharmacovigilance database. Fundam Clin Pharmacol 2014;28: 230–5.
24. Lapi F, Azoulay L, Yin H, et al. Concurrent use of diuretics, angiotensin converting enzyme inhibitors, and angiotensin receptor blockers with non-steroidal anti-inflammatory drugs and risk of acute kidney injury: nested case-control study. BMJ 2013;346:e8525.
25. Smithburger PL, Seybert AL, Armahizer MJ, et al. QT prolongation in the intensive care unit: commonly used medications and the impact of drug-drug interactions. Expert Opin Drug Saf 2010;9:699–712.
26. Burgess LD, Drew RH. Comparison of the incidence of vancomycin-induced nephrotoxicity in hospitalized patients with and without concomitant piperacillin-tazobactam. Pharmacotherapy 2014;34:670–6.
27. Deray G. Amphotericin B nephrotoxicity. J Antimicrob Chemother 2002;49(suppl 1): 37–41.
28. Kane-Gill SL, Sileanu FE, Murugan R, et al. Risk factors for acute kidney injury in older adults with critical illness: a retrospective cohort study. Am J Kidney Dis 2014. http://dx.doi.org/10.1053/j.ajkd.2014.10.018.
29. Hanrahan TP, Harlow G, Hutchinson J, et al. Vancomycin-associated nephrotoxicity in the critically ill: a retrospective multivariate regression analysis. Crit Care Med 2014;42:2527–36.
30. Handler SM, Kane-Gill SL, Kellum JA. Optimal and early detection of acute kidney injury requires effective clinical decision support systems. Nephrol Dial Transplant 2014;29:1802–3.
31. Resar RK, Rozich JD, Simmonds T, et al. trigger tool to identify adverse events in the intensive care unit. Jt Comm J Qual Patient Saf 2006;32:585–90.

32. Selby NM, Crowley L, Fluck RJ, et al. Use of electronic results reporting to diagnose and monitor AKI in hospitalized patients. Clin J Am Soc Nephrol 2012;7: 533–40.

33. Chertow GM, Lee J, Kuperman GJ, et al. Guided medication dosing for inpatients with renal insufficiency. JAMA 2001;286:2839–44.

34. McCoy AB, Waitman LR, Gadd CS, et al. A computerized provider order entry intervention for medication safety during acute kidney injury: a quality improvement report. Am J Kidney Dis 2010;56:832–41.

35. Colpaert K, Hoste E, Van Hoecke S, et al. Implementation of a real-time electronic alert based on the RIFLE criteria for acute kidney injury in ICU patients. Acta Clin Belg Suppl 2007;(2):322–5.

36. Colpaert K, Hoste EA, Steurbaut K, et al. Impact of real-time electronic alerting of acute kidney injury on therapeutic intervention and progression of RIFLE class. Crit Care Med 2012;40:1164–70.

37. Matheny ME, Miller RA, Ikizler TA, et al. Development of inpatient risk stratification models of acute kidney injury for use in electronic health records. Med Decis Making 2010;30:639–50.

38. Goldstein SL, Kirkendall E, Nguyen H, et al. Electronic health record identification of nephrotoxin exposure and associated acute kidney injury. Pediatrics 2013;132: e756–67.

39. Moffett BS, Goldstein SL. Acute kidney injury and increasing nephrotoxic-medication exposure in noncritically-ill children. Clin J Am Soc Nephrol 2011;6: 856–63.

40. Zappitelli M, Moffett BS, Hyder A, et al. Acute kidney injury in non-critically ill children treated with aminoglycoside antibiotics in a tertiary healthcare centre: a retrospective cohort study. Nephrol Dial Transplant 2011;26:144–50.

41. Kirkendall ES, Spires WL, Mottes TA, et al. Development and performance of electronic acute kidney injury triggers to identify pediatric patients at risk for nephrotoxic medication-associated harm. Appl Clin Inform 2014;5:313–33.

42. Schaffzin JK, Dodd CN, Nguyen H, et al. Administrative data misclassifies and fails to identify nephrotoxin-associated acute kidney injury in hospitalized children. Hosp Pediatr 2014;4:159–66.

43. Downes KJ, Rao MB, Kahill L, et al. Daily serum creatinine monitoring promotes earlier detection of acute kidney injury in children and adolescents with cystic fibrosis. J Cyst Fibros 2014;13:435–41.

44. Rewa O, Bagshaw SM. Acute kidney injury-epidemiology, outcomes and economics. Nat Rev Nephrol 2014;10:193–207.

45. Wilson FP, Shashaty M, Testani J, et al. Automated, electronic alerts for acute kidney injury: a single-blind, parallel-group, randomised controlled trial. Lancet 2015;385(9981):1966–74.

46. Stockwell DC, Kane-Gill SL. Developing a patient specific surveillance system to identify adverse events in the intensive care unit. Crit Care Med 2010;38: S117–25.

47. Zhou H, Hewitt SM, Yuen PST, et al. Acute kidney injury biomarker- needs, present status, and future promise. Nephrol Self Assess Program 2006;5: 63–71.

48. Kellum JA, Sileanu F, Murugan R, et al. Classifying AKI by urine output versus serum creatinine level. J Am Soc Nephrol 2015. [Epub ahead of print].

49. McWilliam SJ, Antoine DJ, Sabbisetti V, et al. Mechanism-based urinary biomarkers to identify the potential for aminoglycoside-induced nephrotoxicity in premature neonates: a proof-of-concept study. PLoS One 2012;7:e43809.

50. Jo SK, Rosner MH, Okusa MD. Pharmacologic treatment of acute kidney injury: why drugs haven't worked and what is on the horizon. Clin J Am Soc Nephrol 2007;2:356–65.
51. Nasiri-Toosi Z, Dashti-Khavidaki S, Khalili H, et al. A review of the potential protective effects of pentoxifylline against drug-induced nephrotoxicity. Eur J Clin Pharmacol 2013;69:1057–73.
52. Chousterman BG, Bouadma L, Moutereau S, et al. Prevention of contrast-induced nephropathy by N-acetylcysteine in critically ill patients: different definitions, different results. J Crit Care 2013;28:701–9.
53. Weisbord SD, Gallagher M, Kaufman J, et al. Prevention of contrast-induced AKI: a review of published trials and the design of the prevention of serious adverse events following angiography (PRESERVE) trial. Clin J Am Soc Nephrol 2013;8:1618–31.
54. Levine GN, Bates ER, Blankenship JC, et al. 2011 ACCF/AHA/SCAI guideline for Percutaneous coronary intervention: a report of the American College of Cardiology Foundation/American Heart Association Task Force on practice guidelines and the Society for Cardiovascular Angiography and Interventions. Circulation 2011;124:e574–651.
55. Kane-Gill SL, Forsberg EA, Verrico MM, et al. Comparison of three pharmacovigilance algorithms in the ICU setting: a retrospective and prospective evaluation of ADRs. Drug Saf 2012;35:645–53.
56. Kane-Gill, Kirisci L, Pathak DS. Are the Naranjo criteria reliable and valid for determination of adverse drug reactions in the intensive care unit? Ann Pharmacother 2005;39:1823–7.
57. Blix HS, Viktil KK, Moger TA, et al. Use of renal risk drugs in hospitalized patients with impaired renal function-an underestimated problem. Nephrol Dial Transplant 2006;21:3164–71.
58. Long CL, Raebel MA, Price DW, et al. Compliance with dosing guidelines in patients with chronic kidney disease. Ann Pharmacother 2004;38:853–8.
59. Mehta RL, Awdishu L, Davenport A, et al. Phenotype standardization for drug-induced kidney disease. Kidney Int 2015. [Epub ahead of print].
60. Alge JL, Arthur JM. Biomarkers of AKI: a review of mechanistic relevance and potential therapeutic implications. Clin J Am Soc Nephrol 2015;10:147–55.

A Clinical Approach to the Acute Cardiorenal Syndrome

Jacob C. Jentzer, MD[a], Lakhmir S. Chawla, MD[b,c],*

KEYWORDS

- Cardiorenal syndrome • Heart failure • Acute kidney injury • Diuretics
- Chronic kidney disease • Ultrafiltration • Acute heart failure syndromes

KEY POINTS

- Acute cardiorenal syndrome represents a unique form of acute kidney injury specific to acute heart failure syndromes that is associated with adverse outcomes.
- Acute cardiorenal syndrome results from renal venous congestion, ineffective forward flow, and impaired renal autoregulation caused by neurohormonal activation.
- Biomarkers reflecting different aspects of acute cardiorenal syndrome pathophysiology may allow patient phenotyping to inform prognosis and treatment.
- Aggressive diuretic therapy to relieve congestion is the cornerstone of treatment in acute cardiorenal syndrome.
- Adjunctive therapies may relieve congestive symptoms and/or improve renal function, but no single therapy has been conclusively shown to reduce mortality in acute cardiorenal syndrome.

INTRODUCTION

The medical community has increasingly recognized the complex relationship between the heart and kidneys over recent years. The term cardiorenal syndromes (CRSs) encompasses a spectrum of disease states involving mutually interacting cardiac and renal dysfunction. CRSs are defined as "disorders of the heart and kidneys

Disclosures: Nothing to disclose (Dr J.C. Jentzer); grants or honoraria from Alere, Astute and Abbott (Dr L.S. Chawla).
[a] Department of Critical Care Medicine, UPMC Presbyterian Hospital, University of Pittsburgh Medical Center, 200 Lothrop Street, Pittsburgh, PA 15213, USA; [b] Division of Intensive Care Medicine, Department of Medicine, Washington DC Veterans Affairs Medical Center, 50 Irving Street, Washington, DC 20422, USA; [c] Division of Nephrology, Department of Medicine, Washington DC Veterans Affairs Medical Center, 50 Irving Street, Washington, DC 20422, USA
* Corresponding author. Division of Nephrology, Department of Medicine, Washington DC Veterans Affairs Medical Center, 50 Irving Street, Washington, DC 20422.
E-mail address: minkchawla@gmail.com

Crit Care Clin 31 (2015) 685–703
http://dx.doi.org/10.1016/j.ccc.2015.06.006
0749-0704/15/$ – see front matter Published by Elsevier Inc.

whereby acute or chronic dysfunction in one organ may induce acute or chronic dysfunction of the other."[1,2] The term cardiorenal applies when cardiac dysfunction drives renal dysfunction, as opposed to renocardiac, in which renal dysfunction drives cardiac dysfunction.[1,2] Patients may develop more than 1 CRS simultaneously because of the bidirectional nature of cardiorenal interactions and shared risk factors for cardiac and renal disease.[3] Acute CRS represents a unique form of acute kidney injury (AKI) developing in patients with acute cardiac dysfunction. For a broader overview of the CRSs, we refer readers to recent comprehensive reviews.[3–5]

EPIDEMIOLOGY OF ACUTE CARDIORENAL SYNDROME

Acute CRS is the best-recognized of the CRSs, and the subtype most frequently encountered in acutely ill patients. Acute CRS was initially described as diuretic-refractory volume overload with worsening renal function (WRF) during treatment of decompensated heart failure (HF), which is considered forme fruste acute CRS. The definition of acute CRS has broadened to include patients with declining glomerular filtration rate (GFR) and increasing serum creatinine levels caused by acutely worsening cardiac function, most often during hospitalization for an acute HF syndrome (AHFS).[1–9] AHFSs are a common and morbid complication of chronic HF, leading to millions of hospitalizations each year worldwide.[10,11] At least one-fourth of patients hospitalized with AHFS may develop WRF, depending on the definition of WRF; an increase in creatinine level greater than or equal to 0.3 mg/dL or greater than or equal to 25% from baseline has been used most commonly.[4,6,7,9,12–15] Not all increases in creatinine level during AHFS have the same prognostic relevance, and we suggest that acute CRS should only include patients with treatment failure and persistent congestion.[7]

Chronic kidney disease (CKD) is present in approximately half of all patients with AHFS, so many patients with acute CRS have concomitant chronic CRS.[6,9,12,16] The most important risk factor for WRF in AHFS is CKD, reflected by reduced GFR with increased serum creatinine and cystatin C levels (**Box 1**).[13–15,17–20] AKI is an important contributor to the progression of CKD and HF, and both AKI and CKD are associated with adverse outcomes in diverse patient populations.[21] Patients with CKD or WRF complicating AHFS have significantly increased mortalities compared with patients with preserved renal function, and renal dysfunction is the most important prognostic marker in AHFS.[12,22–28] WRF during AHFS portends an adverse prognosis independently of baseline renal function, and mortality increases progressively with incremental increases in serum creatinine.[1,2,6,7,12,26–29] The adverse prognosis conferred by baseline renal dysfunction seems greater than the effect of WRF.[12,23,26–31] Transient WRF reflecting a reversible reduction in GFR seems less harmful than persistent WRF suggesting established AKI, but even decreases in creatinine during hospitalization representing WRF on presentation may be associated with adverse outcomes.[5,32,33]

BIOMARKERS IN ACUTE CARDIORENAL SYNDROME

Cardiorenal biomarkers reflecting different aspects of cardiac and renal dysfunction predict acute CRS outcomes, but there are no definitive diagnostic tests for acute CRS.[36] Four major groups of cardiorenal biomarkers have been studied in acute CRS, including clearance biomarkers reflecting GFR, natriuretic peptides reflecting congestion, tubular injury biomarkers, and miscellaneous biomarkers reflecting neurohormonal and/or inflammatory activation (**Box 2**). Levels of cardiac injury biomarkers

> **Box 1**
> **Risk factors for WRF in acute HF syndromes**
>
> Chronic kidney disease[a]
>   Reduced baseline GFR
>   Increased serum creatinine level
>   Increased serum cystatin C level
> Diuretic resistance[a]
>   Higher loop diuretic doses
> Congestion[a]
>   Increased central venous pressure or right atrial pressure
>   Pulmonary edema
> Increased HF severity
>   Increased New York Heart Association class
>   Increased number of HF exacerbations
>   Hypotension[a]
>   Hyponatremia
>   Atrial fibrillation
> Risk factors for renal disease
>   Older age
>   Hypertension
>   Diabetes mellitus
> Magnitude of blood pressure reduction[a]
>   Use of vasodilators
>   Increased admission blood pressure
>
> [a] Commonly described risk factors.
>   *Data from* Refs.[13–15,17–20,34,35]

such as troponin may be increased in the setting of AHFS and acute CRS and carry an adverse prognosis.[37]

Patients with acute CRS have increased levels of clearance biomarkers, including creatinine, cystatin C, and blood urea nitrogen (BUN) from GFR reduction caused by the combined effects of underlying CKD with chronic nephron loss, acute tubular injury, and direct influence of AHFS.[5] Acute CRS typically produces a gradual increase in serum creatinine level corresponding with stage I AKI, whereas abrupt increases meeting criteria for stage II or III AKI suggest severe HF or an intrinsic renal process with higher risk of mortality.[7,28–30,38–40] Increases in creatinine during aggressive volume removal and effective decongestive therapy have not been associated with a higher risk of adverse outcomes, suggesting that WRF itself may not be an independent contributor to adverse outcomes.[23,41–44] Lack of an adverse effect of WRF without residual congestion suggests that congestion is the primary determinant of AHFS outcomes and that renal dysfunction contributes to adverse outcomes by causing persistent congestion.[41,43–46] Cystatin C may have higher sensitivity for reduced GFR and AKI, so estimation of GFR using cystatin C may provide greater prognostic value than creatinine-based estimates.[22,46,47] BUN is the most strongly

---

Box 2
Selected prognostic biomarkers in CRS

Renal clearance markers

  Creatinine

  Cystatin C

  Blood urea nitrogen

  Uric acid

Natriuretic peptides

  B-type natriuretic peptide (BNP)

  N-terminal pro-BNP

  Mid-proANP

Tubular injury markers

  Neutrophil gelatin-associated lipocalin

  KIM-1

  L-FABP

  TIMP2

  IGFBP7

Neurohormonal/inflammatory markers

  GDF-15

  FGF-23

  Soluble ST2

  Galectin-3

  CA-125

  Midproadrenomedullin

Abbreviations: CA, cancer antigen; FGF-23, fibroblast growth factor; GDF, growth differentiation factor; IGFBP, insulin-like growth factor binding protein; L-FABP, liver-type fatty acid binding protein; KIM, kidney injury marker; Mid-proANP, midregional pro-A-type (atrial) natriuretic peptide; TIMP-2, tissue inhibitor of metalloproteinases.

  Data from Forni LG, Chawla LS. Biomarkers in cardiorenal syndrome. Blood Purif 2014;37 Suppl 2:14–9.

---

prognostic of the clearance biomarkers, reflecting the combined effects of reduced GFR and neurohormonal activation.[24,25,30] An increased BUN/creatinine ratio suggests neurohormonal activation caused by decreased effective renal perfusion from severe HF and carries adverse prognostic value in AHFS.[43,48]

Levels of tubular injury biomarkers, such as neutrophil gelatin-associated lipocalin (NGAL), become increased early during AKI, and may differentiate true AKI with tubular injury from reversible reductions in GFR without tubular injury.[49–53] Increases in levels of tubular injury biomarkers precede increases in clearance biomarker levels during AKI and predict declines in GFR, allowing clinicians to recognize developing AKI earlier.[5,49–53] Plasma/serum NGAL predicts WRF and adverse outcomes in patients with AHFS, but showed only modest predictive value in some studies.[5,54–58] Urinary tubular injury biomarkers seem to have greater predictive accuracy for AKI than plasma/serum NGAL, but have not been studied systemically in patients with AHFS.[53]

The combined use of both clearance and tubular injury biomarkers can define various AKI subgroups with different renal outcomes and pathophysiology (**Fig. 1**).[49–52] Patients with normal levels of both biomarkers do not have AKI and are at low risk of developing AKI. Patients with increased levels of tubular injury biomarkers in the absence of increased clearance biomarker levels may have early AKI that poses a risk for worsening GFR. Patients with acutely increased levels of clearance biomarkers without increased levels of tubular injury biomarkers may have a potentially transient or reversible change in GFR not associated with tubular injury.[52] Patients with increased levels of both biomarkers have established AKI with an increased risk of severe, progressive, and/or persistent AKI and adverse outcomes.[52]

Natriuretic peptides such as B-type natriuretic peptide (BNP) and N-terminal pro-BNP (NT-proBNP) are significantly increased in acute CRS because of the combined effects of both congestion and reduced GFR. Normal natriuretic peptide levels suggest a cause of AKI other than typical acute CRS (ie, volume depletion). Natriuretic peptide levels cannot distinguish between CRS subtypes and can be increased in patients with severely reduced GFR but no prior cardiac dysfunction (acute renocardiac syndrome).[40,59] Increased natriuretic peptide levels are prognostic in patients with AHFS with or without acute CRS, and the degree of natriuretic peptide increase may modify the relationship between WRF and adverse outcomes.[43,44,46,60,61] Increased natriuretic peptide levels can identify residual congestion as a target for therapy.[61] Patients with AHFS with persistent congestion and increased natriuretic peptide levels at hospital discharge have worse outcomes, especially in the presence of acute CRS and/or WRF; WRF seems benign when natriuretic peptide levels are normal.[43–46,62] Other biomarkers reflecting neurohormonal and inflammatory pathways may provide insight into the underlying pathophysiology of acute CRS, but they are outside the scope of this article.[36]

We propose a multibiomarker approach to acute CRS phenotyping using congestion biomarkers (such as natriuretic peptide levels) and neurohormonal activation biomarkers (such as BUN/creatinine ratio) to define each patient's pathophysiology (**Fig. 2**).[43] Patients with low levels of both biomarkers are in compensated HF and do not have acute

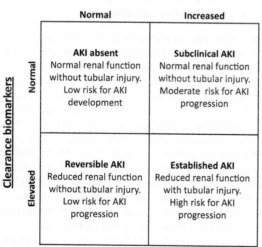

Fig. 1. AKI subtyping based on clearance and tubular injury biomarkers. (*Data from* Refs.[49–52])

Congestion biomarkers

		Normal	Elevated
Neurohormonal activation biomarkers	**Normal**	**Chronic CRS** Compensated HF with CKD causing low GFR. Treat with standard chronic HF therapy	**Congestive CRS** Congestion leading to reduced GFR. Treat with volume removal alone
	Increased	**Hypovolemic AKI** Volume depletion leading to reduced GFR. Treat with diuretic withdrawal and fluids	**Refractory CRS** Advanced HF causing severe CRS. Treat with volume removal and consider advanced therapies

Fig. 2. Proposed acute CRS phenotyping based on biomarkers reflecting congestion and neurohormonal activation. (*Data from* Testani JM, Damman K, Brisco MA, et al. A combined-biomarker approach to clinical phenotyping renal dysfunction in heart failure. J Cardiac Fail 2014;20:912–9.)

CRS. Patients with low natriuretic peptide levels and increased markers of neurohormonal activation likely have hypovolemia (true prerenal AKI). Patients with increased natriuretic peptide levels without increased markers of neurohormonal activation have uncomplicated congestive acute CRS. Patients with increased levels of both biomarkers have persistent congestion and marked neurohormonal activation, reflecting refractory acute CRS, whereby congestion is severe enough to impair renal perfusion.[43] This classification could be further refined using tubular injury biomarkers suggesting AKI, and must be subjected to further investigation before it can be accepted.

PATHOPHYSIOLOGY OF CARDIORENAL SYNDROME

The mechanisms by which cardiac and renal dysfunction can interact to produce progressive bidirectional organ injury are reviewed elsewhere.[3–5,8] Acute CRS results from the interaction between renal venous congestion, reduced renal blood flow, and impaired renal autoregulation; inflammatory pathways contribute to bidirectional cardiac and renal dysfunction.[8,9] Renal congestion is central to acute CRS and distinguishes acute CRS from other causes of AKI. Patients with HF decompensate because of various triggering insults, leading to neurohormonal activation and fluid retention that produce congestion, which in turn impairs renal function and aggravates neurohormonal activation leading to a vicious cycle of fluid retention and worsening congestion.[8] Triggering insults include reductions in cardiac output from deteriorating cardiac function and/or worsening sodium retention from a variety of causes. Neurohormonal activation with sympathetic nervous system activation, renin-angiotensin-aldosterone system (RAAS) activation, and nonosmotic vasopressin release occurs in response to stimuli that are detected by the kidneys as a reduction in perfusion pressure, including reduced cardiac output and/or increased venous congestion.[8]

Effective renal perfusion is decreased in AHFS because of reduced forward flow from impaired cardiac function coupled with increased renal venous pressure, triggering glomerular hemodynamic changes and sodium retention from neurohormonal activation.[9] Most patients with AHFS have adequate cardiac output to maintain renal blood flow in the setting of preserved renal autoregulatory capacity and normal renal venous pressure. Truly low cardiac output with inadequate renal perfusion from hypovolemia or severe pump failure is an infrequent cause of renal dysfunction in AHFS.[33,34,63,64]

Impaired renal autoregulation is a major contributor to GFR reductions that occur despite adequate cardiac output during AHFS treatment.[9] The kidney normally maintains GFR despite reduced renal perfusion by autoregulation of glomerular arteriolar tone; without normal renal autoregulation, the kidney cannot maintain GFR when blood pressure is therapeutically reduced to normal levels.[19,65–67] Drugs that antagonize renal autoregulation include loop diuretics, nonsteroidal antiinflammatory drugs, and RAAS inhibitors.[68,69] Loop diuretics increase tubular flow rate and trigger tubuloglomerular feedback, whereby adenosine binding to adenosine A1 receptors reversibly decreases GFR to prevent excessive urine fluid and electrolyte loss via a manner reversible by adenosine A1 receptor antagonism.[68,70]

Systemic venous congestion is the major driver of acute CRS, especially with severely increased central venous pressures from right ventricular dysfunction and/or tricuspid regurgitation.[8,9,34,63,64,71] Increased central venous pressure reduces glomerular perfusion pressure despite adequate cardiac output and renal blood flow, triggering neurohormonal activation with sodium retention, diuretic resistance, and an increased BUN/creatinine ratio.[43,48] Increased intra-abdominal pressure can compress the renal veins and renal parenchyma, impairing renal perfusion in patients with significant ascites.[72–74]

CLINICAL ASSESSMENT OF CARDIORENAL SYNDROME

Volume overload and congestion are central to typical acute CRS, and we recommend patients excluding hypovolemic and euvolemic patients from the definition of acute CRS, which implies residual congestion.[7] The cause of WRF developing early in the course of AHFS treatment may be different from WRF episodes occurring later.[9] Of patients with AHFS developing WRF, one-third present with WRF, one-half develop WRF during the first 48 hours of treatment, and the rest develop WRF after 48 hours.[29,30,58] Late-onset WRF (developing after day 4) is associated with worse outcomes than earlier WRF, and patients may be at risk for further deterioration in renal function after hospital discharge.[23,30,39,75]

Most patients with WRF on presentation have typical congestive CRS caused by renal venous congestion and/or intra-abdominal hypertension from volume overload, suggested by increased jugular or central venous pressure with a dilated inferior vena cava lacking respiratory variation on echocardiography.[35,61,76] Patients with inadequate renal perfusion and clinical evidence of low cardiac output from severe pump failure (low-output CRS) have true renal hypoperfusion requiring specialized therapy and should be distinguished from most patients who have adequate renal blood flow. When the severity of AKI seems out of proportion to the severity of HF, consider acute renocardiac syndrome with primary AKI producing volume overload and resultant cardiac dysfunction.[40]

During the first few days of ongoing AHFS treatment, patients with congestive CRS often develop WRF as the result of impaired renal autoregulation in the setting of blood pressure reduction from diuretic and/or vasodilator therapy.[19,66,67] Episodes of WRF occurring during effective decongestive therapy may not reflect true acute CRS, which implies persistent congestion with WRF despite AHFS treatment.[7] Episodes of modest WRF during successful AHFS treatment seem benign, especially when accompanied by an increase in hemoglobin level, hematocrit, or serum protein or albumin levels (hemoconcentration) resulting from effective diuresis.[41,66,69]

If a patient remains volume overloaded, then overdiuresis as the cause of WRF is unlikely in the absence of signs of hypovolemia. Overdiuresis may occur in patients with hypoalbuminemia and/or cirrhosis, who may be edematous despite normal filling pressures. Patients with significant left ventricular hypertrophy and diastolic dysfunction are prone to reductions in cardiac output with excessive reduction of filling pressures. Inadequate cardiac output may mimic overdiuresis with low blood pressure, poor diuretic response, and progressive WRF, often with a high/increasing BUN/creatinine ratio and worsening hyponatremia despite positive fluid balance. Objective assessment of cardiac output and filling pressures may be required to differentiate overdiuresis from occult low-output CRS.

The need for hemodynamic assessment increases in proportion to the severity of illness, and exclusion of low-output CRS is appropriate in critically ill patients. Transthoracic Doppler echocardiography can noninvasively estimate cardiac filling pressures and cardiac output to identify occult congestion or hypoperfusion.[35,61,76] A dilated inferior vena cava, implying significant central venous congestion, seems to predict WRF in patients with AHFS.[35] The ESCAPE (Evaluation Study of Congestive Heart Failure and Pulmonary Artery Catheterization Effectiveness) study failed to show an improvement in clinical or renal outcomes with pulmonary artery catheter–guided therapy in patients with AHFS who were not critically ill, but does not exclude a role for invasive hemodynamic monitoring in patients with medically refractory acute CRS.[31]

TREATMENT OF CARDIORENAL SYNDROME

No treatment has unequivocally improved short-term or long-term clinical outcomes in patients with AHFS and/or acute CRS.[10,11] Recent AHFS trials have included significant numbers of patients with renal dysfunction, with a few studies focusing on patients with acute CRS as defined by WRF in the setting of AHFS with persistent volume overload.[77–82] Many studies use diuretic resistance as a proxy for acute CRS, reflecting a narrower definition of acute CRS.[83–86] Studies of acute CRS treatment have been limited by small sample size, and in several cases the promising results of pilot studies were not confirmed in a larger study.[42,68,77–80,87–92] Relief of congestion remains the primary treatment goal in patients with acute CRS, so modest WRF should be tolerated during effective decongestive therapy.[10,11,61] WRF developing during successful volume removal seems benign, and renal dysfunction in patients with AHFS who are free from congestion has minimal adverse prognostic impact.[41–46]

Patients with typical congestive CRS with systemic congestion and volume overload have an improvement in renal function with volume removal alone, although transient WRF often occurs and must be tolerated if the patient is responding appropriately. Patients with excessive diuretic intake, gastrointestinal fluid losses, and/or poor fluid intake who have clinical signs of hypovolemia, such as orthostatic hypotension, require diuretic withdrawal and careful administration of isotonic intravenous fluids. In the presence of persistent congestion and volume overload, holding diuretics and administering fluids to correct WRF leads to a futile cycle of worsening volume overload and congestive renal dysfunction. The few patients with advanced HF resulting in low-output CRS require vasoactive drug support to improve forward flow, restore renal function, and allow adequate decongestion. Patients with forme fruste acute CRS showing diuretic resistance and WRF despite persistent volume overload remain the greatest challenge, warranting aggressive decongestive therapy and exclusion of low-output CRS (**Fig. 3, Table 1**).

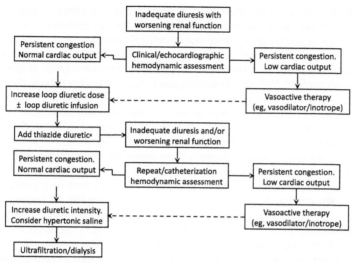

Fig. 3. Suggested approach to acute CRS therapy in the setting of acute HF. [a] Consider substituting vasopressin-2 antagonist if significant hyponatremia is present.

Diuretic Therapy

Loop diuretics are the first-line therapy for relief of volume overload and congestion in patients with AHFS with or without acute CRS.[10,11] Loop diuretic resistance is a common problem in acute CRS and patients who require higher diuretic doses are a high-risk population with poor outcomes, presumably because of the presence of

Table 1
Potential treatments studied in AHFS and/or acute CRS

	Symptoms	Creatinine	Adverse Events
Fluid Removal Therapies			
High-dose loop diuretics[42,91]	↓	↑	↔
Continuous loop diuretic infusion[42,93,94]	↔	↔	↔
Combination diuretic therapy[78,86,95]	?	?	↑
Vasopressin receptor antagonists[81,96]	↓	↔	↔
Adenosine receptors antagonists[77,89,97]	↔	↔	↔
Ultrafiltration/hemodialysis[78,88,98–100]	↓	↑	↑
Peritoneal dialysis/paracentesis[74,101]	↓	?	?
Glucocorticoids[83,84]	↓	↓	?
Hypertonic saline[85,102]	↓	↓	?
Vasoactive Therapies			
Milrinone[24,103]	↔	↓	↑
Dopamine[80,90,91,94]	↔	↔	↔
Nitroglycerin[92]	↓	↔	?
Nitroprusside[104,105]	↓	↔	?
Nesiritide[79,80,87,92,106,107]	↔	↔	↔
Other natriuretic peptides[96,108–110]	↓	↔	?
Serelaxin[82,111]	↓	↓	↓

Question marks (?) denote insufficient evidence from adequately powered randomized trials.

advanced HF and/or CKD rather than a directly harmful effect of higher diuretic doses.[43,112–114] The DOSE (Diuretic Optimization Strategies Evaluation) study showed improved diuresis and better symptom relief with 2.5-fold higher loop diuretic doses.[42] Patients receiving higher diuretic doses had more frequent WRF, which was reversible and not associated with an adverse clinical outcome, as seen in other studies of high-dose diuretics in AHFS.[42,91] Aggressive stepped diuretic algorithms have shown favorable safety and efficacy for the management of volume overload in AHFS and acute CRS.[78] Continuous infusion of loop diuretics improved natriuretic effects in some studies, but DOSE did not show any difference in diuresis or renal function between continuous and bolus loop diuretics at the same total daily dose.[42,93] We use continuous loop diuretic infusions when patients have marginal hemodynamics and/or require very high diuretic doses, being sure to use the minimum possible infusion volume.

Overcoming loop diuretic resistance is often the primary treatment goal in patients with acute CRS with persistent congestion despite WRF (see **Fig. 3**). Adding a thiazide diuretic can augment diuresis and overcome diuretic resistance in AHFS, particularly in patients who have been exposed to prolonged and/or high-dose loop diuretic therapy.[86] The effects of combination diuretic therapy on AHFS outcomes remains uncertain, but patients receiving combination diuretic therapy seem more prone to true overdiuresis and electrolyte disturbances.[86,95] The stepped diuretic algorithm from CARRESS-HF (Cardiorenal Rescue Study in Acute Decompensated Heart Failure) showed good safety and efficacy using escalating doses of continuous furosemide infusion (up to 30 mg/h) plus oral metolazone (up to 10 mg/d).[78] Vasopressin-2 receptor antagonists such as tolvaptan can augment diuresis, ameliorate hyponatremia, and improve symptoms in patients with AHFS, but are not currently approved by the US Food and Drug Administration for AHFS and do not seem to improve renal function.[81,96] Selective adenosine A1 antagonists can augment diuresis and prevent the decrease in GFR caused by loop diuretics.[68,70,89] The PROTECT (Placebo-Controlled Randomized Study of the Selective A1 Adenosine Receptor Antagonist Rolofylline for Patients Hospitalized with Acute Decompensated Heart Failure and Volume Overload to Assess Treatment Effect on Congestion and Renal Function) study failed to show improvement in renal function or clinical outcomes with the adenosine A1 antagonist rolofylline in patients with acute CRS, despite promising preliminary studies.[77,89,97] Glucocorticoids reversed diuretic resistance and improved renal function in small studies of acute CRS, supporting a role for inflammation in the pathophysiology of acute CRS.[83,84]

Hypertonic saline seems to improve the response to high-dose loop diuretics in patients with AHFS with refractory diuretic resistance with or without hyponatremia.[102] Hypertonic saline may improve cardiovascular function and relieve excess neurohormonal activation to reverse the profoundly sodium-avid state that drives diuretic resistance in patients with acute CRS.[85] Studies have shown improvements in diuresis, natriuretic peptide levels, and renal function in patients treated with low-volume hypertonic saline plus high-dose furosemide.[85,102] The largest of these studies showed improved clinical outcomes by adding 150 mL of intravenous 3% sodium chloride twice daily to intravenous furosemide 250 mg twice daily, arguing for less-stringent sodium restriction in patients with acute CRS.[85]

Vasoactive Drugs

A minority of patients have low-output CRS with severely impaired forward flow from advanced HF, requiring vasoactive therapy to normalize renal perfusion (see **Fig. 3**).[10,11,115] Critically ill patients whose WRF is caused by low cardiac output may have dramatic improvements in renal function with inotropic support, explaining why low cardiac index did not predict WRF in patients with AHFS.[34] Inotropes produce serious adverse effects in AHFS, arguing strongly against the empiric use of inotropic drugs in acute CRS without objective evidence of low cardiac output and systemic hypoperfusion.[115] In the OPTIME-HF (Outcomes of a Prospective Trial of Intravenous Milrinone for Exacerbations of Chronic Heart Failure) study, milrinone failed to improve symptoms or clinical outcomes in normotensive patients with AHFS, despite a minor improvement in renal function.[24,103] Prior studies suggested improvements in diuresis and/or renal function when low-dose dopamine was added to loop diuretics.[90,94] Subsequent studies failed to show any benefit of adding dopamine at 2 to 5 µg/kg/min to loop diuretic therapy in terms of renal function, diuresis, or clinical outcomes.[80,91] This mirrors the failure of renal dose dopamine to improve outcomes in critically ill patients with AKI.[116]

Vasodilators are preferred to inotropes for AHFS, but likewise have not been shown to improve renal function or outcomes.[10,11,115] Vasodilators may improve forward flow and renal perfusion in patients with impaired cardiac output, but may potentially worsen renal function by reducing blood pressure in hypertensive patients with impaired renal autoregulation.[65,66,104,105] RAAS inhibitors that improve long-term outcomes in chronic HF should be maintained during AHFS treatment whenever possible and/or started before discharge.[10,11] The optimal approach to WRF in patients on RAAS inhibitors remains uncertain, but temporarily holding these drugs in the setting of significant WRF is reasonable (especially when blood pressure is low). A reduction in GFR is expected after starting an RAAS inhibitor, and an increase in creatinine up to 30% is acceptable and seems to be benign.[69] Progressive renal dysfunction and hypotension after starting an RAAS inhibitor is concerning for advanced HF progressing toward end stage, potentially warranting hemodynamic assessment.[117]

Nesiritide (recombinant human BNP) is the most extensively studied vasoactive drug in AHFS, with early studies showing reductions in symptoms and congestion.[92] Meta-analysis of early studies suggested higher rates of WRF with nesiritide in AHFS, a finding that has not been confirmed in subsequent studies.[87,106,107] The large ASCEND study failed to show a meaningful benefit of nesiritide for improving symptoms, clinical outcomes, or renal function in AHFS.[79,107] Small studies in patients with acute CRS similarly failed to show any clinical or renal outcomes benefit with nesiritide.[80,106] Other recombinant natriuretic peptides remain under investigation for management of AHFS and acute CRS.[96,108–110] Serelaxin (recombinant human relaxin-2) may be the first drug shown to improve outcomes in a randomized controlled trial of patients with AHFS.[82,111] In the RELAX-AHF (RELAXin in Acute Heart Failure) trial, serelaxin improved symptoms and reduced the secondary end point of mortality at 180 days, with improvement in markers of renal and hepatic function.[82,111] Further study is required to confirm the efficacy of this promising new vasodilator therapy in AHFS and acute CRS.

Extracorporeal Volume Removal

Ultrafiltration involves removal of fluid and electrolytes directly from the bloodstream using a standard dialysis machine or a miniaturized device. Early studies, such as UNLOAD (Ultrafiltration versus Intravenous Diuretics for Patients Hospitalized for Acute Decompensated Congestive Heart Failure), suggested that ultrafiltration could improve volume removal compared with diuretics as first-line therapy, with more favorable effects on renal function and clinical outcomes.[88] The subsequent CARRESS study found that ultrafiltration did not improve volume removal or clinical outcomes compared with an aggressive stepped diuretic algorithm when used as first-line therapy in acute CRS.[78] CARRESS showed a greater increase in creatinine level and more adverse events with ultrafiltration compared with diuretic therapy, arguing against the use of ultrafiltration as a first-line modality for fluid removal in acute

CRS.[78] Meta-analysis of studies comparing ultrafiltration with diuretic therapy in AHFS suggests improved fluid removal with ultrafiltration without an increased risk of adverse events, but the heterogeneity of the included studies and lack of aggressive standardized combination diuretic regimens reduces the ability to generalize.[99] Given the results of CARRESS, we recommend the use of a stepped combination diuretic algorithm as first-line therapy for volume overload in AHFS including diuretic-responsive patients with acute CRS who are diuretic responsive, reserving ultrafiltration for refractory diuretic resistance (see **Fig. 3**).[78]

Ultrafiltration can be an effective rescue therapy for patients with refractory volume overload resistant to medical therapy, albeit at risk of further WRF and in some cases progression to dialysis dependence.[98,118] Patients with refractory acute CRS requiring ultrafiltration as rescue therapy have high short-term and long-term mortalities, in addition to significant rates of dialysis dependence that may support early dialysis initiation in eligible patients.[98,100] Several nonrandomized studies have found peritoneal dialysis to be an effective alternative method of volume removal in acute CRS with refractory diuretic resistance.[101] Drainage of tense ascites may improve renal function when intra-abdominal hypertension is contributing to WRF.[73,74] Extracorporeal volume removal can restore diuretic responsiveness in some patients by relieving congestive renal dysfunction.[72,73,88,99,101]

SUMMARY

Development of WRF in the setting of AHFS can occur from acute CRS and disease processes mimicking acute CRS. Acute CRS results from relative decreases in renal blood flow, deranged renal blood flow autoregulation, and renal venous congestion. Congestion is central to the pathophysiology of AHFS and drives acute CRS in most patients, distinguishing acute CRS from typical causes of AKI. We think that acute CRS should only apply to patients with persistent congestion and WRF during AHFS therapy. An accurate assessment of volume status and cardiac output may distinguish true acute CRS from acute CRS mimics. Patients with low cardiac output are less common than patients whose acute CRS is congestive and requires specialized therapy. No specific treatment of acute CRS exists, so optimal management of AHFS including adequate decongestive therapy remains essential. Volume removal is needed to relieve symptoms of congestion and typically resolves congestive CRS. Various adjuncts and alternatives to loop diuretics have been explored in an attempt to improve volume removal, renal function, and/or outcomes, but none has shown unequivocal efficacy. Given the lack of effective therapies, the outcomes of patients with refractory CRS remain poor. Further study is needed to validate promising early studies and identify new therapies for this high-risk population.

REFERENCES

1. House AA, Anand I, Bellomo R, et al. Definition and classification of cardio-renal syndromes: workgroup statements from the 7th ADQI Consensus Conference. Nephrol Dial Transplant 2010;25:1416–20.
2. Ronco C, McCullough P, Anker SD, et al. Cardio-renal syndromes: report from the consensus conference of the acute dialysis quality initiative. Eur Heart J 2010;31:703–11.
3. Ronco C, Di Lullo L. Cardiorenal syndrome. Heart Fail Clin 2014;10:251–80.
4. McCullough PA, Kellum JA, Haase M, et al. Pathophysiology of the cardiorenal syndromes: executive summary from the eleventh consensus conference of the Acute Dialysis Quality Initiative (ADQI). Contrib Nephrol 2013;182:82–98.

5. Legrand M, Mebazaa A, Ronco C, et al. When cardiac failure, kidney dysfunction, and kidney injury intersect in acute conditions: the case of cardiorenal syndrome. Crit Care Med 2014;42:2109–17.
6. Bagshaw SM, Cruz DN, Aspromonte N, et al. Epidemiology of cardio-renal syndromes: workgroup statements from the 7th ADQI Consensus Conference. Nephrol Dial Transplant 2010;25:1406–16.
7. Damman K, Tang WH, Testani JM, et al. Terminology and definition of changes renal function in heart failure. Eur Heart J 2014;35:3413–6.
8. Ronco C, Cicoira M, McCullough PA. Cardiorenal syndrome type 1: pathophysiological crosstalk leading to combined heart and kidney dysfunction in the setting of acutely decompensated heart failure. J Am Coll Cardiol 2012;60: 1031–42.
9. Haase M, Muller C, Damman K, et al. Pathogenesis of cardiorenal syndrome type 1 in acute decompensated heart failure: workgroup statements from the eleventh consensus conference of the Acute Dialysis Quality Initiative (ADQI). Contrib Nephrol 2013;182:99–116.
10. Writing Committee Members, Yancy CW, Jessup M, et al. 2013 ACCF/AHA guideline for the management of heart failure: a report of the American College of Cardiology Foundation/American Heart Association Task Force on Practice Guidelines. Circulation 2013;128:e240–327.
11. McMurray JJ, Adamopoulos S, Anker SD, et al. ESC guidelines for the diagnosis and treatment of acute and chronic heart failure 2012: the Task Force for the Diagnosis and Treatment of Acute and Chronic Heart Failure 2012 of the European Society of Cardiology. Developed in collaboration with the Heart Failure Association (HFA) of the ESC. Eur Heart J 2012;33:1787–847.
12. Damman K, Valente MA, Voors AA, et al. Renal impairment, worsening renal function, and outcome in patients with heart failure: an updated meta-analysis. Eur Heart J 2014;35:455–69.
13. Forman DE, Butler J, Wang Y, et al. Incidence, predictors at admission, and impact of worsening renal function among patients hospitalized with heart failure. J Am Coll Cardiol 2004;43:61–7.
14. Cowie MR, Komajda M, Murray-Thomas T, et al. Prevalence and impact of worsening renal function in patients hospitalized with decompensated heart failure: results of the Prospective Outcomes Study in Heart Failure (POSH). Eur Heart J 2006;27:1216–22.
15. Belziti CA, Bagnati R, Ledesma P, et al. Worsening renal function in patients admitted with acute decompensated heart failure: incidence, risk factors and prognostic implications. Rev Esp Cardiol 2010;63:294–302.
16. Cruz DN, Schmidt-Ott KM, Vescovo G, et al. Pathophysiology of cardiorenal syndrome type 2 in stable chronic heart failure: workgroup statements from the eleventh consensus conference of the Acute Dialysis Quality Initiative (ADQI). Contrib Nephrol 2013;182:117–36.
17. Butler J, Forman DE, Abraham WT, et al. Relationship between heart failure treatment and development of worsening renal function among hospitalized patients. Am Heart J 2004;147:331–8.
18. Breidthardt T, Socrates T, Noveanu M, et al. Effect and clinical prediction of worsening renal function in acute decompensated heart failure. Am J Cardiol 2011;107:730–5.
19. Dupont M, Mullens W, Finucan M, et al. Determinants of dynamic changes in serum creatinine in acute decompensated heart failure: the importance of blood pressure reduction during treatment. Eur J Heart Fail 2013;15:433–40.

20. Wang YN, Cheng H, Yue T, et al. Derivation and validation of a prediction score for acute kidney injury in patients hospitalized with acute heart failure in a Chinese cohort. Nephrology (Carlton) 2013;18:489–96.

21. Chawla LS, Eggers PW, Star RA, et al. Acute kidney injury and chronic kidney disease as interconnected syndromes. N Engl J Med 2014;371:58–66.

22. Tang WH, Dupont M, Hernandez AF, et al. Comparative assessment of short-term adverse events in acute heart failure with cystatin C and other estimates of renal function: results from the ASCEND-HF trial. JACC Heart Fail 2014;3(1):40–9.

23. Blair JE, Pang PS, Schrier RW, et al. Changes in renal function during hospitalization and soon after discharge in patients admitted for worsening heart failure in the placebo group of the EVEREST trial. Eur Heart J 2011;32:2563–72.

24. Klein L, Massie BM, Leimberger JD, et al. Admission or changes in renal function during hospitalization for worsening heart failure predict postdischarge survival: results from the Outcomes of a Prospective Trial of Intravenous Milrinone for Exacerbations of Chronic Heart Failure (OPTIME-CHF). Circ Heart Fail 2008; 1:25–33.

25. Fonarow GC, Adams KF Jr, Abraham WT, et al. Risk stratification for in-hospital mortality in acutely decompensated heart failure: classification and regression tree analysis. JAMA 2005;293:572–80.

26. Abraham WT, Fonarow GC, Albert NM, et al. Predictors of in-hospital mortality in patients hospitalized for heart failure: insights from the Organized Program to Initiate Lifesaving Treatment in Hospitalized Patients with Heart Failure (OPTI-MIZE-HF). J Am Coll Cardiol 2008;52:347–56.

27. Damman K, Navis G, Voors AA, et al. Worsening renal function and prognosis in heart failure: systematic review and meta-analysis. J Card Fail 2007;13:599–608.

28. Smith GL, Vaccarino V, Kosiborod M, et al. Worsening renal function: what is a clinically meaningful change in creatinine during hospitalization with heart failure? J Card Fail 2003;9:13–25.

29. Gottlieb SS, Abraham W, Butler J, et al. The prognostic importance of different definitions of worsening renal function in congestive heart failure. J Card Fail 2002;8:136–41.

30. Givertz MM, Postmus D, Hillege HL, et al. Renal function trajectories and clinical outcomes in acute heart failure. Circ Heart Fail 2014;7:59–67.

31. Nohria A, Hasselblad V, Stebbins A, et al. Cardiorenal interactions: insights from the ESCAPE trial. J Am Coll Cardiol 2008;51:1268–74.

32. Aronson D, Burger AJ. The relationship between transient and persistent worsening renal function and mortality in patients with acute decompensated heart failure. J Card Fail 2010;16:541–7.

33. Testani JM, McCauley BD, Kimmel SE, et al. Characteristics of patients with improvement or worsening in renal function during treatment of acute decompensated heart failure. Am J Cardiol 2010;106:1763–9.

34. Mullens W, Abrahams Z, Francis GS, et al. Importance of venous congestion for worsening of renal function in advanced decompensated heart failure. J Am Coll Cardiol 2009;53:589–96.

35. Lee HF, Hsu LA, Chang CJ, et al. Prognostic significance of dilated inferior vena cava in advanced decompensated heart failure. Int J Cardiovasc Imaging 2014; 30:1289–95.

36. Forni LG, Chawla LS. Biomarkers in cardiorenal syndrome. Blood Purif 2014; 37(Suppl 2):14–9.

37. Newby LK, Jesse RL, Babb JD, et al. ACCF 2012 expert consensus document on practical clinical considerations in the interpretation of troponin elevations: a

report of the American College of Cardiology Foundation task force on Clinical Expert Consensus Documents. J Am Coll Cardiol 2012;60:2427–63.

38. Roy AK, Mc Gorrian C, Treacy C, et al. A Comparison of Traditional and Novel Definitions (RIFLE, AKIN, and KDIGO) of Acute Kidney Injury for the Prediction of Outcomes in Acute Decompensated Heart Failure. Cardiorenal Med 2013;3: 26–37.

39. Shirakabe A, Hata N, Kobayashi N, et al. Prognostic impact of acute kidney injury in patients with acute decompensated heart failure. Circ J 2013;77: 687–96.

40. Bagshaw SM, Hoste EA, Braam B, et al. Cardiorenal syndrome type 3: pathophysiologic and epidemiologic considerations. Contrib Nephrol 2013;182: 137–57.

41. Testani JM, Chen J, McCauley BD, et al. Potential effects of aggressive decongestion during the treatment of decompensated heart failure on renal function and survival. Circulation 2010;122:265–72.

42. Felker GM, Lee KL, Bull DA, et al. Diuretic strategies in patients with acute decompensated heart failure. N Engl J Med 2011;364:797–805.

43. Testani JM, Damman K, Brisco MA, et al. A combined-biomarker approach to clinical phenotyping renal dysfunction in heart failure. J Card Fail 2014;20: 912–9.

44. Metra M, Davison B, Bettari L, et al. Is worsening renal function an ominous prognostic sign in patients with acute heart failure? The role of congestion and its interaction with renal function. Circ Heart Fail 2012;5:54–62.

45. van Kimmenade RR, Januzzi JL Jr, Baggish AL, et al. Amino-terminal pro-brain natriuretic Peptide, renal function, and outcomes in acute heart failure: redefining the cardiorenal interaction? J Am Coll Cardiol 2006;48:1621–7.

46. Ruan ZB, Zhu L, Yin YG, et al. Cystatin C, N-terminal probrain natriuretic peptides and outcomes in acute heart failure with acute kidney injury in a 12-month follow-up: Insights into the cardiorenal syndrome. J Res Med Sci 2014;19: 404–9.

47. Manzano-Fernandez S, Flores-Blanco PJ, Perez-Calvo JI, et al. Comparison of risk prediction with the CKD-EPI and MDRD equations in acute decompensated heart failure. J Card Fail 2013;19:583–91.

48. Brisco MA, Coca SG, Chen J, et al. Blood urea nitrogen/creatinine ratio identifies a high-risk but potentially reversible form of renal dysfunction in patients with decompensated heart failure. Circ Heart Fail 2013;6:233–9.

49. Endre ZH, Kellum JA, Di Somma S, et al. Differential diagnosis of AKI in clinical practice by functional and damage biomarkers: workgroup statements from the tenth Acute Dialysis Quality Initiative Consensus Conference. Contrib Nephrol 2013;182:30–44.

50. McCullough PA, Bouchard J, Waikar SS, et al. Implementation of novel biomarkers in the diagnosis, prognosis, and management of acute kidney injury: executive summary from the tenth consensus conference of the Acute Dialysis Quality Initiative (ADQI). Contrib Nephrol 2013;182:5–12.

51. McCullough PA, Shaw AD, Haase M, et al. Diagnosis of acute kidney injury using functional and injury biomarkers: workgroup statements from the tenth Acute Dialysis Quality Initiative Consensus Conference. Contrib Nephrol 2013;182: 13–29.

52. Basu RK, Wong HR, Krawczeski CD, et al. Combining functional and tubular damage biomarkers improves diagnostic precision for acute kidney injury after cardiac surgery. J Am Coll Cardiol 2014;64:2753–62.

53. Kashani K, Al-Khafaji A, Ardiles T, et al. Discovery and validation of cell cycle arrest biomarkers in human acute kidney injury. Crit Care 2013;17:R25.

54. Maisel AS, Mueller C, Fitzgerald R, et al. Prognostic utility of plasma neutrophil gelatinase-associated lipocalin in patients with acute heart failure: the NGAL EvaLuation Along with B-type NaTriuretic Peptide in acutely decompensated heart failure (GALLANT) trial. Eur J Heart Fail 2011;13:846–51.

55. Aghel A, Shrestha K, Mullens W, et al. Serum neutrophil gelatinase-associated lipocalin (NGAL) in predicting worsening renal function in acute decompensated heart failure. J Card Fail 2010;16:49–54.

56. De Berardinis B, Gaggin HK, Magrini L, et al. Comparison between admission natriuretic peptides, NGAL and sST2 testing for the prediction of worsening renal function in patients with acutely decompensated heart failure. Clin Chem Lab Med 2014;53(4):613–21.

57. Palazzuoli A, Ruocco G, Beltrami M, et al. Admission plasma neutrophil gelatinase associated lipocalin (NGAL) predicts worsening renal function during hospitalization and post discharge outcome in patients with acute heart failure. Acute Card Care 2014;16:93–101.

58. Breidthardt T, Socrates T, Drexler B, et al. Plasma neutrophil gelatinase-associated lipocalin for the prediction of acute kidney injury in acute heart failure. Crit Care 2012;16:R2.

59. Chawla LS, Herzog CA, Costanzo MR, et al. Proposal for a functional classification system of heart failure in patients with end-stage renal disease: proceedings of the acute dialysis quality initiative (ADQI) XI workgroup. J Am Coll Cardiol 2014;63:1246–52.

60. Waldo SW, Beede J, Isakson S, et al. Pro-B-type natriuretic peptide levels in acute decompensated heart failure. J Am Coll Cardiol 2008;51:1874–82.

61. Gheorghiade M, Follath F, Ponikowski P, et al. Assessing and grading congestion in acute heart failure: a scientific statement from the acute heart failure committee of the heart failure association of the European Society of Cardiology and endorsed by the European Society of Intensive Care Medicine. Eur J Heart Fail 2010;12:423–33.

62. Kociol RD, McNulty SE, Hernandez AF, et al. Markers of decongestion, dyspnea relief, and clinical outcomes among patients hospitalized with acute heart failure. Circ Heart Fail 2013;6:240–5.

63. Testani JM, Khera AV, St John Sutton MG, et al. Effect of right ventricular function and venous congestion on cardiorenal interactions during the treatment of decompensated heart failure. Am J Cardiol 2010;105:511–6.

64. Damman K, Navis G, Smilde TD, et al. Decreased cardiac output, venous congestion and the association with renal impairment in patients with cardiac dysfunction. Eur J Heart Fail 2007;9:872–8.

65. Abuelo JG. Normotensive ischemic acute renal failure. N Engl J Med 2007;357:797–805.

66. Testani JM, Coca SG, McCauley BD, et al. Impact of changes in blood pressure during the treatment of acute decompensated heart failure on renal and clinical outcomes. Eur J Heart Fail 2011;13:877–84.

67. Voors AA, Davison BA, Felker GM, et al. Early drop in systolic blood pressure and worsening renal function in acute heart failure: renal results of Pre-RELAX-AHF. Eur J Heart Fail 2011;13:961–7.

68. Gottlieb SS, Brater DC, Thomas I, et al. BG9719 (CVT-124), an A1 adenosine receptor antagonist, protects against the decline in renal function observed with diuretic therapy. Circulation 2002;105:1348–53.

69. Testani JM, Kimmel SE, Dries DL, et al. Prognostic importance of early worsening renal function after initiation of angiotensin-converting enzyme inhibitor therapy in patients with cardiac dysfunction. Circ Heart Fail 2011;4: 685–91.

70. Givertz MM, Massie BM, Fields TK, et al. The effects of KW-3902, an adenosine A1-receptor antagonist,on diuresis and renal function in patients with acute decompensated heart failure and renal impairment or diuretic resistance. J Am Coll Cardiol 2007;50:1551–60.

71. Maeder MT, Holst DP, Kaye DM. Tricuspid regurgitation contributes to renal dysfunction in patients with heart failure. J Card Fail 2008;14:824–30.

72. Mullens W, Abrahams Z, Skouri HN, et al. Elevated intra-abdominal pressure in acute decompensated heart failure: a potential contributor to worsening renal function? J Am Coll Cardiol 2008;51:300–6.

73. Verbrugge FH, Dupont M, Steels P, et al. Abdominal contributions to cardiorenal dysfunction in congestive heart failure. J Am Coll Cardiol 2013;62:485–95.

74. Mullens W, Abrahams Z, Francis GS, et al. Prompt reduction in intra-abdominal pressure following large-volume mechanical fluid removal improves renal insufficiency in refractory decompensated heart failure. J Card Fail 2008;14: 508–14.

75. Takaya Y, Yoshihara F, Yokoyama H, et al. Impact of onset time of acute kidney injury on outcomes in patients with acute decompensated heart failure. Heart Vessels 2014. [Epub ahead of print].

76. Tsutsui RS, Borowski A, Tang WH, et al. Precision of echocardiographic estimates of right atrial pressure in patients with acute decompensated heart failure. J Am Soc Echocardiogr 2014;27:1072–8.e2.

77. Massie BM, O'Connor CM, Metra M, et al. Rolofylline, an adenosine A1-receptor antagonist, in acute heart failure. N Engl J Med 2010;363:1419–28.

78. Bart BA, Goldsmith SR, Lee KL, et al. Ultrafiltration in decompensated heart failure with cardiorenal syndrome. N Engl J Med 2012;367:2296–304.

79. O'Connor CM, Starling RC, Hernandez AF, et al. Effect of nesiritide in patients with acute decompensated heart failure. N Engl J Med 2011;365:32–43.

80. Chen HH, Anstrom KJ, Givertz MM, et al. Low-dose dopamine or low-dose nesiritide in acute heart failure with renal dysfunction: the ROSE acute heart failure randomized trial. JAMA 2013;310:2533–43.

81. Gheorghiade M, Konstam MA, Burnett JC Jr, et al. Short-term clinical effects of tolvaptan, an oral vasopressin antagonist, in patients hospitalized for heart failure: the EVEREST Clinical Status Trials. JAMA 2007;297:1332–43.

82. Teerlink JR, Cotter G, Davison BA, et al. Serelaxin, recombinant human relaxin-2, for treatment of acute heart failure (RELAX-AHF): a randomised, placebo-controlled trial. Lancet 2013;381:29–39.

83. Liu C, Liu G, Zhou C, et al. Potent diuretic effects of prednisone in heart failure patients with refractory diuretic resistance. Can J Cardiol 2007;23:865–8.

84. Liu C, Liu K, Group C-AS. Cardiac outcome prevention effectiveness of glucocorticoids in acute decompensated heart failure: COPE-ADHF study. J Cardiovasc Pharmacol 2014;63:333–8.

85. Paterna S, Fasullo S, Parrinello G, et al. Short-term effects of hypertonic saline solution in acute heart failure and long-term effects of a moderate sodium restriction in patients with compensated heart failure with New York Heart Association class III (Class C) (SMAC-HF Study). Am J Med Sci 2011;342:27–37.

86. Jentzer JC, DeWald TA, Hernandez AF. Combination of loop diuretics with thiazide-type diuretics in heart failure. J Am Coll Cardiol 2010;56:1527–34.

87. Sackner-Bernstein JD, Skopicki HA, Aaronson KD. Risk of worsening renal function with nesiritide in patients with acutely decompensated heart failure. Circulation 2005;111:1487–91.

88. Costanzo MR, Guglin ME, Saltzberg MT, et al. Ultrafiltration versus intravenous diuretics for patients hospitalized for acute decompensated heart failure. J Am Coll Cardiol 2007;49:675–83.

89. Cotter G, Dittrich HC, Weatherley BD, et al. The PROTECT pilot study: a randomized, placebo-controlled, dose-finding study of the adenosine A1 receptor antagonist rolofylline in patients with acute heart failure and renal impairment. J Card Fail 2008;14:631–40.

90. Giamouzis G, Butler J, Starling RC, et al. Impact of dopamine infusion on renal function in hospitalized heart failure patients: results of the Dopamine in Acute Decompensated Heart Failure (DAD-HF) Trial. J Card Fail 2010;16:922–30.

91. Triposkiadis FK, Butler J, Karayannis G, et al. Efficacy and safety of high dose versus low dose furosemide with or without dopamine infusion: the Dopamine in Acute Decompensated Heart Failure II (DAD-HF II) trial. Int J Cardiol 2014;172:115–21.

92. Publication Committee for the VI. Intravenous nesiritide vs nitroglycerin for treatment of decompensated congestive heart failure: a randomized controlled trial. JAMA 2002;287:1531–40.

93. Wu MY, Chang NC, Su CL, et al. Loop diuretic strategies in patients with acute decompensated heart failure: a meta-analysis of randomized controlled trials. J Crit Care 2014;29:2–9.

94. Aziz EF, Alviar CL, Herzog E, et al. Continuous infusion of furosemide combined with low-dose dopamine compared to intermittent boluses in acutely decompensated heart failure is less nephrotoxic and carries a lower readmission at thirty days. Hellenic J Cardiol 2011;52:227–35.

95. Ng TM, Konopka E, Hyderi AF, et al. Comparison of bumetanide- and metolazone-based diuretic regimens to furosemide in acute heart failure. J Cardiovasc Pharmacol Ther 2013;18:345–53.

96. Suzuki S, Yoshihisa A, Yamaki T, et al. Acute heart failure volume control multicenter randomized (AVCMA) trial: comparison of tolvaptan and carperitide. J Clin Pharmacol 2013;53:1277–85.

97. Voors AA, Dittrich HC, Massie BM, et al. Effects of the adenosine A1 receptor antagonist rolofylline on renal function in patients with acute heart failure and renal dysfunction: results from PROTECT (Placebo-Controlled Randomized Study of the Selective Adenosine A1 Receptor Antagonist Rolofylline for Patients Hospitalized with Acute Decompensated Heart Failure and Volume Overload to Assess Treatment Effect on Congestion and Renal Function). J Am Coll Cardiol 2011;57:1899–907.

98. Patarroyo M, Wehbe E, Hanna M, et al. Cardiorenal outcomes after slow continuous ultrafiltration therapy in refractory patients with advanced decompensated heart failure. J Am Coll Cardiol 2012;60:1906–12.

99. Wen H, Zhang Y, Zhu J, et al. Ultrafiltration versus intravenous diuretic therapy to treat acute heart failure: a systematic review. Am J Cardiovasc Drugs 2013;13:365–73.

100. Wehbe E, Patarroyo M, Taliercio JJ, et al. Renal failure requiring dialysis complicating slow continuous ultrafiltration in acute heart failure: importance of systolic perfusion pressure. J Card Fail 2014;21(2):108–15.

101. Broekman KE, Sinkeler SJ, Waanders F, et al. Volume control in treatment-resistant congestive heart failure: role for peritoneal dialysis. Heart Fail Rev 2014;19:709–16.

102. Gandhi S, Mosleh W, Myers RB. Hypertonic saline with furosemide for the treatment of acute congestive heart failure: a systematic review and meta-analysis. Int J Cardiol 2014;173:139–45.

103. Cuffe MS, Califf RM, Adams KF Jr, et al. Short-term intravenous milrinone for acute exacerbation of chronic heart failure: a randomized controlled trial. JAMA 2002;287:1541–7.

104. Mullens W, Abrahams Z, Francis GS, et al. Sodium nitroprusside for advanced low-output heart failure. J Am Coll Cardiol 2008;52:200–7.

105. Schwartzenberg S, Redfield MM, From AM, et al. Effects of vasodilation in heart failure with preserved or reduced ejection fraction implications of distinct pathophysiologies on response to therapy. J Am Coll Cardiol 2012;59:442–51.

106. Witteles RM, Kao D, Christopherson D, et al. Impact of nesiritide on renal function in patients with acute decompensated heart failure and pre-existing renal dysfunction a randomized, double-blind, placebo-controlled clinical trial. J Am Coll Cardiol 2007;50:1835–40.

107. van Deursen VM, Hernandez AF, Stebbins A, et al. Nesiritide, renal function, and associated outcomes during hospitalization for acute decompensated heart failure: results from the Acute Study of Clinical Effectiveness of Nesiritide and Decompensated Heart Failure (ASCEND-HF). Circulation 2014;130:958–65.

108. Hata N, Seino Y, Tsutamoto T, et al. Effects of carperitide on the long-term prognosis of patients with acute decompensated chronic heart failure: the PROTECT multicenter randomized controlled study. Circ J 2008;72:1787–93.

109. Luss H, Mitrovic V, Seferovic PM, et al. Renal effects of ularitide in patients with decompensated heart failure. Am Heart J 2008;155(1012):e1–8.

110. Chan WY, Frampton CM, Crozier IG, et al. Urocortin-2 infusion in acute decompensated heart failure: findings from the UNICORN study (urocortin-2 in the treatment of acute heart failure as an adjunct over conventional therapy). JACC Heart Fail 2013;1:433–41.

111. Metra M, Cotter G, Davison BA, et al. Effect of serelaxin on cardiac, renal, and hepatic biomarkers in the Relaxin in Acute Heart Failure (RELAX-AHF) development program: correlation with outcomes. J Am Coll Cardiol 2013;61:196–206.

112. Singh D, Shrestha K, Testani JM, et al. Insufficient natriuretic response to continuous intravenous furosemide is associated with poor long-term outcomes in acute decompensated heart failure. J Card Fail 2014;20:392–9.

113. Testani JM, Brisco MA, Turner JM, et al. Loop diuretic efficiency: a metric of diuretic responsiveness with prognostic importance in acute decompensated heart failure. Circ Heart Fail 2014;7:261–70.

114. Valente MA, Voors AA, Damman K, et al. Diuretic response in acute heart failure: clinical characteristics and prognostic significance. Eur Heart J 2014;35:1284–93.

115. Abraham WT, Adams KF, Fonarow GC, et al. In-hospital mortality in patients with acute decompensated heart failure requiring intravenous vasoactive medications: an analysis from the Acute Decompensated Heart Failure National Registry (ADHERE). J Am Coll Cardiol 2005;46:57–64.

116. Kellum JA, Decker JM. Use of dopamine in acute renal failure: a meta-analysis. Crit Care Med 2001;29:1526–31.

117. Kittleson M, Hurwitz S, Shah MR, et al. Development of circulatory-renal limitations to angiotensin-converting enzyme inhibitors identifies patients with severe heart failure and early mortality. J Am Coll Cardiol 2003;41:2029–35.

118. Dev S, Shirolkar SC, Stevens SR, et al. Reduction in body weight but worsening renal function with late ultrafiltration for treatment of acute decompensated heart failure. Cardiology 2012;123:145–53.

Acute Kidney Injury in the Surgical Patient

Charles Hobson, MD, MHA[a,b], Girish Singhania, MD[c], Azra Bihorac, MD, MS[c,d],*

KEYWORDS

- Perioperative • Acute kidney injury • Chronic kidney disease • Complications

KEY POINTS

- Acute and chronic kidney injury and dysfunction play important roles in affecting perioperative outcomes.
- AKI is a common complication after surgery and mild to moderate AKI is more common than severe AKI.
- All stages of AKI severity are associated with increased short- and long-term morbidity and mortality.
- Clinical risk factors for AKI are similar but not identical in different surgical populations.

INTRODUCTION

Perioperative acute kidney injury (AKI), characterized by persistent oliguria or an increase in serum creatinine levels, is a common perioperative complication and is associated with up to a 10-fold increase in hospital cost and mortality, decreased long-term survival, and an increased risk for chronic kidney disease (CKD) and hemodialysis after discharge.[1–11] Depending on the type of surgical procedure that a patient undergoes, AKI complicates the perioperative hospital stay for up to 50% of surgical patients.[1,2,12–16] Nevertheless, AKI remains among the most underdiagnosed postoperative complications despite increasing understanding of its epidemiology and

Conflicts of Interest and Source of Funding: A. Bihorac is supported by Center for Sepsis and Critical Illness Award P50 GM-111152 from the National Institute of General Medical Sciences and has received research grants from the Society of Critical Care Medicine and Astute Medical, Inc.
a Department of Surgery, Malcom Randall VA Medical Center, NF/SG VAMC, Gainesville, FL 32608, USA; b Department of Health Services Research, Management, and Policy, University of Florida, Gainesville, FL, USA; c Department of Medicine, University of Florida, PO Box 100254, Gainesville, FL 32610-0254, USA; d Department of Anesthesiology, University of Florida, PO Box 100254, Gainesville, FL 32610-0254, USA
* Corresponding author. Department of Anesthesiology, PO Box 100254, Gainesville, FL 32610-0254.
E-mail address: abihorac@anest.ufl.edu

Crit Care Clin 31 (2015) 705–723
http://dx.doi.org/10.1016/j.ccc.2015.06.007
0749-0704/15/$ – see front matter
criticalcare.theclinics.com

outcomes. Considering the high prevalence of AKI and the deleterious effect when it occurs, efforts must focus on AKI prevention, mitigation of further injury when AKI has already occurred, treatment of negative effects on other organs, and facilitation of renal recovery in patients with established AKI. Although the understanding of the mechanisms of AKI has grown substantially, and the emergence of new biomarkers and imaging techniques has provided new tools for early risk stratification and diagnosis, the translation of these discoveries into clinical practice has been slow. The well-defined timing of surgical physiologic stress on the kidney in the perioperative period provides a unique opportunity for early risk stratification to guide perioperative assessment and preventive therapies to achieve these goals.

DEFINITIONS, EPIDEMIOLOGY, AND OUTCOMES ASSOCIATED WITH PERIOPERATIVE ACUTE KIDNEY INJURY

Before 2004, the reported incidence of hospital-acquired AKI varied significantly from 1% to 31% due to the incoherent criteria used to define AKI and the focus placed on the most severe AKI defined either by a large increase in serum creatinine or by the need for renal replacement therapy (RRT).[17,18] In 2004, the Acute Dialysis Quality Initiative published Risk, Injury, Failure, Loss, and End-stage Kidney (RIFLE), a consensus definition for AKI, that for the first time included less severe AKI stages and provided a structured classification for severity and recovery.[19] The recent Kidney Disease: Improving Global Outcomes (KDIGO) guidelines have expanded the AKI criteria to include changes as small as 0.3 mg/dL.[20] The reported epidemiology and outcomes of AKI have been under rapid evolution since the publication of these new definitions.

Surgical societies and registries have been slow in adopting these new definitions. The American College of Surgeons (ACS) Committee on Trauma defines acute renal failure as a serum creatinine increase greater than or equal to 3.5 mg/dL, but in a large multicenter trauma study, only 15% of all patients with AKI defined by RIFLE criteria had a peak creatinine value greater than 3 mg/dL.[2] The ACS National Surgical Quality Improvement Project (NSQIP) is the largest existing prospective surgical database that quantifies 30-day risk-adjusted surgical outcomes for patients undergoing major surgery, and it defines AKI as an increase in serum creatinine greater than 2 mg/dL from the patient's baseline or as the acute need for RRT.[21] Not surprisingly, studies using the ACS NSQIP database have demonstrated a substantial 30-day mortality associated with AKI and an incidence as low as 1%, creating the perception that postoperative AKI is a rare and often fatal complication after surgery.[22] In a recent single-center cohort study of greater than 20,000 postoperative patients, the ACS NSQIP definition for AKI severely underestimated the incidence of AKI defined by consensus criteria.[12]

The incidence of AKI in recent studies using the current consensus criteria ranges from 25% for trauma patients[2] to as high as 50% for patients undergoing aortic surgery or liver transplantation.[23,24] AKI has been demonstrated to be a common and serious postoperative complication associated with increased risk for short- and long-term mortality, increased incidence of CKD, increased incidence of other postoperative complications, and much higher resource utilization compared with patients with no postoperative AKI.[3,5,12,25–33] The risk-adjusted association between postoperative change in serum creatinine and adverse clinical outcomes is continuous and observed at even lower cutoffs than in the original RIFLE definition,[12,34] and it has been shown that the adverse effects of AKI, as defined by consensus criteria, persist for years even for those patients considered to have partial or even full recovery by the time of hospital discharge.[3,4] The risk-adjusted average cost of care for these patients was $42,600 for patients with any AKI compared with $26,700 for patients without AKI.[1] Thus, prevention of postoperative AKI should be seen as an important target in standardized surgical practice and in studies focusing on quality measures that could translate into improved care for the surgical patient.

RISK FACTORS FOR ACUTE KIDNEY INJURY

Several preoperative and intraoperative factors have emerged as important and common predictors for AKI across different surgical populations (**Table 1**). Scoring systems have been used for years in an attempt to measure risk factors for adverse outcomes after surgery. Several existing scoring systems that measure the risk for AKI after cardiac surgery rely mostly on preoperative variables (reviewed in[35]). More novel preoperative factors such as total lymphocyte count less than 1500 cells/μL and elevated C-reactive protein were identified to be associated with AKI after cardiac surgery.[36,37] Genetic polymorphisms for selected inflammatory and vasoconstrictor genes (alleles angiotensinogen 842C and interleukin 6-572C in Caucasians, and endothelial nitric oxide synthase 894T and angiotensin-converting enzyme deletion and insertion in African Americans) provided 2-to 4-fold improvement over clinical factors alone in explaining postcardiac surgery AKI.[38] For patients undergoing noncardiac surgery, preoperative factors unique for the surgery type need to be considered.[39] Women undergoing surgery for any type of cancer, and especially those with metastatic cancer, had significantly higher odds of developing AKI.[14] Among patients undergoing orthotopic liver transplantation, the Model for End-Stage Liver Disease score, but not pretransplantation creatinine values, was predictive of AKI.[40] A low Norton scale score (a measure of a patient's risk for developing a pressure ulcer) and preoperative use of diuretics and nonsteroidal anti-inflammatory drugs (NSAIDs) were all associated with AKI following total hip arthroplasty.[41,42] Among patients undergoing endovascular abdominal aortic aneurysm repair, the use of fenestrated grafts and increasing contrast dose carried a higher risk for AKI.[43] In a large prospective study of severe trauma patients, any increase in serum creatinine on admission greater than that expected (based on a patients age, gender, and race), an increase in lactic acid, low body temperature, and any transfusion of packed red blood cells and cryoprecipitate within the first 24 hours of trauma were associated with the increased risk for subsequent AKI.[2] Attempting to create a meaningful risk calculation for AKI from these disparate factors has been challenging.

Although some of these factors are unavoidable, others are both preventable and largely ignored in routine clinical practice. Preoperative assessment of kidney health using readily available clinical tests—urinary albuminuria and estimated glomerular filtration rate (eGFR) using serum creatinine—is one of the least used yet most valuable clinical resources not only for the assessment of the risk for AKI but also for the overall risk for postoperative morbidity and mortality. CKD affects 5% of the US population[44] and is an independent predictor of mortality and cardiovascular events.[45] A systematic review of 31 cohort studies of patients undergoing elective surgery demonstrated a graded relationship between CKD severity and postoperative death, comparable to that seen with diabetes, stroke, and coronary disease.[46] In a recent analysis of the ACS NSQIP database, the adjusted hazard ratio for 30-day mortality ranged from 2.30 for stage 3 CKD to 3.05 for stage 5 CKD compared with no CKD.[47] Furthermore, preoperative proteinuria, independent of preoperative eGFR and other comorbidities, was not only associated with the risk of AKI but also a powerful independent risk factor for long-term all-cause mortality and end-stage

Table 1
Risk factors for acute kidney injury

Type of Surgery	Preoperative Risk Factors	Intraoperative Risk Factors
Cardiac surgery	Advanced age	Emergent reoperation
	Female sex	Valve replacement surgery
	Baseline renal function	Surgery on the thoracic aorta
	Diabetes mellitus	Deep hypothermic circulatory arrest
	Poor glycemic control	Low-output syndrome
	Congestive heart failure	Vasopressors needed before cardiopulmonary bypass
	Low ejection fraction	Use of cardiopulmonary bypass
	Peripheral vascular disease	Volume of blood transfusion
	Intra-aortic balloon pump use	Intraoperative nadir hemoglobin level
	Chronic obstructive pulmonary disease	Intraoperative hypotension (<50 mm Hg)
	Peripheral vascular disease	Urine output
	Hypertension	Surgery requiring cardiopulmonary bypass
	Lower preoperative hemoglobin	Cardiopulmonary bypass duration
	Atrial fibrillation	Low pump flow
	Preoperative total lymphocyte count <1500 cells/μL	Low perfusion pressure
	Gene polymorphisms (Alleles angiotensinogen 842C and interleukin 6-572C in Caucasians; alleles endothelial nitric oxide synthase 894T and angiotensin-converting enzyme deletion and insertion in African Americans)	Severe hemodilution
		Low oxygen delivery (DO_2) and low DO_2/VCO_2 ratios
		Hyperthermia (the arterial outlet temperature >37°C)
		Intraoperative inotropes
		Furosemide administration
	Elevated preoperative C-reactive protein	ICU admission temperature after CPB
		Aprotinin use
Noncardiac surgery	Advanced age	Emergent surgery
	Male sex	High-risk surgery
	Baseline renal function	Reoperation
	Diabetes mellitus	Open vascular surgery procedure
	Liver disease	Surgery for malignant gynecologic tumors
	Peripheral vascular disease	Prolonged surgical times (>4 h)
	Chronic obstructive pulmonary disease	Aortic cross-clamp time
	Left ventricular dysfunction	Fenestrated grafts and contrast dose for endovascular procedures
	High body mass index	Intraoperative hypotension
	American Society of Anesthesiologists physical status	Intraoperative vasopressor use
	Preoperative albumin <3.2	Number of transfused packed red blood cells
	Preoperative anemia	Prolonged dopamine use
	Use of hydroxyethyl starch fluids	Lactic acidosis
	Model for end-stage liver disease score, hepatorenal syndrome type II, and hepatitis C (orthotopic liver transplantation)	Lateral decubitus positioning in laparoscopic surgery
		Administration of furosemide or mannitol
	Low Norton scores (performed by nurses) and preoperative diuretics and NSAIDS (total hip arthroplasty)	Duration of anhepatic phase (orthotopic liver transplantation)

renal disease after cardiac surgery.[48,49] However, the importance of CKD as a peri-operative risk factor is still not widely appreciated among physicians involved in peri-operative decision-making.

Some perioperative risk indicators consider CKD an important prognostic factor in postoperative risk assessment,[50–52] whereas others do not.[53,54] One difficulty in increasing the awareness of CKD as an important perioperative risk factor is the complicated relationship between serum creatinine and eGFR calculated with commonly used estimation equations such as the Chronic Kidney Disease Epidemiology Collaboration equation.[55] Especially among women and the elderly, the serum creatinine alone may not give an accurate picture of CKD because creatinine values within normal limits may correspond to a low eGFR. Thus, in the perioperative setting, use of estimation equations to assess eGFR, rather than relying on serum creatinine values alone, is a strategy to assure that CKD is appropriately assessed as a risk factor for not only AKI but also overall postoperative mortality.

One factor that has received intense interest recently has been the possible effect of preoperative medications on preoperative complications. Statins (or HMG-CoA reductase inhibitors) have received the most attention because of their important pleiotropic effects, including reduced vascular inflammation and improved endothelial function.[56] The data on preoperative statin use and risk for AKI are evolving and contradictory. The subgroup analysis of a systematic review of preoperative use of statins among cardiac surgery patients (including 4 studies with a total of 367 patients, including 19 patients with renal failure) demonstrated no benefit from preoperative statin use.[57] A study from The Cleveland Clinic reporting no difference in AKI or hospital mortality between 4683 statin users propensity matched with 22,000 non-statin users was limited to elective surgery cases and reported a very low incidence of AKI (6%), hospital mortality (0.6%), and need for dialysis (0.05%), rendering it difficult to compare to other studies. In a small cohort of 151 vascular surgery patients, Kor and colleagues[58] found no difference with preoperative statin use using moderate to severe AKI (incidence 7%), need for RRT (3%), and mortality (5%) as endpoints.[57] In contrast, a population-based Canadian retrospective cohort study including 213,347 older patients who underwent major elective surgery demonstrated 16% lower odds of severe AKI, 17% lower odds of acute dialysis, and 21% lower odds of mortality for patients on a preoperative statin.[59] In a retrospective cohort of 98,939 patients undergoing a major open abdominal, cardiac, thoracic, or vascular procedure, preoperative statin use was associated with a 20% to 26% reduction in the incidence of postoperative AKI defined by consensus criteria.[60] These retrospective results, and the intriguing pleiotropic actions of statins, have prompted several prospective trials on the effect of statins on perioperative complications.

Several modifiable intraoperative factors have been identified as risk factors for AKI for both cardiac and noncardiac surgery, including use of cardiopulmonary bypass (CPB), hemodilution, intraoperative transfusion and hemoglobin levels, hypotension, oxygen delivery and any use of diuretics, vasopressors, and inotropes.[61–64] Rewarming after CPB and hyperthermic perfusion during CPB are novel risk factors for AKI after cardiac surgery.[65,66] A recent systematic review of perioperative interventions aimed to optimize global blood flow showed no difference in mortality, but the rates of renal failure (relative risk 0.71, 95% confidence interval [CI] 0.57–0.90) were reduced.[67] Goal-directed intraoperative management to reduce the risk of postoperative AKI through optimizing renal perfusion is both feasible and underused.

RISK STRATIFICATION FOR ACUTE KIDNEY INJURY

Given that AKI is common after surgery, and associated with significant morbidity and cost, the ability to detect AKI within hours of onset would likely be helpful in implementing measures to protect the kidney from further injury and to preserve renal function. In the presence of common clinical risk factors for perioperative AKI, such as hypotension or hypoxemia or certain comorbidities, it is difficult to discriminate those who will imminently develop AKI from those who will not before change in creatinine or urine output is measurable. Widespread adoption of effective preventive interventions is only likely with the assistance of a test or tests that can be quickly done at the bedside and that reliably discern those patients at increased risk for AKI from those at low risk.

Use of Imaging Techniques

Ultrasound and Doppler imaging of the kidney have been used for years in the assessment of CKD in the transplanted kidney and in renal artery stenosis. Doppler imaging detects macroscopic vascular abnormalities as well as microvascular changes in blood flow in the kidney. Renal resistive index (RRI), determined by Doppler ultrasonography, quantifies changes in renal vascular resistance, and recent studies have shown that an elevated RRI is associated with an increased risk for AKI.[68] In patients with septic shock, an increased RRI has been shown to be associated with AKI.[69–71] The RRI, when used in the immediate postoperative period after cardiac surgery with cardiopulmonary bypass, predicts delayed AKI and its severity.[72] When measured using intraoperative transesophageal echocardiography, for patients undergoing cardiac surgery, the predictive results for AKI are comparable to RRI obtained via translumbar ultrasound.[73] The association between elevated RRI and AKI holds for noncardiac surgeries like orthopedic surgeries and in critically ill patients in the medical intensive care unit (ICU).[74,75] RRI has also been shown to be helpful in predicting the progression of postoperative AKI after cardiac surgery.[76] Although RRI is closely related to renal vascular resistance, it has become clear in recent studies that there are other factors that affect RRI especially in the unstable patient, and the indications and utility of the test for predicting AKI are still unresolved.[77,78] Another newly developed technique for assessing renal microvasculature is contrast-enhanced ultrasonography (CEUS) to assess renal perfusion.[79] A recent study of patients undergoing elective cardiac surgery, who were considered to be at risk of AKI and were studied with CEUS, showed that renal perfusion decreased within 24 hours after surgery. The technique of CEUS has been validated in the quantification of microcirculatory flow in the liver and the heart and shows early promise in assessing the risk of AKI.[80]

MRI is another emerging modality in the early diagnosis of AKI. Newer and less toxic contrast agents, including ultrasmall particles of iron oxide, are being studied for imaging renal blood flow and volume.[81] Blood oxygenation level dependent (BOLD) MRI, which uses deoxyhemoglobin as an endogenous contrast agent for the noninvasive assessment of tissue oxygen bioavailability, has been used to evaluate intrarenal oxygenation.[82] Changes in medullary blood flow related to the use of nephrotoxic agents, including NSAIDs, intravenous contrast agents, and calcineurin inhibitors, are effectively demonstrated with BOLD MRI.[83] It has recently been used to study changes in medullary blood flow associated with hypertension and CKD.[84–86] BOLD MRI has been used to study renal oxygenation and function in animal models of AKI[87,88]; however, one recent study using BOLD MRI in patients with AKI found no correlation between MRI findings and GFR.[89] As with the Doppler ultrasound-derived

RRI, the indications and utility of BOLD MRI for predicting AKI in surgical patients are still unresolved.

Use of Urine and Plasma Biomarkers

Another approach for rapid diagnosis of organ injury is the analysis of serum or urine biomarkers that reveal early evidence of cellular stress or injury. Biomarkers for cardiac injury, such as serum troponin, are useful in the evaluation and treatment of patients with chest pain because they help clinicians identify those patients who have undergone recent myocardial injury. Many serum and urine biomarkers have been studied for their ability to predict AKI (reviewed in[90–94]). Difficulties in finding biomarkers with good predictive power include the variable time from insult to the development of AKI, the association of biomarkers with both CKD and AKI, and their association with the diverse underlying disease processes that can cause AKI. Furthermore, surgical and critically ill patients are exposed to systemic inflammation with cellular stress and injuries in several organs, repetitive exposure to invasive procedures and hemodynamic perturbations requiring fluid therapy and vasopressor support, blood transfusion, and nephrotoxic drugs. The abundance of these potential mediators and confounders of AKI may cause nonspecific increases in biomarkers reflecting overall illness severity rather than specific organ damage.

Among surgical patients, the use of biomarkers for AKI prediction was most studied after cardiac procedures with the most promising results demonstrated for the use of plasma and urine neutrophil gelatinase-associated lipocalin (NGAL) (reviewed in[94,95]). Systemic inflammation induces NGAL synthesis by extrarenal tissues and the release of NGAL from neutrophils mainly in the dimeric form. A recent systematic review summarized studies that measured NGAL in more than 7000 patients after cardiac surgery and showed moderate overall discriminatory ability with area under the receiver operating characteristic curve (ROC-AUC) between 0.82 and 0.83. Studies including more than 8500 critically ill patients, mostly recruited from mixed medical/surgical ICU populations, demonstrated similar overall predictive performance with ROC-AUC between 0.79 and 0.80.[96,97] The inability to distinguish systemic inflammatory effects from organ-specific increases in NGAL, and the lack of a diagnostic platform to differentiate specific biological forms of NGAL, has hampered widespread clinical use of this biomarker.

Cystatin C (CyC) is the most studied novel functional kidney biomarker.[92] This cysteine protease inhibitor is produced by all nucleated cells of the body, released into the bloodstream at a constant rate, excreted through glomerular filtration into primary urine, and subsequently completely reabsorbed and catabolized in proximal renal tubules. As a consequence, CyC is not normally found in urine in significant amounts, and urinary CyC may reflect tubular damage. Because of the constant rate of its production, plasma CyC concentrations may be a better marker of GFR than creatinine in surgical patients. However, its ability to provide early risk stratification for postoperative AKI or RRT requirement remains uncertain among surgical patients.[92]

Recently, 2 urinary biomarkers, tissue inhibitor of metalloproteinases-2 (TIMP-2) and insulin-like growth factor binding protein 7 (IGFBP7), have been validated as markers of risk for AKI.[98,99] These markers were recently approved for use by the US Food and Drug Administration, becoming the first AKI biomarkers to do so. A multicenter study involving 420 patients found that urinary [TIMP-2]•[IGFBP7] was predictive of moderate to severe AKI in critically ill patients within 12 hours. Unlike prior studies evaluating these markers or others for AKI,[98] the endpoint was adjudicated by a committee of 3 independent experts who were blinded to the results of the test. The ROC-AUC for the urinary [TIMP-2]•[IGFBP7] test was 0.82 (95% CI 0.76–0.88) and was superior to simultaneously measured serum creatinine and other existing biomarkers for predicting the risk of imminent AKI. Patients with a urinary test result higher than the prespecified high sensitivity cutoff value of 0.3 (ng/mL)^2/1000 had 7 times the risk for AKI (95% CI 4–22). Meersch and colleagues[100] examined the sensitivity and specificity of the [TIMP-2]•[IGFBP7] test for any AKI stage among patients undergoing cardiac surgery and found a sensitivity of 0.92 and specificity of 0.81 for a cutoff value of 0.5 (ROC-AUC of 0.84) using the highest urinary [TIMP-2]•[IGFBP7] achieved in the first 24 hours following surgery. Interestingly, TIMP-2 and IGFBP7 are both associated with G1 cell-cycle arrest, an epithelial cellular protective mechanism, rather than with cellular necrosis or apoptosis. Epithelial cells, by virtue of their anatomy and function, are susceptible to multiple environmental stressors: toxin exposure, oxidative stress, and inflammation among others. When DNA may be damaged, or when bioenergetic resources are scarce, epithelial cells may enter cell-cycle arrest to protect themselves, and TIMP-2 and IGFBP7 become elevated. Thus, these urinary biomarkers may indicate risk for injury before any actual AKI takes place.

Use of Clinical Prediction Scores

One very different approach toward early diagnosis and prediction of organ injury is automated analysis of the large amounts of clinical data obtained during routine care to detect critical incidents or trends that might be predictive of injury. Accurate risk stratification of patients in real time could enable the selection of optimal therapy in a timely fashion to prevent AKI altogether, or to mitigate the effects of the complication even before signs and symptoms arise, and could be tailored to a patient's personal clinical profile. Despite the acquisition of multiple continuously recorded physiologic signals during modern perioperative management, the use of these data for the development of risk and prediction models has been limited to the prediction of broad outcomes such as postoperative mortality rather than to specific morbidity events including AKI.[101–103] Most of the predictive scores and algorithms have been limited either to a specific type of surgery or to preoperative risk factors only, or have used the occurrence of the most severe AKI as an endpoint while excluding the more prevalent mild and moderate AKI.

Most of the studies that developed and validated predictive models or clinical scores for AKI were performed among cardiac surgery patients. A recent systematic review[35] evaluated the available risk models for AKI after cardiac surgery and reported 4 clinical risk scores for AKI requiring dialysis,[104–107] and 3 scores to predict a broader definition of AKI.[108–110] These scores predicted a probability of severe AKI between less than 1% and greater than 20%, with the ROC-AUC varying between 0.77 and 0.84. For patients undergoing noncardiac surgery, a few predictive models, developed in small cohorts using limited intraoperative data or in larger cohorts but using only severe AKI as an endpoint, are further limited by the lack of validation studies and provide only modest predictive accuracy.[22,111–113] Recently, the UK AKI in Cardiac Surgery Collaborators group have developed and validated a new risk prediction score for any stage AKI after cardiac surgery with ROC-AUC of 0.74, providing better discrimination compared with previously published scores.[114]

The volume of physiologic data routinely acquired during intraoperative hemodynamic monitoring is rarely used in published risk scores and, when used, it is usually summarized by some reductionist approach (mean, lowest value) rather than applied in their continuity and complexity and almost never in automatized fashion.[13,22,105,111,112,115–120] Lack of sophistication in both data collection and analysis of real-time physiologic data has limited this approach. Automated risk scores, developed using machine learning to automatically analyze physiologic time series data, have already been shown to predict neonatal clinical outcomes more accurately than can be achieved with any pre-existing scoring system.[121] Machine learning applied to the automated, rapid, noninvasive measurements obtained in the operating room and ICU raises the prospect of real-time risk prediction for perioperative AKI and studies using them are starting to emerge.[34,122–124]

PREVENTION AND TREATMENT OF PERIOPERATIVE ACUTE KIDNEY INJURY

One of the challenges in managing AKI is the paucity of interventions to treat it once it occurs. Given that reality, prevention of AKI is of paramount importance. Many interventions have been studied in an attempt to prevent or ameliorate perioperative AKI.[13,15,16] Although patients with CKD have a higher risk for adverse perioperative events, preoperative optimization of renal function using pharmacologic therapy, such as angiotensin converting enzyme inhibitors (ACE-I), diuretic therapy, or regular visits to a nephrologist, to prevent a decline in kidney function around the time of surgery was not proven to mitigate the risk of AKI.[112,125] Some investigators advocate avoidance of ACE-I or angiotensin receptor blocker therapies around the time of surgery, especially when hypotension is anticipated.[125,126] Multiple pharmacologic therapies have been unsuccessfully tested for the prevention of perioperative AKI, including scavengers of oxygen free radicals such as mannitol and N-acetylcysteine, dopamine, fenoldapam, loop diuretics, and atrial natriuretic peptide (reviewed in[13,15,16,127]). A recent systematic review and meta-analysis including 1079 patients in 5 randomized control trials demonstrated no benefit for the prophylactic perioperative use of sodium bicarbonate for prevention of AKI after cardiac surgery. In contrast, the use of sodium bicarbonate prolonged the duration of mechanical ventilation and ICU length of stay and increased the risk of alkalemia.[128] A recent large randomized clinical trial of patients undergoing noncardiac surgery found that neither aspirin nor clonidine administered perioperatively reduced the risk of AKI (13.4% for aspirin vs 12.3% for placebo; 13.0% for clonidine vs 12.7% for placebo), whereas both aspirin and clonidine were associated with clinically important adverse effects.[129]

Some aspects of perioperative management do appear to have an important effect on kidney function. The use of off-pump technique in cardiac surgery has demonstrated benefit in randomized control trials and meta-analyses.[115] Two large meta-analyses and a systematic review have showed that intraoperative interventions associated with goal-directed fluid management were associated with a significant reduction in the incidence of all severity stages of AKI.[67,130] Initiating appropriate hemodynamic monitoring to allow the anesthesiologist to optimize intravascular volume, cardiac output, or oxygen delivery in high-risk patients resulted in a decreased risk of perioperative AKI if started preoperatively (odds ratio 0.70, 95% CI 0.53–0.94; $P = .02$) or intraoperatively (OR 0.47, 95% CI 0.27–0.81; $P = .006$).[130] One contentious and unresolved issue in goal-directed fluid management and resuscitation is the optimal endpoint and how to measure it. An optimal mean arterial pressure (MAP) for the kidney at risk for AKI is unknown and may be different from that obtained peripherally.[80] The ability to assess renal perfusion at the bedside using Doppler ultrasound may provide better fluid and vasoactive medication management for the unstable patient at risk for AKI. One study in patients with septic shock showed that RRI decreased significantly when MAP was increased using norepinephrine from 65 to 75 mm Hg.[69] Another prospective study of patients who had experienced sustained hypotension showed that an average MAP between 72 and 82 mm Hg during the first 3 days after hypotension was associated with a lower incidence of RIFLE-AKI compared with patients with an average MAP less than 72 mm Hg.[131] Further studies exploring the optimal resuscitation endpoints for the kidney to prevent AKI, and how to measure those endpoints, are needed. Another interesting meta-analysis involving 1600 patients in 10 trials demonstrated that volatile anesthetics may provide renal protection in patients undergoing cardiac surgery and supports the notion that further research of high methodologic quality is needed to define optimal intraoperative management of patients at high risk of AKI.[132]

Another evolving concept is the use of remote ischemic preconditioning to prevent AKI in certain patient populations. Ischemia reperfusion injury occurs whenever a tissue bed becomes temporarily ischemic and is then restored to normal perfusion. The kidneys are particularly sensitive to ischemia reperfusion injury due to their high metabolic and oxygen demands and complex microvasculature.[68] However, in addition to causing injury, programmed brief and intermittent ischemia is known to have cytoprotective effects. Local ischemic preconditioning has been shown to be effective against various types of AKI.[133,134] Remote ischemic preconditioning, involving programmed brief and repeated ischemia of a remote tissue such as limb skeletal muscle, has been shown to be as effective as local ischemic preconditioning in preventing cellular damage. It is thought to attenuate injury through upregulation of a variety of intracellular kinases, resulting in modification of mitochondrial function, metabolic downregulation, and temporary cell-cycle arrest.[135] Recently, in a randomized controlled trial, remote ischemic preconditioning was found to be protective against contrast medium–induced AKI for patients undergoing elective coronary angiography and who were judged to be at high risk for AKI.[133] Similar results were found in a randomized controlled trial of 120 patients undergoing elective cardiac surgery, in which the patients randomized to remote ischemic preconditioning had significantly less risk of postoperative AKI.[129] Although these early trials provide the promise of a novel, noninvasive, and virtually morbidity-free therapy to prevent AKI, further investigation is needed to define the indications and utility of this approach.

One important potential method of limiting the consequences of AKI in surgical patients is early and continued involvement of a nephrologist. A study from 2 hospitals in the United Kingdom with no on-site nephrology services showed that, compared with hospitals with nephrology consultation available, there were significant shortcomings in AKI recognition and management that were associated with poor survival and increased rates of CKD.[136] In prospective observational studies of the patient admitted to the ICU, it has been shown that delayed nephrology consultation was associated with higher mortality[137,138] and increased dialysis-dependence rates at hospital discharge.[138] In a recent prospective controlled nonrandomized study, patients in an early nephrology consultation group (seen within 18 hours of onset of AKI) had significantly lower risk of further decrease in kidney function.[139]

Nephrology referral has also been shown to be important in follow-up care after an episode of AKI. A study of patients who sustained AKI between 2003 and 2008 in a Veterans Administration hospital, and were considered to be at risk for subsequent worsening of renal function, showed that the cumulative incidence of outpatient nephrology referrals for these patients was only 8.5%.[140] Another more recent study of Veterans Administration patients admitted to the hospital with AKI showed that measurement of serum creatinine during outpatient follow-up was common, but measurement of proteinuria, parathyroid hormone, or serum phosphorus was rare.[141] The importance of this low referral rate is emphasized in a cohort study of hospitalized adults with AKI who received temporary inpatient dialysis and survived for 90 days following discharge, in which patients with early nephrology follow-up had significantly lower all-cause mortality.[142]

Given the association between AKI and the later development of CKD and other complications, follow-up care for patients who sustain AKI in the hospital could have important public health and socioeconomic impact.[143,144] In 2012, the KDIGO AKI work group released guidelines recommending that patients be evaluated 3 months after AKI for the new onset of CKD or worsening of any pre-existing CKD.[145] Patients with CKD are to be managed according to the Kidney Disease Outcome Quality Initiative (KDOQI) CKD guidelines, and patients with no CKD are to be managed according to the KDOQI guidelines for patients at risk for CKD. Finally, in addition to nephrology consultation for the patient who has sustained AKI, it is imperative that primary care practitioners understand the risks associated with even mild degrees of AKI suffered by their patients, both to initiate timely nephrology involvement and to optimally manage patients at risk for the development of CKD.[146–148] The current attempts at better coordinating care for the patient with chronic disease, including the patient-centered medical home and accountable-care organizations with robust electronic medical record-keeping, may help improve the care of patients who have sustained AKI.[149–151]

SUMMARY

Acute and chronic kidney injury and dysfunction play important roles in affecting perioperative outcomes. AKI is a common complication after surgery and mild to moderate AKI is more common than severe AKI. All stages of AKI severity are associated with increased short- and long-term morbidity and mortality. Clinical risk factors for AKI are similar but not identical in different surgical populations. There seems to be no single therapy that will prevent perioperative AKI. Considering the high prevalence of AKI and the deleterious effect when it occurs, effort must focus on prevention of AKI, mitigation of further injury when AKI has already occurred, treatment of negative effects on other organs, and facilitation of renal recovery in patients with established AKI. This clinical pathway requires a medical team of experts, including all primary health care providers who manage surgical and critically ill patients, backed up by bedside nurses, pharmacists, and nephrologists. Every patient admitted needs a comprehensive and systematic assessment of kidney health. Current strategies should focus on better management of the preoperative risks and susceptibilities for AKI by more accurate assessment of the patient's renal reserve and susceptibility to new injury. A standardized approach for intraoperative management for patients at high risk for AKI needs to focus on avoidance of hemodynamic derangements that have been shown to impact renal function. In the early postoperative period, the magnitude of exposures to insult and the extent of the sustained renal distress or damage need to be evaluated using a combination of clinical parameters, novel biomarkers, and evolving imaging techniques. The determination of potential causes of AKI, the initiation of treatment, and then continued reassessment in response to that therapy should follow promptly afterward with the early involvement of nephrology teams.

REFERENCES

1. Hobson C, Ozrazgat-Baslanti T, Kuxhausen A, et al. Cost and mortality associated with postoperative acute kidney injury. Ann Surg 2014;261(6):1207–14.

2. Bihorac A, Delano MJ, Schold JD, et al. Incidence, clinical predictors, genomics, and outcome of acute kidney injury among trauma patients. Ann Surg 2010;252:158–65.

3. Hobson CE, Yavas S, Segal MS, et al. Acute kidney injury is associated with increased long-term mortality after cardiothoracic surgery. Circulation 2009; 119:2444–53.

4. Bihorac A, Yavas S, Subbiah S, et al. Long-term risk of mortality and acute kidney injury during hospitalization after major surgery. Ann Surg 2009;249: 851–8.

5. Wald R, Quinn RR, Luo J, et al. Chronic dialysis and death among survivors of acute kidney injury requiring dialysis. JAMA 2009;302:1179–85.

6. van Kuijk JP, Flu WJ, Chonchol M, et al. Temporary perioperative decline of renal function is an independent predictor for chronic kidney disease. Clin J Am Soc Nephrol 2010;5:1198–204.

7. Ishani A, Nelson D, Clothier B, et al. The magnitude of acute serum creatinine increase after cardiac surgery and the risk of chronic kidney disease, progression of kidney disease, and death. Arch Intern Med 2011;171:226–33.

8. James MT, Ghali WA, Knudtson ML, et al. Associations between acute kidney injury and cardiovascular and renal outcomes after coronary angiography. Circulation 2011;123:409–16.

9. Thakar CV, Christianson A, Himmelfarb J, et al. Acute kidney injury episodes and chronic kidney disease risk in diabetes mellitus. Clin J Am Soc Nephrol 2011;6:2567–72.

10. Coca SG, Singanamala S, Parikh CR. Chronic kidney disease after acute kidney injury: a systematic review and meta-analysis. Kidney Int 2012;81:442–8.

11. Chawla LS, Amdur RL, Shaw AD, et al. Association between AKI and long-term renal and cardiovascular outcomes in United States veterans. Clin J Am Soc Nephrol 2014;9:448–56.

12. Bihorac A, Brennan M, Ozrazgat Baslanti T, et al. National surgical quality improvement program underestimates the risk associated with mild and moderate postoperative acute kidney injury. Crit Care Med 2013;41: 2570–83.

13. Borthwick E, Ferguson A. Perioperative acute kidney injury: risk factors, recognition, management, and outcomes. BMJ 2010;341:c3365.

14. Vaught A, Ozrazgat-Baslanti T, Javed A, et al. Acute kidney injury in major gynaecological surgery: an observational study. BJOG 2014. [Epub ahead of print].

15. Calvert S, Shaw A. Perioperative acute kidney injury. Perioper Med (Lond) 2012;1:6.

16. Thakar CV. Perioperative acute kidney injury. Adv Chronic Kidney Dis 2013;20: 67–75.

17. Hoste EA, Kellum JA. Incidence, classification, and outcomes of acute kidney injury. Contrib Nephrol 2007;156:32–8.

18. Ricci Z, Cruz DN, Ronco C. Classification and staging of acute kidney injury: beyond the RIFLE and AKIN criteria. Nat Rev Nephrol 2011;7:201–8.

19. Bellomo R, Ronco C, Kellum JA, et al. Acute renal failure - definition, outcome measures, animal models, fluid therapy and information technology needs: the Second International Consensus Conference of the Acute Dialysis Quality Initiative (ADQI) Group. Crit Care 2004;8:R204–12.

20. Kidney Disease: Improving Global Outcomes (KDIGO) Acute Kidney Injury Work Group. KDIGO Clinical Practice Guideline for Acute Kidney Injury. Kidney Inter 2012;2(Suppl):1-138.

21. American College of Surgeons National Surgical Quality Improvement Program. User guide for the 2010 participant use data file. Chicago: American College of Surgeons; 2010. p. 60611–3211.
22. Kheterpal S, Tremper KK, Heung M, et al. Development and validation of an acute kidney injury risk index for patients undergoing general surgery: results from a national data set. Anesthesiology 2009;110:505–15.
23. Arnaoutakis GJ, Bihorac A, Martin TD, et al. RIFLE criteria for acute kidney injury in aortic arch surgery. J Thorac Cardiovasc Surg 2007;134:1554–61.
24. Kundakci A, Pirat A, Komurcu O, et al. Rifle criteria for acute kidney dysfunction following liver transplantation: incidence and risk factors. Transplant Proc 2010; 42:4171–4.
25. Bihorac A, Schold JD, Hobson CE. Long-term mortality associated with acute kidney injury requiring dialysis. JAMA 2010;303:229 [author reply: 229–30].
26. Hobson C, Ozrazgat-Baslanti T, Kuxhausen A, et al. Cost and mortality associated with postoperative acute kidney injury. Annals of Surgery 2015;261(6):1207–14.
27. Dimick JB, Pronovost PJ, Cowan JA, et al. Complications and costs after high-risk surgery: where should we focus quality improvement initiatives? J Am Coll Surg 2003;196:671–8.
28. Dimick JB, Chen SL, Taheri PA, et al. Hospital costs associated with surgical complications: a report from the private-sector National Surgical Quality Improvement Program. J Am Coll Surg 2004;199:531–7.
29. Thakar CV, Christianson A, Freyberg R, et al. Incidence and outcomes of acute kidney injury in intensive care units: a Veterans Administration study. Crit Care Med 2009;37:2552–8.
30. Duran PA, Concepcion LA. Survival after acute kidney injury requiring dialysis: long-term follow up. Hemodial Int 2014;18:S1–6.
31. Coca SG, Yusuf B, Shlipak MG, et al. Long-term risk of mortality and other adverse outcomes after acute kidney injury: a systematic review and meta-analysis. Am J Kidney Dis 2009;53:961–73.
32. Lafrance J-P, Miller DR. Acute kidney injury associates with increased long-term mortality. J Am Soc Nephrol 2010;21:345–52.
33. Amdur RL, Chawla LS, Amodeo S, et al. Outcomes following diagnosis of acute renal failure in U.S. veterans: focus on acute tubular necrosis. Kidney Int 2009; 76:1089–97.
34. Ozrazgat Baslanti T, Korenkevych D, Momcilovic P, et al. Mathematical modeling of the association between the pattern of change in postoperative serum creatinine and hospital mortality. Crit Care Med 2012;40(12):U131.
35. Huen SC, Parikh CR. Predicting acute kidney injury after cardiac surgery: a systematic review. Ann Thorac Surg 2012;93:337–47.
36. Lomivorotov VV, Efremov SM, Boboshko VA, et al. Preoperative total lymphocyte count in peripheral blood as a predictor of poor outcome in adult cardiac surgery. J Cardiothorac Vasc Anesth 2011;25:975–80.
37. Kim DH, Shim JK, Hong SW, et al. Predictive value of C-reactive protein for major postoperative complications following off-pump coronary artery bypass surgery: prospective and observational trial. Circ J 2009;73:872–7.
38. Stafford-Smith M, Podgoreanu M, Swaminathan M, et al. Association of genetic polymorphisms with risk of renal injury after coronary bypass graft surgery. Am J Kidney Dis 2005;45:519–30.
39. van Kuijk JP, Flu WJ, Valentijn TM, et al. Preoperative left ventricular dysfunction predisposes to postoperative acute kidney injury and long-term mortality. J Nephrol 2011;24:764–70.

40. Romano TG, Schmidtbauer I, Silva FM, et al. Role of MELD score and serum creatinine as prognostic tools for the development of acute kidney injury after liver transplantation. PLoS One 2013;8:e64089.

41. Asleh K, Sever R, Hilu S, et al. Association between low admission Norton scale scores and postoperative complications after elective THA in elderly patients. Orthopedics 2012;35:e1302–6.

42. Aveline C, Leroux A, Vautier P, et al. Risk factors for renal dysfunction after total hip arthroplasty. Ann Fr Anesth Reanim 2009;28:728–34 [in French].

43. Brooks CE, Middleton A, Dhillon R, et al. Predictors of creatinine rise post-endovascular abdominal aortic aneurysm repair. ANZ J Surg 2011;81:827–30.

44. Lamb EJ, Levey AS, Stevens PE. The Kidney Disease Improving Global Outcomes (KDIGO) guideline update for chronic kidney disease: evolution not revolution. Clin Chem 2013;59:462–5.

45. Matsushita K, van der Velde M, Astor BC, et al. Association of estimated glomerular filtration rate and albuminuria with all-cause and cardiovascular mortality in general population cohorts: a collaborative meta-analysis. Lancet 2010;375: 2073–81.

46. Mathew A, Devereaux PJ, O'Hare A, et al. Chronic kidney disease and postoperative mortality: a systematic review and meta-analysis. Kidney Int 2008;73: 1069–81.

47. Gaber AO, Moore LW, Aloia TA, et al. Cross-sectional and case-control analyses of the association of kidney function staging with adverse postoperative outcomes in general and vascular surgery. Ann Surg 2013;258:169–77.

48. Wu VC, Huang TM, Wu PC, et al. Preoperative proteinuria is associated with long-term progression to chronic dialysis and mortality after coronary artery bypass grafting surgery. PLoS One 2012;7:e27687.

49. Huang TM, Wu VC, Young GH, et al. Preoperative proteinuria predicts adverse renal outcomes after coronary artery bypass grafting. J Am Soc Nephrol 2011; 22:156–63.

50. Fleisher LA, Eagle KA. Clinical practice. Lowering cardiac risk in noncardiac surgery. N Engl J Med 2001;345:1677–82.

51. Kertai MD, Boersma E, Klein J, et al. Optimizing the prediction of perioperative mortality in vascular surgery by using a customized probability model. Arch Intern Med 2005;165:898–904.

52. Lee TH, Marcantonio ER, Mangione CM, et al. Derivation and prospective validation of a simple index for prediction of cardiac risk of major noncardiac surgery. Circulation 1999;100:1043–9.

53. Detsky AS, Abrams HB, McLaughlin JR, et al. Predicting cardiac complications in patients undergoing non-cardiac surgery. J Gen Intern Med 1986;1:211–9.

54. Goldman L, Caldera DL, Nussbaum SR, et al. Multifactorial index of cardiac risk in noncardiac surgical procedures. N Engl J Med 1977;297:845–50.

55. Levey AS, Stevens LA, Schmid CH, et al. A new equation to estimate glomerular filtration rate. Ann Intern Med 2009;150:604–12.

56. Davignon J. Beneficial cardiovascular pleiotropic effects of statins. Circulation 2004;109:III39–43.

57. Liakopoulos OJ, Kuhn EW, Slottosch I, et al. Preoperative statin therapy for patients undergoing cardiac surgery. Cochrane Database Syst Rev 2012;(4):CD008493.

58. Kor DJ, Brown MJ, Iscimen R, et al. Perioperative statin therapy and renal outcomes after major vascular surgery: a propensity-based analysis. J Cardiothorac Vasc Anesth 2008;22:210–6.

59. Molnar AO, Coca SG, Devereaux PJ, et al. Statin use associates with a lower incidence of acute kidney injury after major elective surgery. J Am Soc Nephrol 2011;22:939–46.
60. Brunelli SM, Waikar SS, Bateman BT, et al. Preoperative statin use and postoperative acute kidney injury. Am J Med 2012;125:1195–204.e3.
61. Karkouti K, Wijeysundera DN, Yau TM, et al. Acute kidney injury after cardiac surgery: focus on modifiable risk factors. Circulation 2009;119:495–502.
62. Haase M, Bellomo R, Story D, et al. Effect of mean arterial pressure, haemoglobin and blood transfusion during cardiopulmonary bypass on post-operative acute kidney injury. Nephrol Dial Transplant 2012;27:153–60.
63. de Somer F, Mulholland J, Bryan M, et al. O2 delivery and CO2 production during cardiopulmonary bypass as determinants of acute kidney injury: time for a goal-directed perfusion management? Crit Care 2011;15:R192.
64. Parolari A, Pesce LL, Pacini D, et al. Risk factors for perioperative acute kidney injury after adult cardiac surgery: role of perioperative management. Ann Thorac Surg 2012;93:584–91.
65. Newland RF, Tully PJ, Baker RA. Hyperthermic perfusion during cardiopulmonary bypass and postoperative temperature are independent predictors of acute kidney injury following cardiac surgery. Perfusion 2013;28:223–31.
66. Boodhwani M, Rubens FD, Wozny D, et al. Effects of mild hypothermia and rewarming on renal function after coronary artery bypass grafting. Ann Thorac Surg 2009;87:489–95.
67. Grocott MPW, Dushianthan A, Hamilton MA, et al. Perioperative increase in global blood flow to explicit defined goals and outcomes following surgery. John Wiley & Sons, Ltd. Cochrane Database Syst Rev 2012;(11):CD004082.
68. Ninet S, Schnell D, Dewitte A, et al. Doppler-based renal resistive index for prediction of renal dysfunction reversibility: a systematic review and meta-analysis. J Crit Care 2015;30(3):629–35.
69. Deruddre S, Cheisson G, Mazoit JX, et al. Renal arterial resistance in septic shock: effects of increasing mean arterial pressure with norepinephrine on the renal resistive index assessed with Doppler ultrasonography. Intensive Care Med 2007;33:1557–62.
70. Lerolle N, Guerot E, Faisy C, et al. Renal failure in septic shock: predictive value of Doppler-based renal arterial resistive index. Intensive Care Med 2006;32:1553–9.
71. Gornik I, Godan A, Gasy C, et al. Renal failure index at ICU admission and its change after 24 hours predict acute kidney injury in sepsis. Crit Care 2014;18:P366.
72. Bossard G, Bourgoin P, Corbeau JJ, et al. Early detection of postoperative acute kidney injury by Doppler renal resistive index in cardiac surgery with cardiopulmonary bypass. Br J Anaesth 2011;107:891–8.
73. Kararmaz A, Kemal Arslantas M, Cinel I. Renal resistive index measurement by transesophageal echocardiography: comparison with translumbar ultrasonography and relation to acute kidney injury. J Cardiothorac Vasc Anesth 2014. [Epub ahead of print].
74. Darmon M, Schortgen F, Vargas F, et al. Diagnostic accuracy of Doppler renal resistive index for reversibility of acute kidney injury in critically ill patients. Intensive Care Med 2011;37:68–76.
75. Marty P, Szatjnic S, Ferre F, et al. Doppler renal resistive index for early detection of acute kidney injury after major orthopaedic surgery: a prospective observational study. Eur J Anaesthesiol 2015;32:37–43.

76. Guinot PG, Bernard E, Abou Arab O, et al. Doppler-based renal resistive index can assess progression of acute kidney injury in patients undergoing cardiac surgery. J Cardiothorac Vasc Anesth 2013;27:890–6.

77. Viazzi F, Leoncini G, Derchi LE, et al. Ultrasound Doppler renal resistive index: a useful tool for the management of the hypertensive patient. J Hypertens 2014; 32:149–53.

78. Dewitte A, Coquin J, Meyssignac B, et al. Doppler resistive index to reflect regulation of renal vascular tone during sepsis and acute kidney injury. Crit Care 2012;16:R165.

79. Mahoney M, Sorace A, Warram J, et al. Volumetric contrast-enhanced ultrasound imaging of renal perfusion. J Ultrasound Med 2014;33:1427–37.

80. Harrois A, Duranteau J. Contrast-enhanced ultrasound: a new vision of microcirculation in the intensive care unit. Crit Care 2013;17:449.

81. Choyke P, Kobayashi H. Functional magnetic resonance imaging of the kidney using macromolecular contrast agents. Abdom Imaging 2006;31:224–31.

82. Prasad PV, Edelman RR, Epstein FH. Noninvasive evaluation of intrarenal oxygenation with BOLD MRI. Circulation 1996;94:3271–5.

83. Hofmann L, Simon-Zoula S, Nowak A, et al. BOLD-MRI for the assessment of renal oxygenation in humans: acute effect of nephrotoxic xenobiotics. Kidney Int 2006;70:144–50.

84. Vink E, Boer A, Verloop W, et al. The effect of renal denervation on kidney oxygenation as determined by BOLD MRI in patients with hypertension. Eur Radiol 2015;25:1984–92.

85. Vink EE, de Boer A, Hoogduin HJ, et al. Renal BOLD-MRI relates to kidney function and activity of the renin-angiotensin-aldosterone system in hypertensive patients. J Hypertens 2015;33(3):597–603.

86. Pruijm M, Hofmann L, Piskunowicz M, et al. Determinants of renal tissue oxygenation as measured with BOLD-MRI in chronic kidney disease and hypertension in humans. PLoS One 2014;9:e95895.

87. Oostendorp M, de Vries EE, Slenter JM, et al. MRI of renal oxygenation and function after normothermic ischemia–reperfusion injury. NMR Biomed 2011; 24:194–200.

88. Li L-P, Lu J, Zhou Y, et al. Evaluation of intrarenal oxygenation in iodinated contrast-induced acute kidney injury–susceptible rats by blood oxygen level–dependent magnetic resonance imaging. Invest Radiol 2014;49:403–10.

89. Inoue T, Kozawa E, Okada H, et al. Noninvasive evaluation of kidney hypoxia and fibrosis using magnetic resonance imaging. J Am Soc Nephrol 2011;22: 1429–34.

90. Vanmassenhove J, Vanholder R, Nagler E, et al. Urinary and serum biomarkers for the diagnosis of acute kidney injury: an in-depth review of the literature. Nephrol Dial Transplant 2013;28:254–73.

91. Ostermann M, Philips BJ, Forni LG. Clinical review: biomarkers of acute kidney injury: where are we now? Crit Care 2012;16:233.

92. Wasung ME, Chawla LS, Madero M. Biomarkers of renal function, which and when? Clin Chim Acta 2015;438:350–7.

93. Charlton JR, Portilla D, Okusa MD. A basic science view of acute kidney injury biomarkers. Nephrol Dial Transplant 2014;29:1301–11.

94. Koyner JL, Parikh CR. Clinical utility of biomarkers of AKI in cardiac surgery and critical illness. Clin J Am Soc Nephrol 2013;8:1034–42.

95. Martensson J, Bellomo R. The rise and fall of NGAL in acute kidney injury. Blood Purif 2014;37:304–10.

96. Haase M, Bellomo R, Devarajan P, et al. Accuracy of neutrophil gelatinase-associated lipocalin (NGAL) in diagnosis and prognosis in acute kidney injury: a systematic review and meta-analysis. Am J Kidney Dis 2009;54:1012–24.
97. Haase-Fielitz A, Haase M, Devarajan P. Neutrophil gelatinase-associated lipocalin as a biomarker of acute kidney injury: a critical evaluation of current status. Ann Clin Biochem 2014;51:335–51.
98. Kashani K, Al-Khafaji A, Ardiles T, et al. Discovery and validation of cell cycle arrest biomarkers in human acute kidney injury. Crit Care 2013;17:R25.
99. Bihorac A, Chawla LS, Shaw AD, et al. Validation of cell-cycle arrest biomarkers for acute kidney injury using clinical adjudication. Am J Respir Crit Care Med 2014;189(8):932–9.
100. Meersch M, Schmidt C, Van Aken H, et al. Urinary TIMP-2 and IGFBP7 as early biomarkers of acute kidney injury and renal recovery following cardiac surgery. PLoS One 2014;9:e93460.
101. Lake AP, Williams EG. ASA classification and perioperative variables: graded anaesthesia score? Br J Anaesth 1997;78:228–9.
102. Copeland GP, Jones D, Walters M. POSSUM: a scoring system for surgical audit. Br J Surg 1991;78:355–60.
103. Gawande AA, Kwaan MR, Regenbogen SE, et al. An Apgar score for surgery. J Am Coll Surg 2007;204:201–8.
104. Chertow GM, Lazarus JM, Christiansen CL, et al. Preoperative renal risk stratification. Circulation 1997;95:878–84.
105. Thakar CV, Arrigain S, Worley S, et al. A clinical score to predict acute renal failure after cardiac surgery. J Am Soc Nephrol 2005;16:162–8.
106. Mehta RH, Grab JD, O'Brien SM, et al. Bedside tool for predicting the risk of postoperative dialysis in patients undergoing cardiac surgery. Circulation 2006;114:2208–16 [quiz: 2208].
107. Wijeysundera DN, Karkouti K, Dupuis JY, et al. Derivation and validation of a simplified predictive index for renal replacement therapy after cardiac surgery. JAMA 2007;297:1801–9.
108. Aronson S, Fontes ML, Miao Y, et al. Risk index for perioperative renal dysfunction/failure: critical dependence on pulse pressure hypertension. Circulation 2007;115:733–42.
109. Palomba H, de Castro I, Neto AL, et al. Acute kidney injury prediction following elective cardiac surgery: AKICS Score. Kidney Int 2007;72:624–31.
110. Brown JR, Cochran RP, Leavitt BJ, et al. Multivariable prediction of renal insufficiency developing after cardiac surgery. Circulation 2007;116:I139–43.
111. Rueggeberg A, Boehm S, Napieralski F, et al. Development of a risk stratification model for predicting acute renal failure in orthotopic liver transplantation recipients. Anaesthesia 2008;63:1174–80.
112. Kheterpal S, Tremper KK, Englesbe MJ, et al. Predictors of postoperative acute renal failure after noncardiac surgery in patients with previously normal renal function. Anesthesiology 2007;107:892–902.
113. Abelha FJ, Botelho M, Fernandes V, et al. Determinants of postoperative acute kidney injury. Crit Care 2009;13:R79.
114. Birnie K, Verheyden V, Pagano D, et al. Predictive models for kidney disease: improving global outcomes (KDIGO) defined acute kidney injury in UK cardiac surgery. Crit Care 2014;18:606.
115. Nigwekar SU, Kandula P, Hix JK, et al. Off-pump coronary artery bypass surgery and acute kidney injury: a meta-analysis of randomized and observational studies. Am J Kidney Dis 2009;54:413–23.

116. Seabra VF, Alobaidi S, Balk EM, et al. Off-pump coronary artery bypass surgery and acute kidney injury: a meta-analysis of randomized controlled trials. Clin J Am Soc Nephrol 2010;5:1734–44.

117. Kolhe NV, Stevens PE, Crowe AV, et al. Case mix, outcome and activity for patients with severe acute kidney injury during the first 24 hours after admission to an adult, general critical care unit: application of predictive models from a secondary analysis of the ICNARC Case Mix Programme database. Crit Care 2008; 12(Suppl 1):S2.

118. Thakar CV, Liangos O, Yared JP, et al. Predicting acute renal failure after cardiac surgery: validation and re-definition of a risk-stratification algorithm. Hemodial Int 2003;7:143–7.

119. Candela-Toha A, Elias-Martin E, Abraira V, et al. Predicting acute renal failure after cardiac surgery: external validation of two new clinical scores. Clin J Am Soc Nephrol 2008;3:1260–5.

120. Josephs SA, Thakar CV. Perioperative risk assessment, prevention, and treatment of acute kidney injury. Int Anesthesiol Clin 2009;47:89–105.

121. Saria S, Rajani AK, Gould J, et al. Integration of early physiological responses predicts later illness severity in preterm infants. Sci Transl Med 2010;2:48ra65.

122. Ng SY, Sanagou M, Wolfe R, et al. Prediction of acute kidney injury within 30 days of cardiac surgery. J Thorac Cardiovasc Surg 2014;147:1875–83.e1.

123. Celi LA, Tang RJ, Villarroel MC, et al. A clinical database-driven approach to decision support: predicting mortality among patients with acute kidney injury. J Healthc Eng 2011;2:97–110.

124. Celi LA, Galvin S, Davidzon G, et al. A database-driven decision support system: customized mortality prediction. J Pers Med 2012;2:138–48.

125. Thakar CV, Kharat V, Blanck S, et al. Acute kidney injury after gastric bypass surgery. Clin J Am Soc Nephrol 2007;2:426–30.

126. Kheterpal S, Khodaparast O, Shanks A, et al. Chronic angiotensin-converting enzyme inhibitor or angiotensin receptor blocker therapy combined with diuretic therapy is associated with increased episodes of hypotension in noncardiac surgery. J Cardiothorac Vasc Anesth 2008;22:180–6.

127. Patel NN, Rogers CA, Angelini GD, et al. Pharmacological therapies for the prevention of acute kidney injury following cardiac surgery: a systematic review. Heart Fail Rev 2011;16:553–67.

128. Tie HT, Luo MZ, Luo MJ, et al. Sodium bicarbonate in the prevention of cardiac surgery-associated acute kidney injury: a systematic review and meta-analysis. Crit Care 2014;18:517.

129. Garg AX, Kurz A, Sessler DI, et al. Perioperative aspirin and clonidine and risk of acute kidney injury: a randomized clinical trial. JAMA 2014;312:2254–64.

130. Brienza N, Giglio MT, Marucci M, et al. Does perioperative hemodynamic optimization protect renal function in surgical patients? A meta-analytic study. Crit Care Med 2009;37:2079–90.

131. Badin J, Boulain T, Ehrmann S, et al. Relation between mean arterial pressure and renal function in the early phase of shock: a prospective, explorative cohort study. Crit Care 2011;15:R135.

132. Cai J, Xu R, Yu X, et al. Volatile anesthetics in preventing acute kidney injury after cardiac surgery: a systematic review and meta-analysis. J Thorac Cardiovasc Surg 2014;148:3127–36.

133. Lee HT, Emala CW. Protective effects of renal ischemic preconditioning and adenosine pretreatment: role of A1 and A3 receptors. Am J Physiol Renal Physiol 2000;278:F380–7.

134. Turman MA, Bates CM. Susceptibility of human proximal tubular cells to hypoxia: effect of hypoxic preconditioning and comparison to glomerular cells. Ren Fail 1997;19:47–60.

135. Kharbanda RK, Nielsen TT, Redington AN. Translation of remote ischaemic preconditioning into clinical practice. Lancet 2009;374:1557–65.

136. Meran S, Wonnacott A, Amphlett B, et al. How good are we at managing acute kidney injury in hospital? Clin Kidney J 2014;7:144–50.

137. Ponce D, Zorzenon Cde P, dos Santos NY, et al. Early nephrology consultation can have an impact on outcome of acute kidney injury patients. Nephrol Dial Transplant 2011;26:3202–6.

138. e Silva VT, Liaño F, Muriel A, et al. Nephrology referral and outcomes in critically ill acute kidney injury patients. PLoS One 2013;8:e70482.

139. Balasubramanian G, Al-Aly Z, Moiz A, et al. Early nephrologist involvement in hospital-acquired acute kidney injury: a pilot study. Am J Kidney Dis 2011;57: 228–34.

140. Siew ED, Peterson JF, Eden SK, et al. Outpatient nephrology referral rates after acute kidney injury. J Am Soc Nephrol 2012;23:305–12.

141. Matheny ME, Peterson JF, Eden SK, et al. Laboratory test surveillance following acute kidney injury. PLoS One 2014;9:e103746.

142. Harel Z, Wald R, Bargman JM, et al. Nephrologist follow-up improves all-cause mortality of severe acute kidney injury survivors. Kidney Int 2013;83:901–8.

143. Lameire NH, Bagga A, Cruz D, et al. Acute kidney injury: an increasing global concern. Lancet 2013;382:170–9.

144. Kirwan C, Prowle J. Acute kidney injury is a chronic disease that requires long-term follow-up. In: Annual update in intensive care and emergency medicine 2013. Berlin: Springer; 2013. p. 723–37.

145. Kellum JA, Lameire N. Diagnosis, evaluation, and management of acute kidney injury: a KDIGO summary (Part 1). Crit Care 2013;17:204.

146. Bowman BT, Kleiner A, Bolton WK. Comanagement of diabetic kidney disease by the primary care provider and nephrologist. Med Clin North Am 2013;97: 157–73.

147. Diamantidis CJ, Powe NR, Jaar BG, et al. Primary care-specialist collaboration in the care of patients with chronic kidney disease. Clin J Am Soc Nephrol 2011; 6(2):334–43.

148. Richards N, Harris K, Whitfield M, et al. Primary care-based disease management of chronic kidney disease (CKD), based on estimated glomerular filtration rate (eGFR) reporting, improves patient outcomes. Nephrol Dial Transplant 2008;23:549–55.

149. Stoves J, Connolly J, Cheung CK, et al. Electronic consultation as an alternative to hospital referral for patients with chronic kidney disease: a novel application for networked electronic health records to improve the accessibility and efficiency of healthcare. Qual Saf Health Care 2010;19:e54.

150. DuBose TD, Behrens MT, Berns A, et al. The patient-centered medical home and nephrology. J Am Soc Nephrol 2009;20:681–2.

151. Chang J, Ronco C, Rosner MH. Computerized decision support systems: improving patient safety in nephrology. Nat Rev Nephrol 2011;7:348–55.

Contrast-associated Acute Kidney Injury

Steven D. Weisbord, MD, MSc[a,b,*], Paul M. Palevsky, MD[b,c]

KEYWORDS

- Contrast • Acute kidney injury • Nephrotoxin • Prevention • Iatrogenic

KEY POINTS

- Chronic kidney disease, particularly in the setting of diabetes, is the principal risk factor for contrast-associated acute kidney injury.
- Contrast-associated acute kidney injury is a common iatrogenic condition.
- Contrast-associated acute kidney injury is associated with serious adverse short-term and long-term outcomes, including increased mortality and progressive chronic kidney disease, although the causal nature of these associations remains unknown.
- Prevention of contrast-associated acute kidney injury includes identification of high-risk patients, withdrawal of potentially nephrotoxic medications, use of low-osmolal or iso-osmolal contrast in the lowest required volume, and expansion of the intravascular space with isotonic intravenous crystalloid.

INTRODUCTION

Contrast-associated acute kidney injury (CAAKI) is a common iatrogenic condition that typically manifests as small transient decrements in kidney function following the intravascular administration of iodinated contrast media.[1,2] Underlying renal impairment is the principal risk factor for CAAKI, whereas the presence of diabetes mellitus amplifies the risk in patients with underlying renal impairment.[3,4] Patients with absolute or effective intravascular volume depletion, in whom there is reduced renal perfusion, are susceptible to renal injury from iodinated contrast. The risk for CAAKI is also associated with the use of larger volumes of contrast as well as intra-arterial (as opposed to intravenous) contrast administration.[5,6] Several observational studies show that CAAKI is associated with increased hospital length of stay, costs, and short-term mortality.[3,7–12] Growing evidence also supports an association of

[a] Renal Section, VA Pittsburgh Healthcare System, Room 7E120 (111F-U), University Drive, Pittsburgh, PA 15240, USA; [b] Renal-Electrolyte Division, University of Pittsburgh School of Medicine, A919 Scaife Hall, 3550 Terrace Street, Pittsburgh, PA 15261, USA; [c] Renal Section, VA Pittsburgh Healthcare System, Room 7E123 (111F-U), University Drive, Pittsburgh, PA 15240, USA
* Corresponding author.
E-mail address: weisbordsd@upmc.edu

Crit Care Clin 31 (2015) 725–735
http://dx.doi.org/10.1016/j.ccc.2015.06.008
0749-0704/15/$ – see front matter Published by Elsevier Inc.

criticalcare.theclinics.com

CAAKI with long-term mortality and acceleration in chronic kidney disease (CKD) progression.[9] However, it remains unknown whether CAAKI is a proximate cause of these adverse short-term and long-term outcomes or represents a marker of patients at heightened risk.

Studies of preventive strategies for CAAKI have focused primarily on the comparative toxicity of different contrast media, the putative benefit of enhanced elimination of contrast using renal replacement therapy, the role of pharmacologic interventions, and the efficacy of periprocedural intravenous (IV) volume expansion with various crystalloid solutions. However, many of these studies enrolled small numbers of patients, which limited statistical power. Most used surrogate biochemical outcomes that may, in some settings, have been directly affected by the intervention, and very few tracked more clinically important events, which precluded definitive determinations of the interventions' efficacy for the prevention of serious outcomes.

This article discusses the risk factors for and incidence of CAAKI; reviews past studies that investigated outcomes associated with CAAKI, including data documenting the underuse of iodinated contrast in high-risk patients; and outlines the current evidence base for interventions to prevent this iatrogenic condition.

RISK FACTORS FOR CONTRAST-ASSOCIATED ACUTE KIDNEY INJURY

Patient-related risk factors for CAAKI can be collectively characterized by pathophysiologic processes that limit the capacity for the kidneys to adequately compensate for the hemodynamic and microcirculatory stress induced by iodinated contrast media administration (**Table 1**). CKD is the principal patient-related risk factor for CAAKI, with lower levels of glomerular filtration associated with escalating levels of risk.[3,13] The presence of diabetes mellitus substantially increases the risk for CAAKI in patients with underlying kidney disease, but is not a strong independent risk factor in patients without renal dysfunction.[4] Patients with absolute or effective intravascular volume depletion and those taking nonsteroidal antiinflammatory agents are at heightened risk because of increased dependence on vasodilatory prostaglandins for adequate intrarenal oxygen delivery.[14] Additional factors that may predispose patients to the development of CAAKI include older age, hypertension, increased serum glucose level, and anemia.[15,16] Of note, recent studies have documented an association of proteinuria with risk for acute kidney injury in general, and following contrast-enhanced procedures.[17,18] However, proteinuria, similar to other patient-related risk factors, is common in patients with CKD; hence, its true association with CAAKI independent of underlying renal impairment remains uncertain.

Certain procedure-related factors also increase CAAKI risk (see **Table 1**). Multiple consecutive procedures and/or the use of large volumes of contrast seem to increase

---

Table 1
Principal risk factors for CAAKI

Patient-related Factors	Procedure-related Factors
Underlying renal insufficiency	Increased contrast volume
Diabetes mellitus[a]	Multiple sequential procedures
Intravascular volume depletion[b]	Intra-arterial contrast administration
Congestive heart failure	High-osmolal contrast

[a] Amplifies risk in the setting of underlying kidney disease.
[b] Absolute or effective.

the risk, although studies to date have been unable to establish a threshold volume of contrast above which the likelihood of renal injury increases substantially. Use of high-osmolal contrast has also been strongly associated with the development of CAAKI.

INCIDENCE OF CONTRAST-ASSOCIATED ACUTE KIDNEY INJURY

The reported incidence of CAAKI in past studies has varied based on the risk profile of the patient population being studied, type of contrast-enhanced procedure performed, criteria used to define renal injury, and timing of assessment of postcontrast renal injury.[13,19–21] D'Elia and colleagues[13] reported that 0.68% of patients without and 17.4% of patients with renal insufficiency experienced CAAKI, defined by an increase in serum creatinine of 1.0 mg/dL, following angiography. A more recent study by Weisbord and colleagues[22] that enrolled patients with CKD who were undergoing coronary angiography, noncoronary angiography, or computed tomography (CT) reported incident rates of CAAKI, defined by an increase in serum creatinine of greater than or equal to 25%, of 13.2%, 8.5%, and 6.5% for each procedure type, respectively. Few patients (<1%) overall experienced an increase in serum creatinine level of greater than or equal to 1.0 mg/dL. Note that determining precise incidence estimates of true renal injury from contrast is confounded by underlying variability in serum creatinine level related to dietary intake, hemodynamic fluctuations that affect renal perfusion, and laboratory variation. This finding was underscored in a study by Bruce and colleagues[23] that examined acute changes in serum creatinine level among patients who underwent 13,274 CT scans, 5790 with and 7484 without iodinated contrast. Among patients with baseline CKD, 8.2% showed an increase in serum creatinine level of greater than or equal to 0.5 mg/dL or decrease in estimated glomerular filtration rate (eGFR) of greater than or equal to 25% after undergoing CT without contrast, whereas just a slightly higher proportion of patients who underwent CT with iso-osmolal contrast (9.3%) manifested these changes in serum creatinine level and eGFR. A subsequent retrospective study by McDonald and colleagues[24] reported similar risks for acute kidney injury following contrast-enhanced and non–contrast-enhanced CT in patients with renal impairment, including stages 3 and 4 CKD. Thus, increases in serum creatinine levels and corresponding decrements in eGFR following contrast-enhanced radiographic procedures may occur independently of iodinated contrast administration. The poor predictive value of serum creatinine level for the diagnosis of true renal injury from iodinated contrast has led to efforts to identify blood and urine biomarkers that are more specific for renal epithelial cell damage and/or reduced glomerular filtration. Preliminary studies suggest that increments in certain biomarkers following contrast administration, including neutrophil gelatinase-associated lipoprotein, hold promise as an alternative means of identifying renal injury.[25,26] Additional studies in large patient populations are needed to better evaluate the role of such biomarkers.

OUTCOMES ASSOCIATED WITH CONTRAST-ASSOCIATED ACUTE KIDNEY INJURY

Several studies have shown an association of CAAKI with increased short-term mortality[3,12,27–30] (**Table 2**). In a study of more than 1800 patients undergoing percutaneous intervention, McCullough and colleagues[3] documented increased in-hospital mortality among patients who developed CAAKI compared with those who did not develop CAAKI (7.1% vs 1.1%; P<.0001). Similarly, a study by Gruberg and colleagues[30] of 439 patients reported that the development of CAAKI was associated with nearly 4-fold increased odds of short-term death following coronary angiography. CAAKI has also been associated with adverse long-term outcomes, including mortality

Table 2
Association of CAAKI with short-term mortality

Study Authors	Number of Patients	Definition of CAAKI	Adjusted OR	95% CI
Bartholomew et al	20,479	↑ Serum creatinine level ≥1.0 mg/dL	22	16–31
From et al	3236	↑ Serum creatinine level ≥25% or ≥0.5 mg/dL	3.4	2.6–4.4
Gruberg et al	439	↑ Serum creatinine level >25%	3.9	2.0–7.6
McCullough et al	1826	↑ Serum creatinine level >25%	6.6	3.3–12.9
Rihal et al	7586	↑ Serum creatinine level >0.5 mg/dL	10.8	6.9–17.0
Weisbord et al	27,608	↑ Serum creatinine level 0.25–0.5 mg/dL	1.8	1.4–2.5

Abbreviations: CI, confidence interval; OR, odds ratio (for death).

and progressive CKD.[7,31–33] Solomon and colleagues[33] documented that CAAKI following angiography was associated with a greater than 3-fold increased risk of death, stroke, myocardial infarction, or end-stage renal disease requiring renal replacement therapy at 1 year of follow up. Goldenberg and colleagues[7] reported that patients who developed transient CAAKI following angiography experienced a larger decline in eGFR over a period of approximately 2 years than patients without CAAKI (Δ eGFR = -20 ± 11 mL/min/1.73 m^2 vs -6 ± 16 mL/min/1.73 m^2; $P = .02$).

Note that the causal nature of these associations of CAAKI with adverse short-term and long-term outcomes remains unknown. Whether CAAKI, defined by small increments in serum creatinine level, is a marker of increased risk for or a mediator of serious adverse outcomes is unknown, because the clinical factors that increase risk for CAAKI are independent risk factors for serious adverse short-term and long-term outcomes (**Fig. 1**). This point is significant because recent research has documented underuse of indicated diagnostic and therapeutic interventions such as angiography in patients with kidney disease because of concern that these procedures are more deleterious (eg, pose undue risk for CAAKI) in this population, a

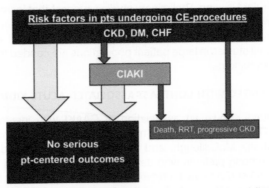

Fig. 1. Patient risk factors and outcomes following contrast-enhanced (CE) procedures. CHF, congestive heart failure; CIAKI, contrast-induced acute kidney injury; DM, diabetes mellitus; pt, patient; RRT, renal replacement therapy.

phenomenon that has been referred to as renalism.[34] Until definitive evidence of a causal relationship between CAAKI and serious adverse outcomes emerges, and in light of renalism having potentially negative effects on patient outcomes, clinically indicated contrast-enhanced procedures should be performed, albeit with the use of evidence-based preventive care.

PREVENTION OF CONTRAST-ASSOCIATED ACUTE KIDNEY INJURY

Preventive interventions for CAAKI that have been investigated can be categorized into 4 principal strategies: (1) use of less nephrotoxic contrast agents, (2) provision of preemptive renal replacement therapy to clear contrast from the circulation, (3) administration of pharmacologic agents to counteract the nephrotoxic effects of contrast media, and (4) provision of IV fluids to expand the intravascular space and enhance diuresis.

Contrast Agents

The forms of intravascular iodinated contrast media currently used include low-osmolal and iso-osmolal agents. Note that the term low osmolal is a misnomer because these compounds have higher osmolality (ie, 600–850 mOsm/kg) than iso-osmolal contrast, but lower osmolality than the original so-called high-osmolal agents. Although some studies document lower risk for CAAKI with iso-osmolal contrast compared with specific low-osmolal agents such as iohexol, there does not seem to be a broad class benefit compared with the other low-osmolal agents.[35–42] The collective findings of multiple trials and meta-analyses comparing contrast agents are reflected in guidelines from the American College of Cardiology/American Heart Association and European Society of Urogenital Radiology, which recommend the use of either low-osmolal or iso-osmolal contrast in patients at increased risk of CAAKI.[43–45]

Renal Replacement Therapies

Extracorporeal renal replacement therapy effectively removes iodinated contrast media from the circulation because of its high solubility in aqueous solution, limited protein binding, and restricted distribution to the extracellular space. Although some trials have shown lower rates of acute kidney injury in patients who receive prophylactic hemodialysis, others reported either no benefit or increased rates of renal injury.[46–49] A meta-analysis by Cruz and colleagues[50] observed a risk ratio for CAAKI of 1.61 (95% confidence interval, 1.13–2.28) associated with prophylactic hemodialysis.[50] Two trials by Marenzi and colleagues[51,52] showed lower risk for CAAKI and death among patients who received continuous venovenous hemofiltration. However, there have been no adequately powered trials that used primary patient-centered outcomes rather than postcontrast change in serum creatinine level (which itself is directly reduced by hemofiltration) to support the role of continuous renal replacement therapy (CRRT) for the prevention of CAAKI. Given the substantial costs and potential infectious and noninfectious risks of administering CRRT, preemptive use of this therapy to reduce the risk of CAAKI is not recommended.

Pharmacologic Agents

Diuretics, dopamine, and fenoldopam are ineffective for the prevention of CAAKI and are potentially deleterious.[19,53–55] Trials of atrial natriuretic peptide, theophylline, and prostaglandins report inconsistent findings. Recent trials suggest that periprocedural statin administration may reduce the risk for CAAKI.[56,57] However, statins may have a direct effect on serum creatinine levels, as shown by an increase in the eGFR following statin administration.[58] Hence, the use of small changes in serum creatinine to define the development of CAAKI in trials of statins could result in the misclassification of patients because of the direct effects of these agents on the end point rather than a renal-protective effect. A multitude of studies and meta-analyses have investigated N-acetylcysteine, an antioxidant with vasodilatory properties, for the prevention of CAAKI.[59–61] Although yielding mixed results, most trials enrolled small numbers of patients, used nominal changes in serum creatinine level as the primary outcome, and/or included patients at very low risk for CAAKI. As a result, no definitive conclusions can be drawn at this time on the benefit of this agent.

Intravenous Fluids

Intravascular volume expansion with IV crystalloid may counteract the intrarenal vasoconstrictive effects of contrast and decrease the concentration and viscosity of contrast media in the tubular lumen, potentially attenuating renal tubular epithelial cell injury.[62] More than 2 decades ago, Solomon and colleagues[19] randomized patients undergoing angiography to receive IV 0.45% NaCl alone or in combination with IV mannitol or furosemide and found a lower incidence of CAAKI with IV fluid alone (11%) than in combination with mannitol (28%) or furosemide (40%). Subsequently, Mueller and colleagues[63] randomized patients undergoing angiography to receive 0.45% or 0.9% sodium chloride and showed that CAAKI developed more commonly in patients administered 0.45% saline compared with 0.9% saline (2% v 0.7%; $P = .04$). Recent research on IV fluid for CAAKI prevention has focused on the comparison of isotonic sodium chloride and isotonic sodium bicarbonate, with a multitude of clinical trials reporting discordant findings.[21,64–68] The resultant clinical equipoise led to the publication of several systematic reviews and meta-analyses, the results of which largely reflect the inconclusive findings of the primary trials.[69–72]

Recent studies showed lower rates of CAAKI with a device that matches IV fluid administration to volume of periprocedural urine output.[65,73] However, use of this device may lead to positive sodium balance compared with the administration of IV fluids alone, resulting in modest intravascular volume expansion and an associated independent decline in serum creatinine, potentially confounding conclusions on its potential benefit.

Current Recommendations for Prevention

The initial step in preventing CAAKI involves identifying high-risk patients, for whom consideration should be given to using alternative imaging procedures that do not require intravascular iodinated contrast but that have comparable diagnostic yield. The use of gadolinium-based contrast is problematic in patients with advanced CKD or in patients with acute kidney injury given the risk for nephrogenic systemic fibrosis.[74] Among at-risk patients who require procedures that use intravascular iodinated contrast, nephrotoxic medications such as nonsteroidal antiinflammatory drugs should be discontinued before the procedure and restarted after there is evidence that CAAKI has not developed. Either isotonic sodium bicarbonate or isotonic sodium chloride should be administered to patients at increased risk. For hospitalized patients and those undergoing nonurgent procedures, 1 mL/kg/h of isotonic crystalloid can be administered for 12 hours before and 12 hours following contrast administration. Alternatively, preprocedural administration of isotonic fluid at a rate of 3 mL/kg/h for 1 hour preprocedure and 1.5 mL/kg/h for 4 to 6 hours postprocedure has been shown to be effective. Note that although heart failure is a recognized risk factor for CAAKI, a recent clinical trial showed that the administration of standard volumes of isotonic IV fluid to patients with increased left ventricular end-diastolic pressures at the time of angiography was effective for the prevention of CAAKI and was associated with low risk for pulmonary compromise.[75] Therefore, IV fluids should not be eschewed in patients with heart failure undergoing contrast-enhanced procedures, but should be used cautiously. Low-osmolal or iso-osmolal contrast in the lowest possible dose should be used and serum creatinine level should be measured approximately 3 to 4 days following the procedure to assess for the development of CAAKI.

SUMMARY

CAAKI, defined by small increments in serum creatinine, is a common iatrogenic condition that has been shown to be independently associated with serious adverse short-term and long-term outcomes. However, the causal nature of these associations is unknown. A growing body of research suggests that contrast-enhanced procedures are less likely to be performed in patients with CKD. Until there is definitive evidence of a causal relationship between CAAKI and adverse patient-centered outcomes, clinically indicated procedures that require intravascular iodinated contrast should not be eschewed in patients with CKD, but should be performed with the implementation of evidence-based preventive care. Notwithstanding a multitude of negative and inconclusive trials of pharmacologic and nonpharmacologic interventions for the prevention of CAAKI, evidence-based recommendations are currently limited to discontinuation of concomitant nephrotoxins, use of low-osmolal or iso-osmolal contrast in the lowest possible doses, and periprocedural administration of isotonic IV sodium chloride or sodium bicarbonate. Large, adequately powered clinical trials that use patient-centered primary outcomes are needed to improve understanding of how to prevent CAAKI in high-risk patients and to elucidate the clinical implications of this common iatrogenic condition.

REFERENCES

1. Parfrey PS, Griffiths SM, Barrett BJ, et al. Contrast material-induced renal failure in patients with diabetes mellitus, renal insufficiency, or both. A prospective controlled study. N Engl J Med 1989;320:143–9.
2. Rudnick MR, Berns JS, Cohen RM, et al. Contrast media-associated nephrotoxicity. Curr Opin Nephrol Hypertens 1996;5:127–33.
3. McCullough PA, Wolyn R, Rocher LL, et al. Acute renal failure after coronary intervention: incidence, risk factors, and relationship to mortality. Am J Med 1997;103: 368–75.
4. Rudnick MR, Goldfarb S, Wexler L, et al. Nephrotoxicity of ionic and nonionic contrast media in 1196 patients: a randomized trial. The Iohexol Cooperative Study. Kidney Int 1995;47:254–61.
5. Cigarroa RG, Lange RA, Williams RH, et al. Dosing of contrast material to prevent contrast nephropathy in patients with renal disease. Am J Med 1989;86:649–52.
6. Manske CL, Sprafka JM, Strony JT, et al. Contrast nephropathy in azotemic diabetic patients undergoing coronary angiography. Am J Med 1990;89:615–20.
7. Goldenberg I, Chonchol M, Guetta V. Reversible acute kidney injury following contrast exposure and the risk of long-term mortality. Am J Nephrol 2009;29: 136–44.
8. James MT, Ghali WA, Knudtson ML, et al. Associations between acute kidney injury and cardiovascular and renal outcomes after coronary angiography. Circulation 2011;123:409–16.

9. James MT, Ghali WA, Tonelli M, et al. Acute kidney injury following coronary angiography is associated with a long-term decline in kidney function. Kidney Int 2010;78:803–9.

10. Levy EM, Viscoli CM, Horwitz RI. The effect of acute renal failure on mortality. A cohort analysis. JAMA 1996;275:1489–94.

11. Subramanian S, Tumlin J, Bapat B, et al. Economic burden of contrast-induced nephropathy: implications for prevention strategies. J Med Econ 2007;10:119–34.

12. Weisbord SD, Chen H, Stone RA, et al. Associations of increases in serum creatinine with mortality and length of hospital stay after coronary angiography. J Am Soc Nephrol 2006;17:2871–7.

13. D'Elia JA, Gleason RE, Alday M, et al. Nephrotoxicity from angiographic contrast material. A prospective study. Am J Med 1982;72:719–25.

14. Taliercio CP, Vlietstra RE, Fisher LD, et al. Risks for renal dysfunction with cardiac angiography. Ann Intern Med 1986;104:501–4.

15. Nikolsky E, Mehran R, Lasic Z, et al. Low hematocrit predicts contrast-induced nephropathy after percutaneous coronary interventions. Kidney Int 2005;67: 706–13.

16. Mehran R, Aymong ED, Nikolsky E, et al. A simple risk score for prediction of contrast-induced nephropathy after percutaneous coronary intervention: development and initial validation. J Am Coll Cardiol 2004;44:1393–9.

17. Hsu RK, Hsu CY. Proteinuria and reduced glomerular filtration rate as risk factors for acute kidney injury. Curr Opin Nephrol Hypertens 2011;20:211–7.

18. He F, Zhang J, Lu ZQ, et al. Risk factors and outcomes of acute kidney injury after intracoronary stent implantation. World J Emerg Med 2012;3:197–201.

19. Solomon R, Werner C, Mann D, et al. Effects of saline, mannitol, and furosemide to prevent acute decreases in renal function induced by radiocontrast agents. N Engl J Med 1994;331:1416–20.

20. Briguori C, Manganelli F, Scarpato P, et al. Acetylcysteine and contrast agent-associated nephrotoxicity. J Am Coll Cardiol 2002;40:298–303.

21. Merten GJ, Burgess WP, Gray LV, et al. Prevention of contrast-induced nephropathy with sodium bicarbonate: a randomized controlled trial. JAMA 2004;291:2328–34.

22. Weisbord SD, Mor MK, Resnick AL, et al. Prevention, incidence, and outcomes of contrast-induced acute kidney injury. Arch Intern Med 2008;168:1325–32.

23. Bruce RJ, Djamali A, Shinki K, et al. Background fluctuation of kidney function versus contrast-induced nephrotoxicity. AJR Am J Roentgenol 2009;192:711–8.

24. McDonald JS, McDonald RJ, Carter RE, et al. Risk of intravenous contrast material-mediated acute kidney injury: a propensity score-matched study stratified by baseline-estimated glomerular filtration rate. Radiology 2014;271:65–73.

25. Bachorzewska-Gajewska H, Malyszko J, Sitniewska E, et al. Neutrophil-gelatinase-associated lipocalin and renal function after percutaneous coronary interventions. Am J Nephrol 2006;26:287–92.

26. Bachorzewska-Gajewska H, Malyszko J, Sitniewska E, et al. NGAL (neutrophil gelatinase-associated lipocalin) and cystatin C: are they good predictors of contrast nephropathy after percutaneous coronary interventions in patients with stable angina and normal serum creatinine? Int J Cardiol 2008;127:290–1.

27. Bartholomew BA, Harjai KJ, Dukkipati S, et al. Impact of nephropathy after percutaneous coronary intervention and a method for risk stratification. Am J Cardiol 2004;93:1515–9.

28. Rihal CS, Textor SC, Grill DE, et al. Incidence and prognostic importance of acute renal failure after percutaneous coronary intervention. Circulation 2002;105: 2259–64.

29. From AM, Bartholmai BJ, Williams AW, et al. Mortality associated with nephropathy after radiographic contrast exposure. Mayo Clin Proc 2008;83:1095–100.

30. Gruberg L, Mintz GS, Mehran R, et al. The prognostic implications of further renal function deterioration within 48 h of interventional coronary procedures in patients with pre-existent chronic renal insufficiency. J Am Coll Cardiol 2000;36:1542–8.

31. Harjai KJ, Raizada A, Shenoy C, et al. A comparison of contemporary definitions of contrast nephropathy in patients undergoing percutaneous coronary intervention and a proposal for a novel nephropathy grading system. Am J Cardiol 2008; 101:812–9.

32. Roghi A, Savonitto S, Cavallini C, et al. Impact of acute renal failure following percutaneous coronary intervention on long-term mortality. J Cardiovasc Med (Hagerstown) 2008;9:375–81.

33. Solomon RJ, Mehran R, Natarajan MK, et al. Contrast-induced nephropathy and long-term adverse events: cause and effect? Clin J Am Soc Nephrol 2009;4:1162–9.

34. Chertow GM, Normand SL, McNeil BJ. "Renalism": inappropriately low rates of coronary angiography in elderly individuals with renal insufficiency. J Am Soc Nephrol 2004;15:2462–8.

35. Heinrich MC, Haberle L, Muller V, et al. Nephrotoxicity of iso-osmolar iodixanol compared with nonionic low-osmolar contrast media: meta-analysis of randomized controlled trials. Radiology 2009;250:68–86.

36. Aspelin P, Aubry P, Fransson SG, et al. Nephrotoxic effects in high-risk patients undergoing angiography. N Engl J Med 2003;348:491–9.

37. Jo SH, Youn TJ, Koo BK, et al. Renal toxicity evaluation and comparison between visipaque (iodixanol) and hexabrix (ioxaglate) in patients with renal insufficiency undergoing coronary angiography: the RECOVER study: a randomized controlled trial. J Am Coll Cardiol 2006;48:924–30.

38. Laskey W, Aspelin P, Davidson C, et al. Nephrotoxicity of iodixanol versus iopamidol in patients with chronic kidney disease and diabetes mellitus undergoing coronary angiographic procedures. Am Heart J 2009;158:822–8.e3.

39. Nguyen SA, Suranyi P, Ravenel JG, et al. Iso-osmolality versus low-osmolality iodinated contrast medium at intravenous contrast-enhanced CT: effect on kidney function. Radiology 2008;248:97–105.

40. Solomon RJ, Natarajan MK, Doucet S, et al. Cardiac Angiography in Renally Impaired Patients (CARE) study: a randomized double-blind trial of contrast-induced nephropathy in patients with chronic kidney disease. Circulation 2007; 115:3189–96.

41. McCullough PA, Bertrand ME, Brinker JA, et al. A meta-analysis of the renal safety of isosmolar iodixanol compared with low-osmolar contrast media. J Am Coll Cardiol 2006;48:692–9.

42. Sharma SK, Kini A. Effect of nonionic radiocontrast agents on the occurrence of contrast-induced nephropathy in patients with mild-moderate chronic renal insufficiency: pooled analysis of the randomized trials. Catheter Cardiovasc Interv 2005;65:386–93.

43. ESUR guidelines on contrast media; 2008.

44. Stacul F, van der Molen AJ, Reimer P, et al. Contrast induced nephropathy: updated ESUR Contrast Media Safety Committee guidelines. Eur Radiol 2011; 21:2527–41.

45. Wright RS, Anderson JL, Adams CD, et al. 2011 ACCF/AHA focused update incorporated into the ACC/AHA 2007 guidelines for the management of patients with unstable angina/non-ST-elevation myocardial infarction: a report of the American College of Cardiology Foundation/American Heart Association Task Force on

Practice Guidelines developed in collaboration with the American Academy of Family Physicians, Society for Cardiovascular Angiography and Interventions, and the Society of Thoracic Surgeons. J Am Coll Cardiol 2011;57:e215–367.

46. Hsieh YC, Ting CT, Liu TJ, et al. Short- and long-term renal outcomes of immediate prophylactic hemodialysis after cardiovascular catheterizations in patients with severe renal insufficiency. Int J Cardiol 2005;101:407–13.

47. Berger ED, Bader BD, Bosker J, et al. Contrast media-induced kidney failure cannot be prevented by hemodialysis. Dtsch Med Wochenschr 2001;126: 162–6 [in German].

48. Frank H, Werner D, Lorusso V, et al. Simultaneous hemodialysis during coronary angiography fails to prevent radiocontrast-induced nephropathy in chronic renal failure. Clin Nephrol 2003;60:176–82.

49. Huber W, Jeschke B, Kreymann B, et al. Haemodialysis for the prevention of contrast-induced nephropathy: outcome of 31 patients with severely impaired renal function, comparison with patients at similar risk and review. Invest Radiol 2002;37:471–81.

50. Cruz DN, Goh CY, Marenzi G, et al. Renal replacement therapies for prevention of radiocontrast-induced nephropathy: a systematic review. Am J Med 2012;125: 66–78.e3.

51. Marenzi G, Lauri G, Campodonico J, et al. Comparison of two hemofiltration protocols for prevention of contrast-induced nephropathy in high-risk patients. Am J Med 2006;119:155–62.

52. Marenzi G, Marana I, Lauri G, et al. The prevention of radiocontrast-agent-induced nephropathy by hemofiltration. N Engl J Med 2003;349:1333–40.

53. Stone GW, McCullough PA, Tumlin JA, et al. Fenoldopam mesylate for the prevention of contrast-induced nephropathy: a randomized controlled trial. JAMA 2003; 290:2284–91.

54. Khoury Z, Schlicht JR, Como J, et al. The effect of prophylactic nifedipine on renal function in patients administered contrast media. Pharmacotherapy 1995;15: 59–65.

55. Abizaid AS, Clark CE, Mintz GS, et al. Effects of dopamine and aminophylline on contrast-induced acute renal failure after coronary angioplasty in patients with preexisting renal insufficiency. Am J Cardiol 1999;83:260–3. A5.

56. Han Y, Zhu G, Han L, et al. Short-term rosuvastatin therapy for prevention of contrast-induced acute kidney injury in patients with diabetes and chronic kidney disease. J Am Coll Cardiol 2014;63:62–70.

57. Leoncini M, Toso A, Maioli M, et al. Early high-dose rosuvastatin for contrast-induced nephropathy prevention in acute coronary syndrome: results from the PRATO-ACS Study (Protective Effect of Rosuvastatin and Antiplatelet Therapy on contrast-induced acute kidney injury and myocardial damage in patients with Acute Coronary Syndrome). J Am Coll Cardiol 2014;63:71–9.

58. Vidt DG, Harris S, McTaggart F, et al. Effect of short-term rosuvastatin treatment on estimated glomerular filtration rate. Am J Cardiol 2006;97:1602–6.

59. Weisbord SD, Gallagher M, Kaufman J, et al. Prevention of contrast-induced AKI: a review of published trials and the design of the Prevention of Serious Adverse Events Following Angiography (PRESERVE) trial. Clin J Am Soc Nephrol 2013;8: 1618–31.

60. Pannu N, Manns B, Lee H, et al. Systematic review of the impact of N-acetylcysteine on contrast nephropathy. Kidney Int 2004;65:1366–74.

61. ACT Investigators. Acetylcysteine for prevention of renal outcomes in patients undergoing coronary and peripheral vascular angiography: main results from the

randomized Acetylcysteine for Contrast-induced Nephropathy Trial (ACT). Circulation 2011;124:1250–9.

62. Weisbord SD, Palevsky PM. Prevention of contrast-induced nephropathy with volume expansion. Clin J Am Soc Nephrol 2008;3:273–80.

63. Mueller C, Buerkle G, Buettner HJ, et al. Prevention of contrast media-associated nephropathy: randomized comparison of 2 hydration regimens in 1620 patients undergoing coronary angioplasty. Arch Intern Med 2002;162:329–36.

64. Brar SS, Shen AY, Jorgensen MB, et al. Sodium bicarbonate vs sodium chloride for the prevention of contrast medium-induced nephropathy in patients undergoing coronary angiography: a randomized trial. JAMA 2008;300:1038–46.

65. Briguori C, Airoldi F, D'Andrea D, et al. Renal insufficiency Following Contrast Media Administration Trial (REMEDIAL): a randomized comparison of 3 preventive strategies. Circulation 2007;115:1211–7.

66. Maioli M, Toso A, Leoncini M, et al. Sodium bicarbonate versus saline for the prevention of contrast-induced nephropathy in patients with renal dysfunction undergoing coronary angiography or intervention. J Am Coll Cardiol 2008;52:599–604.

67. Recio-Mayoral A, Chaparro M, Prado B, et al. The reno-protective effect of hydration with sodium bicarbonate plus N-acetylcysteine in patients undergoing emergency percutaneous coronary intervention: the RENO Study. J Am Coll Cardiol 2007;49:1283–8.

68. Adolph E, Holdt-Lehmann B, Chatterjee T, et al. Renal Insufficiency Following Radiocontrast Exposure Trial (REINFORCE): a randomized comparison of sodium bicarbonate versus sodium chloride hydration for the prevention of contrast-induced nephropathy. Coron Artery Dis 2008;19:413–9.

69. Brar SS, Hiremath S, Dangas G, et al. Sodium bicarbonate for the prevention of contrast induced-acute kidney injury: a systematic review and meta-analysis. Clin J Am Soc Nephrol 2009;4:1584–92.

70. Hogan SE, L'Allier P, Chetcuti S, et al. Current role of sodium bicarbonate-based preprocedural hydration for the prevention of contrast-induced acute kidney injury: a meta-analysis. Am Heart J 2008;156:414–21.

71. Hoste EA, De Waele JJ, Gevaert SA, et al. Sodium bicarbonate for prevention of contrast-induced acute kidney injury: a systematic review and meta-analysis. Nephrol Dial Transplant 2009;25(3):747–58.

72. Navaneethan SD, Singh S, Appasamy S, et al. Sodium bicarbonate therapy for prevention of contrast-induced nephropathy: a systematic review and meta-analysis. Am J Kidney Dis 2009;53:617–27.

73. Marenzi G, Ferrari C, Marana I, et al. Prevention of contrast nephropathy by furosemide with matched hydration The MYTHOS (Induced Diuresis With Matched Hydration Compared to Standard Hydration for Contrast Induced Nephropathy Prevention) trial. JACC Cardiovasc Interv 2012;5:90–7.

74. Cowper SE. Nephrogenic systemic fibrosis: an overview. J Am Coll Radiol 2008; 5:23–8.

75. Brar SS, Aharonian V, Mansukhani P, et al. Haemodynamic-guided fluid administration for the prevention of contrast-induced acute kidney injury: the POSEIDON randomised controlled trial. Lancet 2014;383:1814–23.

Acute Kidney Injury in Cirrhosis

Constantine J. Karvellas, MD, SM, FRCPC[a,b], Francois Durand, MD[c,d],
Mitra K. Nadim, MD[e,*]

KEYWORDS

- Acute on chronic liver failure (ACLF) • Acute kidney injury • Cirrhosis
- Hepatorenal syndrome • Acute dialysis quality initiative • Acute kidney injury network

KEY POINTS

- Evaluation of renal function and identification of the cause of acute kidney injury (AKI) in cirrhotic patients remains a challenge.
- Serum creatinine (sCr) remains the most commonly used clinical index of kidney function; however, it is influenced by a variety of factors.
- Given the limitations of calculating glomerular filtration rate (GFR) with current laboratory techniques, neutrophil gelatinase-associated lipocalin (NGAL), cystatin C, and other novel biomarkers potentially may in the future assist in differentiating hepatorenal syndrome (HRS)-AKI from structural kidney damage.
- Vasoconstrictor therapy (noradrenalin and terlipressin) is the primary therapy in HRS-AKI, although without a demonstrated mortality benefit.
- Predicting renal recovery post–liver transplant (LT) based on current criteria (time on renal replacement therapy [RRT], biomarkers) remains controversial.

Funding sources: Dr C.J. Karvellas: Alberta Transplant Fund, Shering-Merck, Gambro; Dr F. Durand: Consultant for Novartis, Gilead, Astellas, BMS; Dr M.K. Nadim: None.
Conflict of interest: None.
[a] Division of Critical Care Medicine, University of Alberta, 1-40 Zeidler Ledcor Building, 8540, 112 Street, Edmonton, Alberta T6G 2X8, Canada; [b] Division of Gastroenterology, Faculty of Medicine and Dentistry, University of Alberta, Edmonton, Alberta, Canada; [c] Service d'Hépatologie & Réanimation Hépatodigestive, Hepatology and Liver Intensive Care Unit, INSERM U773, Université Paris VII Hôpital Beaujon, 100 Boulevard du Général Leclerc, Clichy 92110, France; [d] INSERM U1149, University Paris VII, Denis Diderot, Paris, France; [e] Division of Nephrology, Department of Medicine, Keck School of Medicine, University of Southern California, Los Angeles, CA, USA
* Corresponding author. USC Vascular Surgery, 1520 San Pablo Street, Suite 4300, Los Angeles, CA 90033-5330.
E-mail address: Mitra.Nadim@med.usc.edu

INTRODUCTION

AKI is a frequent complication of end-stage liver disease, especially in those with acute-on-chronic liver failure (ACLF), occurring in up to 50% of hospitalized patients with cirrhosis.[1–5] The high incidence of AKI is due to the combination of an impaired effective arterial blood volume secondary to arterial vasodilation, with increased intra-renal vasoconstriction and impaired renal autoregulation that predisposes to renal dysfunction, and several precipitating factors related to cirrhosis, typically bacterial infections and gastrointestinal bleeding.[6–8] There is no specific blood or urine biomarker that can reliably identify the cause of AKI in cirrhotic patients. Traditional diagnostic criteria focused particular attention on HRS and its physiology of renal vasoconstriction and splanchnic vasodilatation[9] with criteria based on elevation in sCr level greater than 50% over baseline with value greater than1.5 mg/dL (133 μmol/L). Initial studies suggested that irreversibility of HRS had a deleterious impact on mortality.[10] However, subsequent studies have questioned these criteria as being narrow and required a broader look at AKI in cirrhosis.[11,12]

EPIDEMIOLOGY

Classification of renal dysfunction in cirrhotic patients can be based on acuity of presentation (acute, chronic, or acute on chronic); however, most cirrhotic patients (~70%) have AKI without structural changes.[13] Causes of AKI include hypovolemia/prerenal azotemia, intrinsic renal/parenchymal disorders (acute tubular necrosis [ATN], interstitial nephritis, glomerular disease), obstructive nephropathy, and HRS.[14]

HRS is a severe complication of advanced cirrhosis. Its clinical manifestations are related to changes in renal, hepatic, and the systemic circulation. HRS is a consequence of intense renal vasoconstriction leading to a reduction in renal perfusion and glomerular filtration. The ability of the kidney to excrete sodium and free water is also severely impaired without histologic changes accounting for this renal impairment. Traditionally, HRS has been described in 2 different clinical patterns, according to intensity and onset of renal failure.[15] Type 1 HRS increasingly represents the severe end of the spectrum of renal failure in cirrhosis. It is characterized by rapidly progressive renal failure with oliguria. It is defined as a doubling of the sCr level to greater than 2.5 mg/dL or a 50% reduction in 24-hour creatinine clearance to a level less than 20 mL/min in less than 2 weeks. Type II HRS progresses slowly and represents a less severe deterioration in renal function that may remain stable for extended periods. The dominant clinical feature of a patient with type II HRS is refractory ascites. This condition is the result of intense sodium retention, reduced glomerular filtration, and marked stimulation of the renin-angiotensin system. The Acute Dialysis Quality Initiative (ADQI) and the International Club of Ascites (ICA) have proposed a revision of these traditional criteria to define HRS and to remove sCr cutoff values to define HRS.[11,12,14,16]

PATHOPHYSIOLOGY OF HEPATORENAL SYNDROME

HRS is derived primarily from circulatory failure. According to the peripheral vasodilatation model, in cirrhosis the decrease in splanchnic and systemic arterial vascular resistance is likely related to increased expression of endothelial nitric oxide synthase and the concentration of nitric oxide and its metabolites in the splanchnic as well as systemic circulation.[17] In contrast, the production of nitric oxide in the intrahepatic circulation is reduced, exacerbating portal hypertension. The resultant decreased mean arterial pressure (MAP) and low total systemic vascular resistance is offset initially in compensated cirrhosis by an increase in cardiac output. In contrast to splanchnic blood flow, other vascular beds such as the cerebral, renal, and hepatic beds demonstrate an increase in resistance. The kidneys are initially able to compensate by increasing production of renal prostaglandins, resulting in renal vasodilation and preservation of renal perfusion and function. When cardiac output can no longer compensate, hypovolemia occurs with subsequent activation of the renin-angiotensin, vasopressin, and sympathetic nervous systems. In particular, angiotensin II plays a central role in stimulating renal vasoconstriction while increasing release of aldosterone, leading to increased sodium retention and ascites. As hepatic failure progresses and splanchnic vasodilation predominates, the heightened effects of potent renal vasoconstrictors (angiotensin II, endothelin, norepinephrine, and arginine-vasopressin) override the effect of local renal prostaglandins. This imbalance eventually results in HRS.[18]

HRS may occur spontaneously with worsening liver function or secondary to a precipitating event, such as spontaneous bacterial peritonitis (SBP). Approximately one-third of patients with SBP develop renal impairment in the absence of nephrotoxic antibiotics and shock. For some of these patients, renal impairment is reversible with appropriate antimicrobial therapy, but for most it is not. Other precipitating causes include large-volume therapeutic paracentesis without albumin replacement, diuretic use in refractory ascites, and gastrointestinal bleeding (especially with shock).[2]

PATHOPHYSIOLOGY OF ACUTE KIDNEY INJURY IN CIRRHOSIS: INFLAMMATION?

Although several publications have made reference to dysregulation of the renin-angiotensin system and sympathetic nervous system and antidiuretic hormone production in the development of AKI and cirrhosis, inflammation in the presence or absence of infection plays a prominent role. Cirrhotic patients are at high risk of bacterial translocation leading to increased circulating levels of lipopolysaccharide-binding protein, increasing production of tumor necrosis factor α, which exacerbates splanchnic vasodilation. Other important immunologic factors triggered by hepatic injury include release of damage-associated molecular pattern (DAMP) compounds, including high-mobility group box 1. This DAMP compound interacts through toll-like receptors 2 and 4 causing subsequent renal tubule injury.[19,20]

ASSESSMENT OF RENAL DYSFUNCTION

Evaluation of renal function in patients with cirrhosis remains a critically important and challenging problem (**Table 1**). sCr remains the most commonly used clinical index of kidney function; however, it is influenced by a variety of factors, including age, muscle mass, gender, and ethnicity. In liver cirrhosis, sCr overestimates renal function because of decreased creatine production by the liver, protein calorie malnutrition, and muscle wasting; thus, a sCr level within the normal range does not exclude significant renal impairment. In addition, sCr values may vary widely in patients with ascites because of dilutional changes in volume status after paracentesis and with the use of diuretics. High serum bilirubin levels may affect the assays used for measurement of sCr, resulting in falsely low sCr concentrations. GFR is considered the best estimate of renal function, although there is no universally accepted gold standard for measurement of GFR. GFR can be measured by creatinine clearance with timed urinary collection and determination of urinary and serum creatinine concentrations. However, in addition to inherent limitations related to inaccurate or incomplete urine collection, increased tubular secretions of creatinine may bias creatinine clearance as GFR declines in cirrhosis.[21,22] In patients with cirrhosis, creatinine clearance tends to

Table 1
Methods of assessing renal function in liver disease

		Advantages	Disadvantages
Serum-based methods	Serum creatinine	• Universally available • Inexpensive • MELD/AKI scores, current HRS definitions use this	• Affected by age, gender, muscle mass, steroids, medications • Decreased generation in liver disease • Bilirubin effect on assay • Lack of standardization of creatinine assays • Slow to increase in AKI
	Serum cystatin C	• Not affected by age, gender, muscle mass, sepsis • Simple blood test • Seems to detect early kidney dysfunction and AKI earlier than serum creatinine	• Underestimates GFR posttransplant • Dilution as with all serum markers • Variable performance of cystatin C • Variable expense • Results may not be available on a timely fashion
Clearance-based methods	Urinary creatinine clearance	• Inexpensive • Avoids dilution issues of serum markers	• Difficult to get accurate collections • Systematically overestimates GFR in liver disease by 10%–15% especially in patients with chronic kidney disease
	Inulin	• Still considered gold standard	• Systematic plasma clearance overestimates GFR • Cumbersome
	Iothalamate	• As good as inulin in most studies	• Significant extrarenal clearance • Shown to overestimate GFR by 10–20 mL/min
	GFR measured by CrEDTA	• As good as inulin in most studies	• Significant extrarenal clearance • Shown to overestimate GFR by 10–20 mL/min
	DcDPTA	• As good as inulin in most studies	• Significant extrarenal clearance

Abbreviations: CrEDTA, (51)Chromium-EDTA clearance; DcDPTA, Technetium-99m-diethylene-triamine-pentaacetate; MELD, Model for End-Stage Liver Disease.

overestimate true GFR. The clearance of exogenous markers such as iothalamate, inulin, or radioisotopes is the most accurate method of GFR assessment. However, they are not routinely used in clinical practice, for reasons of cost, convenience, and availability. The Modified Diet in Renal Disease (MDRD)[23] equations are widely used to estimate GFR in the general population, but MDRD-4 consistently overestimates GFR in cirrhotic patients.[22,24] Among creatinine-based equations, it has been shown that MDRD-6 is the most accurate in cirrhosis.[25] However, in contrast to MDRD-4, MDRD-6 may underestimate true GFR, discordances being more pronounced in old patients and patients with low serum sodium. Other indirect markers of renal function such as cystatin C are available; however, they are costly and not widely available, and recent studies have shown that similar to sCr, cystatin C level is affected by muscle mass and liver disease and overestimates renal function in patients with cirrhosis.[26,27] Equations based on cystatin C, with or without creatinine, may be superior to creatinine-based equation.[28,29] Again, the performance of current cystatin C–based equations (ie, chronic kidney disease epidemiology collaboration [CKD-EPI] creatinine-cystatin C equation) in patients with cirrhosis is inferior to that observed in the general population. In more than 20% of cirrhotic patients, a discordance of more than 30% is observed between cystatin C–based equations and true GFR.[28]

ACUTE KIDNEY INJURY IN PATIENTS WITH LIVER DISEASE: DIAGNOSIS AND DEFINITIONS

In 2004, the ADQI Workgroup developed a consensus definition and classification for AKI known as the risk, injury, failure, loss, end-stage renal disease (RIFLE) criteria, which stratified acute renal dysfunction into grades of increasing severity based on changes in sCr levels and/or urine output.[30] Subsequently, the Acute Kidney Injury Network (AKIN) proposed to broaden the definition of AKI to include an absolute increase in sCr level of 0.3 mg/dL or more (26 μmol/L) when documented to occur within 48 hours.[31] Once AKI is established, a staging system then defines the severity of the AKI. These criteria were then adopted by the international multidisciplinary Kidney Disease: Improving Global Outcomes (KDIGO) in their 2012 clinical practice guideline[32] (**Table 2**). In 2010, the ADQI workgroup along with several members of the ICA recommended adaptation of the modified RIFLE criteria to define AKI in patients with cirrhosis instead of the traditional definition using a fixed sCr cutoff value of greater than 1.5 mg/dL.[11,12] These criteria are irrespective of whether the presumed cause of the acute deterioration in renal function is related to a functional or structural disorder. As such, HRS type 1 was categorized as a specific type of AKI and HRS type 2 as a form of acute-on-chronic kidney disease, and the term hepatorenal disorders was proposed to encompass the full range of conditions in which liver and kidney disease coexist. Since then, the use of AKIN criteria in predicting mortality has been validated in several studies of hospitalized patients with cirrhosis, including those in the intensive care units.[2,3,33,34]

ACUTE KIDNEY INJURY IN CIRRHOSIS: NOVEL BIOMARKERS

Given the limitations of calculating GFR with currently available laboratory tests and techniques, other novel renal biomarkers have been investigated not only to diagnose AKI earlier and more accurately but potentially also to shed light on the cause (ie, differentiating ATN vs HRS-AKI).[35–37] There are several urinary biomarkers associated with tubular damage. Neutrophil gelatinase-associated lipocalin (NGAL), interleukin (IL)-18, kidney injury molecule-1 (KIM-1), and liver-type fatty acid–binding protein (L-FABP) are associated with renal tubular injury. In a study of 110 cirrhotic patients with AKI who were retrospectively identified as having prerenal azotemia, HRS, or ATN, levels of NGAL, KIM-1, IL-17, and L-FABP were significantly higher in patients with ATN than in those with HRS/prerenal azotemia.[35] This finding suggests that these tubular biomarkers may identify patients who are less likely to benefit from volume resuscitation and vasopressor therapy, although one caveat is that urinary tract infection may confound NGAL levels.[38]

Renal biomarkers predictive of recovery from AKI after LT could enhance decision algorithms regarding the need for liver-kidney transplant or renal sparing regimens. Levitsky and colleagues[39] published a pilot study of 16 patients, which showed that the levels of plasma proteins osteopontin, NGAL, cystatin C, TFF3 (Trefoil factor 3), tissue inhibitor of metalloproteinases (TIMP)-1, β-2 microglobulin

Table 2
Kidney Disease: Improving Global Outcomes 2012 criteria

AKI Definition	AKI Stage Serum Creatinine Criteria			AKI Stage Urine Output Criteria		
	1 (Risk)	2 (Injury)	3 (Failure)	1 (Risk)	2 (Injury)	3 (Failure)
RIFLE (2004)[69] ↑ sCr ≥1.5 × baseline, within 7 d; or GFR ↑ >25%; or urine output (UO) <0.5 mL/kg/h × 6 h	↑ 1.5 × baseline or GFR ↑>25%	↑ 2 × baseline or GFR ↑>50%	↑ 3 × baseline or sCr >4 mg/dL (>354 μmol/L) with an acute increase >0.5 mg/dL (44 μmol/L) or GFR ↑>75%	<0.5 mL/kg/h × 6–12 h	<0.5 mL/kg/h × 12 h	<0.3 mL/kg/h × 24 h or anuria × 12 h
AKIN (2007)[31] ↑ sCr ≥0.3 mg/dL (26.5 μmol/L) within 48 h; or ↑ sCr ≥1.5 × baseline within 48 h; or UO <0.5 mL/kg/h × 6 h	↑ ≥0.3 mg/dL (>26.5 μmol/L) within 48 h or ↑ sCr ≥1.5–2 × baseline	↑ 2–3 × baseline	↑ 3 × baseline or sCr >4 mg/dL (>354 μmol/L) with an acute increase >0.5 mg/dL (44 μmol/L) or on RRT	<0.5 mL/kg/h × 6–12 h	<0.5 mL/kg/h × 12 h	<0.3 mL/kg/h × 24 h or anuria × 12 h
KDIGO (2012)[70] ↑ sCr ≥0.3 mg/dL (26.5 μmol/L) within 48 h; or ↑ sCr ≥1.5 × baseline, which is known or presumed to have occurred within the prior 7 d; or UO <0.5 mL/kg/h for 6 h	↑ ≥0.3 mg/dL (>26.5 μmol/L) within 48 h or ↑ sCr ≥1.5–2 × baseline	↑ 2–3 × baseline	↑ 3 × baseline or sCr >4 mg/dL (>354 μmol/L) with an acute increase >0.5 mg/dL (44 μmol/L) or on RRT	<0.5 mL/kg/h × 6–12 h	<0.5 mL/kg/h × 12 h	<0.3 mL/kg/h × 24 h or anuria × 12 h
ADQI (2010)[12] AKI in cirrhosis ↑ sCr ≥0.3 mg/dL (26.5 μmol/L) within 48 h; or ↑ sCr ≥1.5 × baseline HRS-1 is a specific form of AKI	↑ ≥0.3 mg/dL (>26.5 μmol/L) within 48 h or ↑ sCr ≥1.5–2 × baseline	↑ 2–3 × baseline	↑ 3 × baseline or sCr >4 mg/dL (>354 μmol/L) with an acute increase >0.5 mg/dL (44 μmol/L) or on RRT	—	—	—
ICA (2015)[16] AKI in cirrhosis ↑ sCr ≥0.3 mg/dL (≥26.5 μmol/L) within 48 h; or ↑ sCr ≥50% from baseline which is known, or presumed, to have occurred within the prior 7 d	↑ ≥0.3 mg/dL (≥26.5 μmol/L) within 48 h or ↑ sCr ≥1.5–2 × baseline	↑ 2–3 × baseline	↑ 3 × baseline or sCr >4 mg/dL (>354 μmol/L) with an acute rise >0.5 mg/dL (44 μmol/L) or on RRT	—	—	—

were higher in patients with reversible AKI post-LT than in patients without AKI (P<.05). Furthermore, in a validation set of 46 patients, levels of osteopontin and TIMP-1 were significantly higher in patients with reversible AKI post-LT than in patients with irreversible AKI post-LT.[39]

THERAPIES: HEPATORENAL SYNDROME

Although LT is the only definitive treatment of HRS, it is clear that patients with renal failure at the time of transplant have poorer outcomes than those without.[40–45] Furthermore, a longer duration of renal dysfunction pretransplant is associated with poorer posttransplant renal recovery. The main purpose of treatments investigated for HRS is to provide a bridge to transplant. To date, therapies that have been evaluated include albumin, vasoconstrictor therapy, transjugular intrahepatic portosystemic shunt (TIPS), and extracorporeal liver support.

ALBUMIN

Administration of albumin in patients with cirrhosis also has been shown to cause arterial vasoconstriction in patients with SBP, possibly due to the ability of albumin to bind vasodilators such as nitric oxide.[46] This condition forms the basis for the use of extracorporeal liver support in HRS (see later discussion). Previous studies have shown that albumin prevented type 1 HRS in patients with SBP with a typical dose of 1 g/kg (20%–25%) on day 1 and then 20 to 60 g/d thereafter.[47] Adding albumin to other pharmacologic therapies likely provides the most benefit.

VASOCONSTRICTOR THERAPY
Vasopressin Analogues

Vasoconstrictor therapies have been well studied in the treatment of HRS and in particular, vasopressin analogues. The high prevalence of V_1 receptors in the splanchnic vasculature makes it especially sensitive to the vasoconstrictive effect of vasopressin analogues, and therefore, it is an important target for HRS therapy. The net theoretic result would be an increase in effective circulating arterial blood volume and suppression of the renin-angiotensin system and the sympathetic nervous system, resulting in renal afferent vasodilatation. Terlipressin has a strong affinity toward the V_1 receptors with a longer half-life and can be dosed intermittently. In 2 randomized controlled studies, in patients with type 1 HRS comparing albumin with terlipressin plus albumin, HRS reversal occurred significantly more frequently in the terlipressin group. Furthermore, survival in patients responding to treatment was longer than in those who did not.[1,48] Furthermore, a meta-analysis of 5 trials evaluating terlipressin for type 1 HRS showed that mortality was 48% in patients who received terlipressin alone or terlipressin with albumin, versus 64% in patients randomized to no intervention, placebo, or albumin alone; it thus reduced mortality with a relative risk of 0.76.[49] The assessment of mortality was limited because of small numbers and a short follow-up (1–6 months). Cardiovascular adverse events were higher in patients administered terlipressin.[49] Finally, a prospective study that included 18 patients with type 1 HRS and sepsis who received terlipressin and albumin showed that there was a significant improvement in arterial blood pressure and suppression of high renin and norepinephrine levels. Improvement of renal function was observed in 67% of the patients and was associated with an improved 3-month survival compared with patients without response. Patients who did not respond had higher Model for End-Stage Liver Disease

(MELD) and Child-Pugh scores and higher CLIF-SOFA (Chronic Liver Failure-Sequential Organ Failure Assessment).[50]

Terlipressin should be dosed progressively, starting at 0.5 mg intravenously every 4 hours. If the sCr does not decrease by 30% in 3 days, the dose should be doubled. In general, a patient not responding to 12 mg/d does not respond to higher doses. In patients who respond to terlipressin, treatment should be continued until normalization of sCr (<1.5 mg/dL).

Noradrenaline

Early uncontrolled pilot data showed that titrating noradrenaline to achieve an MAP increase of 10 mm Hg was associated with improved urine output, sodium excretion, and creatinine clearance. Four controlled studies have compared the efficacy of noradrenaline with that of terlipressin.[51–54] In one study of 22 patients with HRS (type I n = 9, type II n = 13), patients received albumin plus norepinephrine, 0.1 to 0.7 μg/kg/min, intravenous infusion or terlipressin, 1 to 2 mg, every 4 hours. Reversal of HRS occurred in 70% of patients receiving noradrenaline versus 83% of patients receiving terlipressin (P = NS).[52] A second study compared albumin with noradrenaline (8–50 μg/min intravenous) or terlipressin (0.5–2.0 mg every 6 hours) in 20 patients with type 1 HRS. The number of patients who responded to therapy did not significantly differ between the 2 groups (50%–40%, P = .7), and furthermore, there was no significant difference in cumulative survival.[51] These results suggest that noradrenaline may be a safe and noninferior alternative to vasopressin analogues in the treatment of HRS. A systematic review examined the major vasoconstrictors available for HRS, focusing on terlipressin and noradrenaline.[55] In this review of 4 studies and a total of 154 patients, terlipressin and noradrenaline seemed to be equivalent in terms of HRS reversal, mortality at 30 days, and recurrence of HRS. Adverse events were less frequent in patients who received noradrenaline.[55]

Midodrine and Octreotide

Midodrine is an orally administered α-adrenergic agonist that seems to be beneficial in HRS. Its oral preparation makes it a feasible option for patients who are not in intensive care but require long-term vasoconstrictor therapy. It is often given in combination with octreotide, a long-acting somatostatin analogue, which reduces portal hypertension and splanchnic hyperemia. It may cause splanchnic vasoconstriction through inhibition of glucagon synthesis or a direct effect on vascular smooth muscle. In a recent observational study, 75 patients received a mean of 8 days of midodrine (7.5–12.5 mg orally 3 times daily), subcutaneous octreotide (100–200 μg subcutaneously 3 times daily), and intravenous albumin (50–100 g intravenous daily). The treatment group was compared with a historical control group of 87 patients with type 1 or 2 HRS who did not receive these therapies. Median survival was significantly improved in both type 1 HRS (40 vs 17 days, P = .007) and type 2 HRS (>12 months vs 22 days P = .0004), with more patients with type 2 HRS in the treatment group undergoing LT (58 vs 25%, P = .04).[56]

TRANSJUGULAR INTRAHEPATIC PORTOSYSTEMIC SHUNT

In theory, the benefit of TIPS is by decreasing portal hypertension with a subsequent decrease in the concentration of vasoconstrictory mediators (vasopressin, norepinephrine, endothelin, and angiotensin II). The role of TIPS has been evaluated in small pilot studies. In 7 cirrhotic patients with type 1 HRS who underwent TIPS, 6 had improvement in sCr and blood urea nitrogen levels at day 30. Reductions in plasma renin and norepinephrine levels were also noted.[57] In a prospective controlled study of 41 cirrhotic patients with HRS (type 1 n = 21, type 2 n = 20) who could not undergo transplant, 31 patients (type 1 n = 14, type 2 n = 17) received TIPS, whereas 10 patients with advanced liver failure were excluded from a shunt (type I, n = 7; type 2, n = 3). TIPS was associated with improved renal function within 2 weeks (creatinine clearance 18–48 mL/min, $P<.001$) and stabilized thereafter. After TIPS, at 3, 6, 12, and 18 months, survival rates were 81%, 71%, 48%, and 35%, respectively. These rates were significantly higher than in the group without shunt (log rank 18.3, $P<.001$).[58] Unfortunately, in most cirrhotic patients with HRS, TIPS is contraindicated because of the severity of hepatic dysfunction (eg, MELD>20) and the risk of further deterioration.

RENAL REPLACEMENT THERAPY

The role of intermittent or continuous RRT in HRS is primarily as a bridge to LT. Observational studies have shown that RRT is not predictive of improved transplant-free survival. The use of RRT in patients with HRS is likely only appropriate in the setting of a patient who is listed for LT or has another indication for RRT (ie, uremia, acidosis, hyperkalemia).[59] Exact timing of initiation of RRT, similar to the general critically ill population, is controversial.[60]

EXTRACORPOREAL LIVER SUPPORT

Extracorporeal albumin dialysis technologies use albumin as a binding and scavenging molecule in the treatment of HRS. Albumin dialysis is based on dialyzing blood against an albumin-containing solution across a highly permeable high-flux membrane. The blood-bound toxins are cleared by diffusion and taken up by the binding sites of the albumin dialysate.

The molecular adsorbent recirculating system (MARS) consists of a blood circuit, an albumin circuit, and a classic renal circuit. Blood is dialyzed across an albumin-impregnated high-flux dialysis membrane; 600 mL of 20% human albumin in the albumin circuit acts as the dialysate. Albumin-bound toxins in blood are released to the membrane. In a controlled pilot study, Mitzner and colleagues[61] reported 13 patients with decompensated cirrhosis and type 1 HRS; 8 were treated with MARS, and 5 received standard medical therapy. They showed a 37.5% absolute survival benefit at day 7 versus 0% in controls. A significant decrease in the levels of creatinine and bilirubin was also noted in the MARS group. A more recent multicenter study (RELIEF trial [Recompensation of Exacerbated Liver Insufficiency With Hyperbilirubinemia and/or Encephalopathy and/or Renal Failure]) by Banares and colleagues[62] failed to show a mortality benefit in patients with ACLF treated with MARS, with a 28-day survival of 60% in both MARS and SMT (Standard Medical Therapy) groups despite biochemical improvement. This study may have been confounded by indication (transplant and nontransplant candidates).

Prometheus (fractionated plasma separation and adsorption) differs from the other technologies in that the patient's plasma is separated across a membrane and then is run over adsorptive columns. An uncontrolled study reported Prometheus use in 10 patients with HRS who underwent 2 consecutive Prometheus treatments.[63] A statistically significant decrease in creatinine and blood urea nitrogen levels and improvement in arterial blood pH was observed. A more recent multicenter study (HELIOS [Prometheus European Liver Disease Outcome Study]) failed to show a mortality benefit in patients with ACLF treated with Prometheus, with a 28-day survival of 65% in both Prometheus and SMT groups despite biochemical improvement.[64] Like RELIEF, this study also was confounded by indication.

TREATMENT: OTHER CAUSES OF ACUTE KIDNEY INJURY

Early treatment of AKI in cirrhosis is important. Multiple therapies may be initiated before an unequivocal diagnosis of the exact cause of AKI. Nephrotoxins such as nonsteroidal anti-inflammatory drugs and angiotensin-converting-enzyme inhibitors should be discontinued in patients taking them. Patients on diuretic therapy who develop AKI should stop loop and potassium-sparing diuretics. In patients with large-volume ascites, paracentesis may still be warranted to reduce the risk of an abdominal compartment syndrome and improve venous return to the right atrium, but intravenous albumin at 8 g/L is required to maintain intravascular volume. In the patient who is hypotensive (MAP <65 mm Hg), it may be reasonable to consider vasoconstrictor therapy and volume resuscitation unless there is evidence of volume overload (eg, echocardiography). Intravascular depletion can be treated with albumin or crystalloid depending on biochemical factors. In the setting of gastrointestinal bleeding, packed red blood cell transfusion less than 7 g/dL has been shown to be noninferior and potentially beneficial over a more liberal transfusion strategy.[65]

NATURAL HISTORY OF ACUTE KIDNEY INJURY: PRETRANSPLANT AND POSTTRANSPLANT OUTCOMES

The identification of novel methods of determining the cause of AKI in cirrhosis is important as the potential for renal recovery is cause dependent.[62] Prerenal azotemia (ie, diuretics, diarrhea) is usually reversible after discontinuation of the precipitating cause.[66] The severity of AKI associated with bacterial infection depends on the resolution of the infection.[67] The cause of AKI also has a significant impact on patient and renal outcomes post-LT. A study from Nadim and colleagues[40] revealed that patient survival and renal outcomes 1 and 5 years after LT were significantly worse for those with ATN.

Intraoperative RRT in critically ill cirrhotic patients undergoing LT has been shown to be feasible with good patient and renal outcomes.[25,68]

Although duration of RRT (4–8 weeks) and GFR have been traditionally used by some centers to determine the need for simultaneous liver kidney (SLK) transplants, evidence-based guidelines for SLK are lacking.[40] Further investigations, particularly focusing on novel renal plasma protein biomarkers may provide further information on prognostication of potential post-LT renal recovery (along with cause of AKI) before making a decision to proceed with SLK transplant.[39]

SUMMARY

AKI causes significant morbidity in cirrhotic patients. Evaluation of renal dysfunction in patients with cirrhosis remains a critically important and challenging problem. Current diagnostic criteria are based on the sCr level, which has limitations in extrapolating GFR in cirrhotic patients. New diagnostic criteria (KDIGO, RIFLE, AKIN) have been integrated with traditional approaches (ICA/HRS/AKI) to potentially identify AKI earlier and improve outcomes. The cause of AKI has a significant impact on the potential of renal recovery. Further work on urinary tubular biomarkers is required to differentiate structural causes of AKI versus HRS-AKI. Conventional therapies for HRS include vasoconstrictor agents and albumin, although in severe cases in which mortality is high, LT is the only effective treatment. Novel renal plasma protein biomarkers may in the future provide further information on the potential of renal recovery post-LT (along with cause) and potentially affect the decision to allocate an SLK.

REFERENCES

1. Sanyal AJ, Boyer T, Garcia-Tsao G, et al. A randomized, prospective, double-blind, placebo-controlled trial of terlipressin for type 1 hepatorenal syndrome. Gastroenterology 2008;134:1360–8.
2. Tsien CD, Rabie R, Wong F. Acute kidney injury in decompensated cirrhosis. Gut 2013;62:131–7.
3. Barreto R, Fagundes C, Guevara M, et al. Type-1 hepatorenal syndrome associated with infections in cirrhosis: natural history, outcome of kidney function, and survival. Hepatology 2014;59:1505–13.
4. Piano S, Rosi S, Maresio G, et al. Evaluation of the Acute Kidney Injury Network criteria in hospitalized patients with cirrhosis and ascites. J Hepatol 2013;59: 482–9.
5. Wong F, O'Leary JG, Reddy KR, et al. New consensus definition of acute kidney injury accurately predicts 30-day mortality in patients with cirrhosis and infection. Gastroenterology 2013;145:1280–8.e1.
6. Adebayo D, Morabito V, Davenport A, et al. Renal dysfunction in cirrhosis is not just a vasomotor nephropathy. Kidney Int 2015;87:509–15.
7. Gines P, Schrier RW. Renal failure in cirrhosis. N Engl J Med 2009;361:1279–90.
8. Stadlbauer V, Wright GA, Banaji M, et al. Relationship between activation of the sympathetic nervous system and renal blood flow autoregulation in cirrhosis. Gastroenterology 2008;134:111–9.
9. Salerno F, Gerbes A, Ginès P, et al. Diagnosis, prevention and treatment of hepatorenal syndrome in cirrhosis. Gut 2007;56:1310–8.
10. Colle I, Durand F, Pessione F, et al. Clinical course, predictive factors and prognosis in patients with cirrhosis and type 1 hepatorenal syndrome treated with terlipressin: a retrospective analysis. J Gastroenterol Hepatol 2002;17:882–8.
11. Wong F, Nadim MK, Kellum JA, et al. Working Party proposal for a revised classification system of renal dysfunction in patients with cirrhosis. Gut 2011;60: 702–9.
12. Nadim MK, Kellum JA, Davenport A, et al. Hepatorenal syndrome: the 8th International Consensus Conference of the Acute Dialysis Quality Initiative (ADQI) Group. Crit Care 2012;16:R23.
13. Warner NS, Cuthbert JA, Bhore R, et al. Acute kidney injury and chronic kidney disease in hospitalized patients with cirrhosis. J Investig Med 2011;59:1244–51.
14. Garcia-Tsao G, Parikh CR, Viola A. Acute kidney injury in cirrhosis. Hepatology 2008;48:2064–77.
15. Salerno F, Gerbes A, Ginès P, et al. Diagnosis, prevention and treatment of hepatorenal syndrome in cirrhosis. Postgrad Med J 2008;84:662–70.
16. Angeli P, Ginès P, Wong F, et al. Diagnosis and management of acute kidney injury in patients with cirrhosis: revised consensus recommendations of the International Club of Ascites. J Hepatol 2015. http://dx.doi.org/10.1016/j.jhep.2014.12.029.
17. Martin PY, Ohara M, Gines P, et al. Nitric oxide synthase (NOS) inhibition for one week improves renal sodium and water excretion in cirrhotic rats with ascites. J Clin Invest 1998;101:235–42.
18. Gines P, Guevara M, Arroyo V, et al. Hepatorenal syndrome. Lancet 2003;362: 1819–27.
19. Biancofiore G, Critchley LA, Lee A, et al. Evaluation of a new software version of the FloTrac/Vigileo (version 3.02) and a comparison with previous data in cirrhotic patients undergoing liver transplant surgery. Anesth Analg 2011;113:515–22.

20. Park SW, Kim M, Brown KM, et al. Paneth cell-derived interleukin-17A causes multiorgan dysfunction after hepatic ischemia and reperfusion injury. Hepatology 2011;53:1662–75.
21. Proulx NL, Akbari A, Garg AX, et al. Measured creatinine clearance from timed urine collections substantially overestimates glomerular filtration rate in patients with liver cirrhosis: a systematic review and individual patient meta-analysis. Nephrol Dial Transplant 2005;20:1617–22.
22. Francoz C, Glotz D, Moreau R, et al. The evaluation of renal function and disease in patients with cirrhosis. J Hepatol 2010;52:605–13.
23. Levey AS, Bosch JP, Lewis JB, et al. A more accurate method to estimate glomerular filtration rate from serum creatinine: a new prediction equation. Modification of Diet in Renal Disease Study Group. Ann Intern Med 1999;130:461–70.
24. Gonwa TA, Jennings L, Mai ML, et al. Estimation of glomerular filtration rates before and after orthotopic liver transplantation: evaluation of current equations. Liver Transpl 2004;10:301–9.
25. Francoz C, Nadim MK, Baron A, et al. Glomerular filtration rate equations for liver-kidney transplantation in patients with cirrhosis: validation of current recommendations. Hepatology 2014;59:1514–21.
26. Gerbes AL, Gülberg V, Bilzer M, et al. Evaluation of serum cystatin C concentration as a marker of renal function in patients with cirrhosis of the liver. Gut 2002; 50:106–10.
27. Davenport A, Cholongitas E, Xirouchakis E, et al. Pitfalls in assessing renal function in patients with cirrhosis–potential inequity for access to treatment of hepatorenal failure and liver transplantation. Nephrol Dial Transplant 2011;26:2735–42.
28. Mindikoglu AL, Dowling TC, Weir MR, et al. Performance of chronic kidney disease epidemiology collaboration creatinine-cystatin C equation for estimating kidney function in cirrhosis. Hepatology 2014;59:1532–42.
29. De Souza V, Hadj-Aissa A, Dolomanova O, et al. Creatinine- versus cystatine C-based equations in assessing the renal function of candidates for liver transplantation with cirrhosis. Hepatology 2014;59:1522–31.
30. Bellomo R, Kellum JA, Ronco C. Defining acute renal failure: physiological principles. Intensive Care Med 2004;30:33–7.
31. Mehta RL, Kellum JA, Shah SV, et al. Acute Kidney Injury Network: report of an initiative to improve outcomes in acute kidney injury. Crit Care 2007;11:R31.
32. Khwaja A. KDIGO clinical practice guidelines for acute kidney injury. Nephron Clin Pract 2012;120:c179–84.
33. Belcher JM, Garcia-Tsao G, Sanyal AJ, et al. Association of AKI with mortality and complications in hospitalized patients with cirrhosis. Hepatology 2013;57: 753–62.
34. de Carvalho JR, Villela-Nogueira CA, Luiz RR, et al. Acute Kidney Injury Network criteria as a predictor of hospital mortality in cirrhotic patients with ascites. J Clin Gastroenterol 2012;46:e21–6.
35. Belcher JM, Sanyal AJ, Peixoto AJ, et al. Kidney biomarkers and differential diagnosis of patients with cirrhosis and acute kidney injury. Hepatology 2014;60: 622–32.
36. Fagundes C, Pépin MN, Guevara M, et al. Urinary neutrophil gelatinase-associated lipocalin as biomarker in the differential diagnosis of impairment of kidney function in cirrhosis. J Hepatol 2012;57:267–73.
37. Verna EC, Brown RS, Farrand E, et al. Urinary neutrophil gelatinase-associated lipocalin predicts mortality and identifies acute kidney injury in cirrhosis. Dig Dis Sci 2012;57:2362–70.

38. Altamirano J, Fagundes C, Dominguez M, et al. Acute kidney injury is an early predictor of mortality for patients with alcoholic hepatitis. Clin Gastroenterol Hepatol 2012;10:65–71.e3.

39. Levitsky J, Baker TB, Jie C, et al. Plasma protein biomarkers enhance the clinical prediction of kidney injury recovery in patients undergoing liver transplantation. Hepatology 2014;60:2017–26.

40. Nadim MK, Genyk YS, Tokin C, et al. Impact of the etiology of acute kidney injury on outcomes following liver transplantation: acute tubular necrosis versus hepatorenal syndrome. Liver Transpl 2012;18:539–48.

41. Bahirwani R, Campbell MS, Siropaides T, et al. Transplantation: impact of pretransplant renal insufficiency. Liver Transpl 2008;14:665–71.

42. Campbell MS, Kotlyar DS, Brensinger CM, et al. Renal function after orthotopic liver transplantation is predicted by duration of pretransplantation creatinine elevation. Liver Transpl 2005;11:1048–55.

43. Gonwa TA, McBride MA, Anderson K, et al. Continued influence of preoperative renal function on outcome of orthotopic liver transplant (OLTX) in the US: where will MELD lead us? Am J Transplant 2006;6:2651–9.

44. Gonwa TA, Morris CA, Goldstein RM, et al. Long-term survival and renal function following liver transplantation in patients with and without hepatorenal syndrome—experience in 300 patients. Transplantation 1991;51:428–30.

45. Gunning TC, Brown MR, Swygert TH, et al. Perioperative renal function in patients undergoing orthotopic liver transplantation. A randomized trial of the effects of verapamil. Transplantation 1991;51:422–7.

46. Fernandez J, Navasa M, Garcia-Pagan JC, et al. Effect of intravenous albumin on systemic and hepatic hemodynamics and vasoactive neurohormonal systems in patients with cirrhosis and spontaneous bacterial peritonitis. J Hepatol 2004;41:384–90.

47. Sort P, Navasa M, Arroyo V, et al. Effect of intravenous albumin on renal impairment and mortality in patients with cirrhosis and spontaneous bacterial peritonitis. N Engl J Med 1999;341:403–9.

48. Martin-Llahi M, Pépin MN, Guevara M, et al. Terlipressin and albumin vs albumin in patients with cirrhosis and hepatorenal syndrome: a randomized study. Gastroenterology 2008;134:1352–9.

49. Gluud LL, Kjaer MS, Christensen E. Terlipressin for hepatorenal syndrome. Cochrane Database Syst Rev 2012;(9):CD005162.

50. Angeli P, Rodríguez E, Piano S, et al. Acute kidney injury and acute-on-chronic liver failure classifications in prognosis assessment of patients with acute decompensation of cirrhosis. Gut 2014. http://dx.doi.org/10.1136/gutjnl-2014-307526.

51. Sharma P, Kumar A, Shrama BC, et al. An open label, pilot, randomized controlled trial of noradrenaline versus terlipressin in the treatment of type 1 hepatorenal syndrome and predictors of response. Am J Gastroenterol 2008;103:1689–97.

52. Alessandria C, Ottobrelli A, Debernardi-Venon W, et al. Noradrenalin vs terlipressin in patients with hepatorenal syndrome: a prospective, randomized, unblinded, pilot study. J Hepatol 2007;47:499–505.

53. Singh V, Ghosh S, Singh B, et al. Noradrenaline vs. terlipressin in the treatment of hepatorenal syndrome: a randomized study. J Hepatol 2012;56:1293–8.

54. Ghosh S, Choudhary NS, Sharma AK, et al. Noradrenaline vs terlipressin in the treatment of type 2 hepatorenal syndrome: a randomized pilot study. Liver Int 2013;33:1187–93.

55. Nassar AP Jr, Farias AQ, D'Albuquerque LA, et al. Terlipressin versus norepinephrine in the treatment of hepatorenal syndrome: a systematic review and meta-analysis. PLoS One 2014;9:e107466.

56. Skagen C, Einstein M, Lucey MR, et al. Combination treatment with octreotide, midodrine, and albumin improves survival in patients with type 1 and type 2 hepatorenal syndrome. J Clin Gastroenterol 2009;43:680–5.

57. Guevara M, Ginès P, Bandi JC, et al. Transjugular intrahepatic portosystemic shunt in hepatorenal syndrome: effects on renal function and vasoactive systems. Hepatology 1998;28:416–22.

58. Brensing KA, Textor J, Perz J, et al. Long term outcome after transjugular intrahepatic portosystemic stent-shunt in non-transplant cirrhotics with hepatorenal syndrome: a phase II study. Gut 2000;47:288–95.

59. Keller F, Heinze H, Jochimsen F, et al. Risk factors and outcome of 107 patients with decompensated liver disease and acute renal failure (including 26 patients with hepatorenal syndrome): the role of hemodialysis. Ren Fail 1995;17:135–46.

60. Karvellas CJ, Farhat MR, Sajjad I, et al. A comparison of early versus late initiation of renal replacement therapy in critically ill patients with acute kidney injury: a systematic review and meta-analysis. Crit Care 2011;15:R72.

61. Mitzner SR, Stange J, Klammt S, et al. Improvement of hepatorenal syndrome with extracorporeal albumin dialysis MARS: results of a prospective, randomized, controlled clinical trial. Liver Transpl 2000;6:277–86.

62. Banares R, Nevens F, Larsen FS, et al. Extracorporeal albumin dialysis with the molecular adsorbent recirculating system in acute-on-chronic liver failure: the RELIEF trial. Hepatology 2013;57:1153–62.

63. Rifai K, Ernst T, Kretschmer U, et al. The Prometheus device for extracorporeal support of combined liver and renal failure. Blood Purif 2005;23:298–302.

64. Kribben A, Gerken G, Haag S, et al. Effects of fractionated plasma separation and adsorption on survival in patients with acute-on-chronic liver failure. Gastroenterology 2012;142:782–9.e3.

65. Villanueva C, Colomo A, Bosch A, et al. Transfusion strategies for acute upper gastrointestinal bleeding. N Engl J Med 2013;368:11–21.

66. Martin-Llahi M, Guevara M, Torre A, et al. Prognostic importance of the cause of renal failure in patients with cirrhosis. Gastroenterology 2011;140:488–96.e4.

67. Follo A, Llovet JM, Navasa M, et al. Renal impairment after spontaneous bacterial peritonitis in cirrhosis: incidence, clinical course, predictive factors and prognosis. Hepatology 1994;20:1495–501.

68. Nadim MK, Annanthapanyasut W, Matsuoka L, et al. Intraoperative hemodialysis during liver transplantation: a decade of experience. Liver Transpl 2014. http://dx.doi.org/10.1002/lt.23867.

69. Bellomo R, Ronco C, Kellum JA, et al. Acute renal failure - definition, outcome measures, animal models, fluid therapy and information technology needs: the Second International Consensus Conference of the Acute Dialysis Quality Initiative (ADQI) Group. Crit Care 2004;8:R204–12.

70. Kidney Disease: Improving Global Outcomes (KDIGO) Acute Kidney Injury Work Group. KDIGO clinical practice guideline for acute kidney injury. Kidney Int 2012; 2(Suppl):1–138.

Short-term Effects of Acute Kidney Injury

Kai Singbartl, MD, MPH[a], Michael Joannidis, MD[b],*

KEYWORDS

- Acute kidney injury • Short term • Uremic toxins • Electrolytes
- Inflammatory mediators • Cytokines • Neutrophils • Immune system

KEY POINTS

- Acute kidney injury (AKI) is a systemic disease.
- Conventional short-term effects of acute kidney injury (eg, fluid, electrolytes, and acid-base abnormalities; and uremic toxin accumulation) respond well to renal replacement therapies. However, this approach is usually reserved for the severest stages of AKI.
- AKI modulates underlying processes by reducing cytokine clearance, triggering enhanced renal cytokine production and contributing to systemic inflammation.
- AKI negatively affects neutrophil recruitment and thereby worsens infections (experimental evidence).

INTRODUCTION

Acute kidney injury (AKI) occurs in more than 30% of critically ill patients.[1,2] Mounting epidemiologic evidence shows that AKI is an independent risk factor for mortality (ie, patients are dying because of, and not simply with, AKI).[1,3–5] This evidence does not only apply to the most severe form of AKI, for which patients are treated with renal replacement therapy (RRT). It also holds true for small declines in renal function, which in turn are associated with increased short-term mortality.[6,7] When the severity of AKI is classified according to current criteria,[8–10] a strong association between the severity of AKI and hospital mortality emerges.[11–14] AKI, at all stages, also affects other outcomes, including the length of hospital stay, readmission rates, and development of end-stage kidney disease.[15–18] These effects cannot solely be attributed to the loss of organ function, because it has been repeatedly been shown that the mortality of critically ill patients with end-stage renal disease is lower than that of patients with

Conflicts of Interest: The authors report no conflicts with regard to this article.
[a] Department of Anesthesiology, Penn State College of Medicine, Milton S. Hershey Medical Center, P.O. Box 850, H187 Hershey, PA 17033, USA; [b] Division of Intensive Care and Emergency Medicine, Department of Internal Medicine, Medical University Innsbruck, Anichstr. 35, Innsbruck A-6020, Austria
* Corresponding author.
E-mail address: michael.joannidis@i-med.ac.at

Crit Care Clin 31 (2015) 751–762
http://dx.doi.org/10.1016/j.ccc.2015.06.010
0749-0704/15/$ – see front matter © 2015 Elsevier Inc. All rights reserved.

criticalcare.theclinics.com

AKI, even when not requiring RRT.[19] Thus, despite extensive data showing the clinical impact of AKI, the exact underlying mechanisms remain largely unknown.

SHORT-TERM EFFECTS OF ACUTE KIDNEY INJURY: THE CONVENTIONAL PERSPECTIVE

The key acute consequences of AKI comprise electrolyte abnormalities, acidosis, and fluid overload (**Fig. 1**), but accumulation of uremic toxins has also been discussed as factor contributing to the increased mortality associated with AKI.[20–23]

Electrolyte Disturbance

Potassium homeostasis mainly relies on renal excretion, therefore hyperkalemia is a commonly encountered finding in AKI. Additional factors contributing to hyperkalemia in critical illness include pH-dependant shifts from the intracellular space and relative insulin resistance. Furthermore, rhabdomyolysis, hemolysis, and the adverse effects of certain drugs (eg, angiotensin-converting enzyme inhibitors, calcineurin inhibitors, cotrimoxazole) may also contribute to hyperkalemia. Hyperkalemia may induce or worsen metabolic acidosis by interfering with renal ammonium excretion ($NH4^+$).[24] Left untreated, hyperkalemia may be fatal, leading to severe cardiac arrhythmias, muscle weakness, paralysis, and change in mental status. Clinical symptoms are usually observed at potassium levels greater than 7.0 mEq/L in chronic hyperkalemia but may occur earlier with rapid changes in serum potassium occurring, which is often the case in AKI. Classic pharmacologic manipulation of potassium levels provides transitory improvement through intracellular potassium shifts. The only effective measures decreasing whole-body potassium load are diuretic therapy (as long as the kidney is responding), enteric potassium-binding resins, and RRT. A specific threshold for

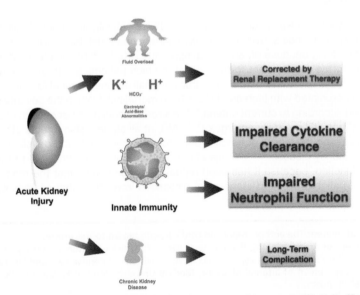

Fig. 1. Clinical effects of AKI. AKI has both short-term and long-term clinical effects. Fluid overload as well as acid-base and electrolyte imbalances are usually well controlled by RRT. The development of chronic kidney disease is a long-term effect of AKI. The effects of AKI on innate immunity have recently emerged as another important short-term factor in the pathophysiology of AKI.

initiation of RRT in hyperkalemia cannot be recommended because this depends on the acuity of serum potassium changes and the observed physiologic effects on the patient. Usually RRT is not commenced at serum potassium values less than 6.5 mmol/L if this is the sole indication.[25]

Both hypernatremia and hyponatremia occur in AKI, being dependent on volume status as well as any remaining effective free-water clearance by the kidneys. If some residual renal function remains it is rarely necessary to start RRT to correct dysnatremias, although RRT may be used as an adjunct to therapy. Severe hypercalcemia may occur in the setting of hyperparathyroidism or malignancy and can lead to crystal nephropathy, tubular obstruction, and subsequent renal failure. In addition to pharmacologic treatments including bisphosphonates, RRT may be considered as a last resort treatment of acute hypercalcemia.[26] Hypocalcemia is a common finding in patients with AKI usually associated with increased phosphorus levels caused by decreased glomerular filtration rate (GFR)[27] or massive release from dying cells (eg, tumor lysis syndrome). Intravenous calcium substitution and application of phosphate binders may be required in symptomatic patients, and treatment with RRT may be necessary in severe hyperphosphatemia.

Acid-Base Disorders

The kidney plays a major role in acid-base regulation. Renal failure results in increasing levels of plasma organic acids and other unmeasured anions through continued fixed acid production of around 50 to 100 mEq H^+/d.[28–30] Rapidly worsening high-anion-gap acidoses in the context of AKI usually result from lactate generation caused by organ hypoperfusion, from ketoacids, or from poisoning, such as ethylene glycol or aspirin intoxication. Acidemia leads to protein catabolism, reduced hepatic blood flow, and hemodynamic instability caused by impairment of myocardial contractility, arteriolar dilatation, venoconstriction, and diminished response to catecholamines.[31,32] In practice, an intractable acidosis with a pH less than 7.1 is usually considered an indication to commence RRT.[33]

Uremia

Accumulation of uremic toxins comprising several small to medium-sized molecules eliminated by the kidneys is considered a major component of uremia in the context of end-stage renal disease.[34,35] Despite full-blown uremic symptoms now being rarely encountered in critically ill patients because of the widespread availability of modern RRT, uremic toxin accumulation may cause significant damage in AKI,[36] such as increasing microvascular permeability,[37] reducing cardiac contractility,[38,39] or leading to bleeding disorders through the functional impairment of platelets.[40] For some molecules, like asymmetrical dimethylarginine, a key role has been established for the development of acute lung injury in the setting of ischemic AKI.[41] At present, there are only limited technologies available for determination of uremic toxins and their specific role in AKI remains to be further defined.[42] Consequently, other low-molecular-weight molecules, such as blood urea nitrogen (BUN), are often used as a surrogate parameter. However, several recent studies questioned the reliability of BUN for this purpose, because the timing of RRT based on BUN levels has not been shown to influence outcome.[33] Creatinine, a nontoxic marker that is useful in chronic kidney disease to estimate glomerular filtration and to determine end-stage renal disease requiring the start RRT, is of even less importance in AKI, because creatinine generation varies substantially in critically ill patients because of excessive muscle wasting[43] or reduced production rate in sepsis.[44]

Fluid Overload

Volume overload caused by salt and water retention frequently complicates AKI, occurring in 30% to 70% of intensive care unit patients.[22,45,46] Fluid overload seems to be a major driving factor of morbidity and mortality in patients with AKI.[47] The cause of fluid overload is multifactorial, resulting from sodium retention caused by renal inflammation[48] and the reduced renal (water) clearance that is already occurring at low stages of AKI, as well as the fluid resuscitation used to treat hemodynamic instability, which may be caused or aggravated by any of the consequences of AKI described earlier. Thus, volume overload may already be seen at early stages of AKI.[46–52] The major pathophysiologic aspect of fluid overload is interstitial edema, which significantly impairs oxygen and metabolite diffusion, distorts tissue architecture, and obstructs capillary blood flow and lymphatic drainage, resulting in disturbed cell-cell interactions and potentially contributing to progressive organ dysfunction. In encapsulated organs, this process increases interstitial pressure. In kidneys with AKI this causes a further reduction of GFR. Similarly, the liver may encounter reduced perfusion. Myocardial edema in the heart can worsen ventricular function, oxygen delivery, and synchronized intraventricular conduction.[49] Most critically, fluid overload of the lungs results in impaired gas exchange early, often requiring mechanical ventilation, which itself must be seen as a proinflammatory intervention contributing to the systemic inflammatory load of critically ill patients.[50,51] In addition, severe volume overload results in visceral edema, causing intra-abdominal hypertension[52] and potentially even reducing cerebral perfusion pressure (cerebral edema). The definition of volume overload usually relies on increase of body weight or cumulative positive fluid balance compared with baseline. Hemodynamic parameters, such as increased global end-diastolic volume, lung water content, or a high central venous pressure, may be helpful for early diagnosis.[53]

Patients who remain responsive to diuretic treatment show outcome benefits,[54] as do patients exposed to restrictive fluid management in acute lung injury.[55,56] Although diuretics are still frequently used in order to prevent oliguria,[57,58] their use has not been translated into any perceived benefit in AKI.[59,60] Consequently, in the presence of refractory, severe volume overload, initiation of RRT seems indicated. In the intensive care setting, initiation of RRT is more frequently triggered by oliguria and is expected to result in volume overload rather than increases in the levels of conventional markers such as creatinine or urea.[61,62]

A few case-control studies have investigated early initiation of RRT using a more functional approach and showed significantly reduced hospital or 30-day mortality in patients in whom RRT was started in the presence of oliguria rather than awaiting increases in BUN or serum creatinine levels.[63–65] However, the only prospective study to date investigating both delivered dose and early versus late initiation of treatment found no difference between starting RRT for oliguria versus waiting for pulmonary edema to occur.[66]

To summarize, although all of the conditions mentioned earlier should hypothetically be treatable by RRT, this method is invasive and the optimal timing of starting treatment is still a matter of debate. Therefore lower stages of AKI are usually treated conservatively.

SHORT-TERM EFFECTS OF ACUTE KIDNEY INJURY: A NEW PERSPECTIVE

Over the past decade, extensive clinical and experimental data have shown that AKI is a systemic disease. In particular, the interactions between AKI and the immune system have become a focus of intense research. These efforts have been fueled by observations that patients with AKI have higher rates of infections such as bacteremia, infections after cardiac surgery, and infections in patients with hematologic malignancies.[67-69] Patients on RRT are particularly affected by infections. Almost half of the infections become apparent shortly before initiation of RRT, 40% during RRT, and approximately 10% in the period following discontinuation of RRT. Similar data have been described for the development of sepsis in AKI.[70] RRT does not seem to alter the AKI-associated risk of infection.[71,72]

Acute Kidney Injury and the Innate Immune System: Proinflammatory Changes

Most of the current knowledge stems from animal studies of the effect of AKI and remote, healthy organs. Almost all studies described models of either renal ischemia-reperfusion or bilateral nephrectomy and subsequent changes in lungs, heart, brain, and intestines.

Acute kidney injury and the lungs
In healthy lungs, ischemia-reperfusion–induced AKI leads to increases in vascular permeability, interstitial edema, wet/dry weight ratio, and expression of proinflammatory mediators and leukocyte adhesion molecules, and eventually interstitial infiltration by leukocytes and macrophages.[73-77] Ischemia-reperfusion injury of the kidney induces enhanced gene expression of proinflammatory mediators in the lung, which is substantially different from the effects of bilateral nephrectomy.[73] However, none of the studies assessed the effect of AKI on clinically relevant parameters (ie, gas exchange or pulmonary function tests). However, in critically ill patients AKI results in significantly longer requirement for mechanical ventilation even without oliguria.[78]

Acute kidney injury and the heart
Similar findings, including upregulation of proinflammatory mediators and recruitment of neutrophils, were found in the healthy rat heart together with cardiac apoptosis.[79] The investigators also showed functional echocardiographic changes such as increases in left ventricular end-diastolic diameter and left ventricular end-systolic diameter, and decreased fractional shortening. Similar to the observed effects in lungs, further analyses revealed that renal ischemia but not bilateral nephrectomy was necessary to induce these changes.

Acute kidney injury and the brain
Exaggerated inflammatory response to renal ischemia/reperfusion has also been detected in the brain, leading to increased vascular permeability, glial fibrillary acid protein expression, and apoptosis in the hippocampus. These changes were associated with significant functional impairment in terms of reaction time.[80]

Acute kidney injury and the gastrointestinal tract
Corresponding changes, including upregulation of inflammatory mediators, increased rate of apoptosis, and vascular permeability, have also been found in the liver and intestines.[81,82]

Acute kidney injury and cytokine homeostasis
All experimental changes described earlier can be attributed to the effect of proinflammatory cytokines. The surgery associated with the induction of experimental postischemic AKI, usually a midline laparotomy, leads to a profound release of proinflammatory cytokines (eg, interleukin-6 or tumor necrosis factor alpha), levels of which usually remain increased for several days. Sham surgery, which is comparable with respect to tissue trauma in these studies, does not lead to such an intense and prolonged cytokine release.[83] Thus, the decline in renal function during AKI is likely to

play a major role in cytokine clearance or lack thereof under these circumstances. In a rat model of rhabdomyolysis-induced AKI, the decline in renal function during AKI was closely followed by a decline in renal clearance of cytokines.[84] This decline in turn led to a sustained increase in plasma cytokine concentrations. Another mechanism by which cytokine levels are increased in AKI may be augmented production of inflammatory mediators by renal tubular cells in response to injury or cytokines,[85,86] which may even stimulate migration of neutrophils across epithelial cell layers.[85,87] Increased renal production rate of mediators leads to a systemic spill-over, which can be derived from systemic cytokine levels being higher after AKI induced by ischemia-reflow than by bilateral nephrectomy.[88] Recent investigations tried to focus on the cytokines causing distant organ effects in AKI. Increased pulmonary cytokine expression and lung injury caused by AKI can be exacerbated by splenectomy and attenuated by administration of interleukin-10.[89]

These experimental data suggest that AKI can modulate an underlying process, such as surgical stress, by reducing cytokine clearance and increasing the systemic load of inflammatory mediators by increased cytokine formation. Specific cytokine intervention may offer therapeutic hope.

Acute Kidney Injury and the Innate Immune System: Impaired Neutrophil Function

Both experimental and clinical data have shown that AKI exerts effects on innate immunity that go beyond modulation of cytokine homeostasis.

Animal studies

In a model of HCl-induced acute lung injury, AKI impairs polymorphonuclear cell (PMN) recruitment into the lungs and thereby improves oxygenation.[90] Only circulating uremic PMNs, but not normal PMNs, circulating in uremic plasma provide protection from acute lung injury. The wet/dry ratios of HCl-injured lungs are not affected by AKI. The effects of AKI on PMN function seem to be restricted to PMN recruitment. Other crucial features, such as apoptosis and production of reactive oxygen species, were not affected by AKI. Another experimental study combining AKI with ventilator-induced lung injury found decreased protein concentrations and PMN counts in the bronchoalveolar lavage fluid during AKI.[91]

A mouse model of *Pseudomonas aeruginosa* pneumonia combined with 2 different models of AKI revealed that AKI can worsen bacterial pneumonia.[92] AKI, in particular, impaired pulmonary recruitment of neutrophils. This impairment was followed by reduced pulmonary clearance of inhaled *P aeruginosa* and ultimately by worse oxygenation.

Further experimental studies revealed more insight into the underlying mechanisms.[93] AKI seems to increase neutrophil rolling velocity and thereby to reduce the number of neutrophils that can interact with the endothelium. Interactions between neutrophils and endothelial cells are essential for subsequent adhesion and transmigration. AKI also seems to negatively affect neutrophil transmigration through the endothelial cell layer directly. Additional experimental data support the notion that these effects are mediated by AKI-induced intracellular changes in F-actin polymerization and phosphorylation of signaling pathways.[92,93]

Clinical studies

A small prospective, observational study in critically ill patients with either sepsis alone or sepsis with severe AKI RIFLE-Failure (RIFLE-F[8]) has provided some evidence to validate the previously mentioned experimental findings at the bedside.[93]

Similar to experimental findings, expression levels of key adhesion molecules were not affected by AKI. Neutrophils from patients with sepsis-induced AKI showed

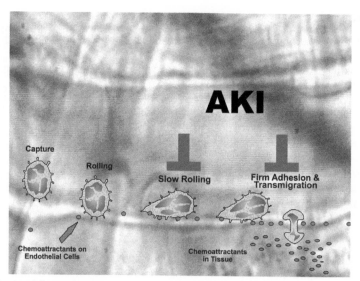

Fig. 2. Neutrophil recruitment cascade and AKI. Neutrophil recruitment into inflamed tissue occurs in a cascadelike fashion, which comprises capture, rolling, slow rolling, firm adhesion, and transmigration. Complex interactions between adhesion molecules and chemoattractant substances mediate each of these steps. AKI negatively affects both slow rolling and transmigration, decreasing overall recruitment of neutrophils.

abolished ex-vivo slow rolling, compared with neutrophils from healthy volunteers and patients with sepsis but no AKI.

The findings that AKI negatively affects PMN recruitment, in particular rolling and transmigration (**Fig. 2**), and subsequently causes higher bacterial load and worse organ function during a bacterial infection provide an excellent rationale for otherwise seemingly unrelated clinical entities. However, despite some observational clinical data supporting this hypothesis,[70] clinical evidence clearly linking AKI and subsequently increased risk for, or rate of, infections is currently missing.

SUMMARY

Over the last decade, AKI has emerged as a systemic disease process with potentially serious outcomes. AKI has both short-term and long-term effects. Some of the short-term effects (e.g. acidosis, hyperkalemia, and fluid overload) usually respond to current forms of RRT. However, all of these well-known short-term effects fail to explain the drastic effects that AKI has on morbidity and mortality.

Extensive evidence from experimental studies as well as some small clinical trials has revealed important interactions between AKI and innate immunity. Two key effects of AKI on innate immunity have been identified so far. AKI decreases cytokine clearance and stimulates renal cytokine production, thereby frequently leading to prolonged increase of proinflammatory cytokine levels in the setting of acute inflammatory processes. AKI also impairs two crucial steps within the leukocyte recruitment cascade. Both slow leukocyte rolling and transmigration are of utmost importance for directing leukocytes to the site of information. There is now experimental evidence that attenuated leukocyte recruitment in the setting of AKI worsens bacterial infections and ultimately organ function.

REFERENCES

1. Hoste EA, Schurgers M. Epidemiology of acute kidney injury: how big is the problem? Crit Care Med 2008;36:S146–51.
2. Singbartl K, Kellum JA. AKI in the ICU: definition, epidemiology, risk stratification, and outcomes. Kidney Int 2012;81:819–25.
3. Joannidis M, Metnitz PG. Epidemiology and natural history of acute renal failure in the ICU. Crit Care Clin 2005;21:239–49.
4. Metnitz PG, Krenn CG, Steltzer H, et al. Effect of acute renal failure requiring renal replacement therapy on outcome in critically ill patients. Crit Care Med 2002;30: 2051–8.
5. Elseviers MM, Lins RL, Van der Niepen P, et al. Renal replacement therapy is an independent risk factor for mortality in critically ill patients with acute kidney injury. Crit Care 2010;14:R221.
6. Chertow GM, Burdick E, Honour M, et al. Acute kidney injury, mortality, length of stay, and costs in hospitalized patients. J Am Soc Nephrol 2005;16: 3365–70.
7. Liangos O, Wald R, O'Bell JW, et al. Epidemiology and outcomes of acute renal failure in hospitalized patients: a national survey. Clin J Am Soc Nephrol 2006;1: 43–51.
8. Bellomo R, Ronco C, Kellum JA, et al. Acute renal failure - definition, outcome measures, animal models, fluid therapy and information technology needs: the Second International Consensus Conference of the Acute Dialysis Quality Initiative (ADQI) Group. Crit Care 2004;8:R204–12.
9. Mehta RL, Kellum JA, Shah SV, et al. Acute Kidney Injury Network: report of an initiative to improve outcomes in acute kidney injury. Crit Care 2007;11:R31.
10. KDIGO clinical practice Guideline for acute kidney injury. Kidney Int 2012;(Suppl 2):1–138.
11. Joannidis M, Metnitz B, Bauer P, et al. Acute kidney injury in critically ill patients classified by AKIN versus RIFLE using the SAPS 3 database. Intensive Care Med 2009;35:1692–702.
12. Ricci Z, Cruz D, Ronco C. The RIFLE criteria and mortality in acute kidney injury: a systematic review. Kidney Int 2008;73:538–46.
13. Hoste EA, Clermont G, Kersten A, et al. RIFLE criteria for acute kidney injury are associated with hospital mortality in critically ill patients: a cohort analysis. Crit Care 2006;10:R73.
14. Thakar CV, Christianson A, Freyberg R, et al. Incidence and outcomes of acute kidney injury in intensive care units: a Veterans Administration study. Crit Care Med 2009;37:2552–8.
15. Ishani A, Xue JL, Himmelfarb J, et al. Acute kidney injury increases risk of ESRD among elderly. J Am Soc Nephrol 2009;20:223–8.
16. Bihorac A, Yavas S, Subbiah S, et al. Long-term risk of mortality and acute kidney injury during hospitalization after major surgery. Ann Surg 2009;249:851–8.
17. Hobson CE, Yavas S, Segal MS, et al. Acute kidney injury is associated with increased long-term mortality after cardiothoracic surgery. Circulation 2009; 119:2444–53.
18. Chawla LS, Amdur RL, Amodeo S, et al. The severity of acute kidney injury predicts progression to chronic kidney disease. Kidney Int 2011;79:1361–9.
19. Clermont G, Acker CG, Angus DC, et al. Renal failure in the ICU: comparison of the impact of acute renal failure and end-stage renal disease on ICU outcomes. Kidney Int 2002;62:986–96.

20. Funk GC, Lindner G, Druml W, et al. Incidence and prognosis of dysnatremias present on ICU admission. Intensive Care Med 2010;36:304–11.
21. Kellum JA, Song M, Li J. Science review: extracellular acidosis and the immune response: clinical and physiologic implications. Crit Care 2004;8:331–6.
22. Payen D, de Pont AC, Sakr Y, et al. A positive fluid balance is associated with a worse outcome in patients with acute renal failure. Crit Care 2008;12:R74.
23. Uchino S, Bellomo R, Ronco C. Intermittent versus continuous renal replacement therapy in the ICU: impact on electrolyte and acid-base balance. Intensive Care Med 2001;27:1037–43.
24. Karet FE. Mechanisms in hyperkalemic renal tubular acidosis. J Am Soc Nephrol 2009;20:251–4.
25. Greenberg A. Hyperkalemia: treatment options. Semin Nephrol 1998;18:46–57.
26. Koo WS, Jeon DS, Ahn SJ, et al. Calcium-free hemodialysis for the management of hypercalcemia. Nephron 1996;72:424–8.
27. Massry SG, Arieff AI, Coburn JW, et al. Divalent ion metabolism in patients with acute renal failure: studies on the mechanism of hypocalcemia. Kidney Int 1974;5:437–45.
28. Forni LG, McKinnon W, Hilton PJ. Unmeasured anions in metabolic acidosis: unravelling the mystery. Crit Care 2006;10:220.
29. Rocktaeschel J, Morimatsu H, Uchino S, et al. Unmeasured anions in critically ill patients: can they predict mortality? Crit Care Med 2003;31:2131–6.
30. Hilton PJ, McKinnon W, Lord GA, et al. Unexplained acidosis of malnutrition: a study by ion-exchange chromatography/mass spectrometry. Biomed Chromatogr 2006;20:1386–9.
31. Kraut JA, Madias NE. Treatment of acute metabolic acidosis: a pathophysiologic approach. Nat Rev Nephrol 2012;8:589–601.
32. Orchard CH, Cingolani HE. Acidosis and arrhythmias in cardiac muscle. Cardiovasc Res 1994;28:1312–9.
33. Joannidis M, Forni LG. Clinical review: timing of renal replacement therapy. Crit Care 2011;15:223.
34. Duranton F, Cohen G, De Smet R, et al. Normal and pathologic concentrations of uremic toxins. J Am Soc Nephrol 2012;23:1258–70.
35. Vanholder R, Baurmeister U, Brunet P, et al. A bench to bedside view of uremic toxins. J Am Soc Nephrol 2008;19:863–70.
36. Herget-Rosenthal S, Glorieux G, Jankowski J, et al. Uremic toxins in acute kidney injury. Semin Dial 2009;22:445–8.
37. Harper SJ, Tomson CR, Bates DO. Human uremic plasma increases microvascular permeability to water and proteins in vivo. Kidney Int 2002;61:1416–22.
38. Lekawanvijit S, Kompa AR, Wang BH, et al. Cardiorenal syndrome: the emerging role of protein-bound uremic toxins. Circ Res 2012;111:1470–83.
39. Bagshaw SM, Hoste EA, Braam B, et al. Cardiorenal syndrome type 3: pathophysiologic and epidemiologic considerations. Contrib Nephrol 2013;182: 137–57.
40. Galbusera M, Remuzzi G, Boccardo P. Treatment of bleeding in dialysis patients. Semin Dial 2009;22:279–86.
41. Ma T, Liu X, Liu Z. Role of asymmetric dimethylarginine in rat acute lung injury induced by acute ischemic kidney injury. Mol Med Rep 2015. http://dx.doi.org/10.3892/mmr.2015.3619.
42. Vanholder R, Boelaert J, Glorieux G, et al. New methods and technologies for measuring uremic toxins and quantifying dialysis adequacy. Semin Dial 2015; 28:114–24.

43. Schetz M, Gunst J, Van den Berghe G. The impact of using estimated GFR versus creatinine clearance on the evaluation of recovery from acute kidney injury in the ICU. Intensive Care Med 2014;40:1709–17.

44. Doi K, Yuen PS, Eisner C, et al. Reduced production of creatinine limits its use as marker of kidney injury in sepsis. J Am Soc Nephrol 2009;20:1217–21.

45. Bouchard J, Soroko SB, Chertow GM, et al. Fluid accumulation, survival and recovery of kidney function in critically ill patients with acute kidney injury. Kidney Int 2009;76:422–7.

46. Sutherland SM, Zappitelli M, Alexander SR, et al. Fluid overload and mortality in children receiving continuous renal replacement therapy: the prospective pediatric continuous renal replacement therapy registry. Am J kidney Dis 2010;55: 316–25.

47. Prowle JR, Kirwan CJ, Bellomo R. Fluid management for the prevention and attenuation of acute kidney injury. Nat Rev Nephrol 2014;10:37–47.

48. Schmidt C, Höcherl K, Schweda F, et al. Regulation of renal sodium transporters during severe inflammation. J Am Soc Nephrol 2007;18:1072–83.

49. Marenzi G, Lauri G, Grazi M, et al. Circulatory response to fluid overload removal by extracorporeal ultrafiltration in refractory congestive heart failure. J Am Coll Cardiol 2001;38:963–8.

50. Sakr Y, Vincent JL, Reinhart K, et al. High tidal volume and positive fluid balance are associated with worse outcome in acute lung injury. Chest 2005;128: 3098–108.

51. Stuber F, Wrigge H, Schroeder S, et al. Kinetic and reversibility of mechanical ventilation-associated pulmonary and systemic inflammatory response in patients with acute lung injury. Intensive Care Med 2002;28:834–41.

52. Kim IB, Prowle J, Baldwin I, et al. Incidence, risk factors and outcome associations of intra-abdominal hypertension in critically ill patients. Anaesth Intensive Care 2012;40:79–89.

53. Legrand M, Dupuis C, Simon C, et al. Association between systemic hemodynamics and septic acute kidney injury in critically ill patients: a retrospective observational study. Crit Care 2013;17:R278.

54. Koyner JL, Davison DL, Brasha-Mitchell E, et al. Furosemide stress test and biomarkers for the prediction of AKI severity. J Am Soc Nephrol 2015. http://dx.doi.org/10.1681/asn.2014060535.

55. Brandstrup B, Tønnesen H, Beier-Holgersen R, et al. Effects of intravenous fluid restriction on postoperative complications: comparison of two perioperative fluid regimens: a randomized assessor-blinded multicenter trial. Ann Surg 2003;238: 641–8.

56. National Heart, Lung, and Blood Institute Acute Respiratory Distress Syndrome (ARDS) Clinical Trials Network, Wiedemann HP, Wheeler AP, et al. Comparison of two fluid-management strategies in acute lung injury. N Engl J Med 2006; 354:2564–75.

57. Mehta RL, Pascual MT, Soroko S, et al. Diuretics, mortality, and nonrecovery of renal function in acute renal failure. JAMA 2002;288:2547–53.

58. Uchino S, Doig GS, Bellomo R, et al. Diuretics and mortality in acute renal failure. Crit Care Med 2004;32:1669–77.

59. Ho KM, Power BM. Benefits and risks of furosemide in acute kidney injury. Anaesthesia 2010;65:283–93.

60. Joannidis M, Druml W, Forni LG, et al. Prevention of acute kidney injury and protection of renal function in the intensive care unit. Expert opinion of the Working Group for Nephrology, ESICM. Intensive Care Med 2010;36:392–411.

61. Uchino S, Bellomo R, Morimatsu H, et al. Continuous renal replacement therapy: a worldwide practice survey. Intensive Care Med 2007;33(9):1563–70.
62. RENAL Replacement Therapy Study Investigators, Bellomo R, Cass A, et al. Intensity of continuous renal-replacement therapy in critically ill patients. N Engl J Med 2009;361:1627–38.
63. Demirkilic U, Kuralay E, Yenicesu M, et al. Timing of replacement therapy for acute renal failure after cardiac surgery. J Card Surg 2004;19:17–20.
64. Elahi MM, Lim MY, Joseph RN, et al. Early hemofiltration improves survival in post-cardiotomy patients with acute renal failure. Eur J Cardiothorac Surg 2004;26:1027–31.
65. Piccinni P, Dan M, Barbacini S, et al. Early isovolaemic haemofiltration in oliguric patients with septic shock. Intensive Care Med 2006;32:80–6.
66. Bouman CS, Oudemans-Van Straaten HM, Tijssen JG, et al. Effects of early high-volume continuous venovenous hemofiltration on survival and recovery of renal function in intensive care patients with acute renal failure: a prospective, randomized trial. Crit Care Med 2002;30:2205–11.
67. Thakar CV, Yared JP, Worley S, et al. Renal dysfunction and serious infections after open-heart surgery. Kidney Int 2003;64:239–46.
68. De Waele JJ, Hoste EA, Blot SI. Blood stream infections of abdominal origin in the intensive care unit: characteristics and determinants of death. Surg Infect (Larchmt) 2008;9:171–7.
69. Tumbarello M, Spanu T, Caira M, et al. Factors associated with mortality in bacteremic patients with hematologic malignancies. Diagn Microbiol Infect Dis 2009;64: 320–6.
70. Mehta RL, Bouchard J, Soroko SB, et al. Sepsis as a cause and consequence of acute kidney injury: program to improve care in acute renal disease. Intensive Care Med 2011;37:241–8.
71. Reynvoet E, Vandijck DM, Blot SI, et al. Epidemiology of infection in critically ill patients with acute renal failure. Crit Care Med 2009;37:2203–9.
72. Hoste EA, Blot SI, Lameire NH, et al. Effect of nosocomial bloodstream infection on the outcome of critically ill patients with acute renal failure treated with renal replacement therapy. J Am Soc Nephrol 2004;15:454–62.
73. Hassoun HT, Grigoryev DN, Lie ML, et al. Ischemic acute kidney injury induces a distant organ functional and genomic response distinguishable from bilateral nephrectomy. Am J Physiol Renal Physiol 2007;293:F30–40.
74. Hassoun HT, Lie ML, Grigoryev DN, et al. Kidney ischemia-reperfusion injury induces caspase-dependent pulmonary apoptosis. Am J Physiol Renal Physiol 2009;297:F125–37.
75. Kramer AA, Postler G, Salhab KF, et al. Renal ischemia/reperfusion leads to macrophage-mediated increase in pulmonary vascular permeability. Kidney Int 1999;55:2362–7.
76. Rabb H, Wang Z, Nemoto T, et al. Acute renal failure leads to dysregulation of lung salt and water channels. Kidney Int 2003;63:600–6.
77. Altmann C, Andres-Hernando A, McMahan RH, et al. Macrophages mediate lung inflammation in a mouse model of ischemic acute kidney injury. Am J Physiol Renal Physiol 2012;302:F421–32.
78. Vieira JM Jr, Castro I, Curvello-Neto A, et al. Effect of acute kidney injury on weaning from mechanical ventilation in critically ill patients. Crit Care Med 2007;35: 184–91.
79. Kelly KJ. Distant effects of experimental renal ischemia/reperfusion injury. J Am Soc Nephrol 2003;14:1549–58.

80. Liu M, Liang Y, Chigurupati S, et al. Acute kidney injury leads to inflammation and functional changes in the brain. J Am Soc Nephrol 2008;19:1360–70.
81. Golab F, Kadkhodaee M, Zahmatkesh M, et al. Ischemic and non-ischemic acute kidney injury cause hepatic damage. Kidney Int 2009;75:783–92.
82. Park SW, Chen SW, Kim M, et al. Cytokines induce small intestine and liver injury after renal ischemia or nephrectomy. Lab Invest 2011;91:63–84.
83. Kelly KJ, Williams WW Jr, Colvin RB, et al. Intercellular adhesion molecule-1-deficient mice are protected against ischemic renal injury. J Clin Invest 1996; 97:1056–63.
84. Zager RA, Johnson AC, Lund S, et al. Acute renal failure: determinants and characteristics of the injury-induced hyperinflammatory response. Am J Physiol Renal Physiol 2006;291:F546–56.
85. Bijuklic K, Sturn DH, Jennings P, et al. Mechanisms of neutrophil transmigration across renal proximal tubular HK-2 cells. Cell Physiol Biochem 2006;17:233–44.
86. Joannidis M, Truebsbach S, Bijuklic K, et al. Neutrophil transmigration in renal proximal tubular LLC-PK1 cells. Cell Physiol Biochem 2004;14:101–12.
87. Bijuklic K, Jennings P, Kountchev J, et al. Migration of leukocytes across an endothelium-epithelium bilayer as a model of renal interstitial inflammation. Am J Physiol Cell Physiol 2007;293:C486–92.
88. Hoke TS, Douglas IS, Klein CL, et al. Acute renal failure after bilateral nephrectomy is associated with cytokine-mediated pulmonary injury. J Am Soc Nephrol 2007;18:155–64.
89. Andres-Hernando A, Altmann C, Ahuja N, et al. Splenectomy exacerbates lung injury after ischemic acute kidney injury in mice. Am J Physiol Renal Physiol 2011;301:F907–16.
90. Zarbock A, Schmolke M, Spieker T, et al. Acute uremia but not renal inflammation attenuates aseptic acute lung injury: a critical role for uremic neutrophils. J Am Soc Nephrol 2006;17:3124–31.
91. Dodd OJ, Hristopoulos M, Scharfstein D, et al. Interactive effects of mechanical ventilation and kidney health on lung function in an in vivo mouse model. Am J Physiol Lung Cell Mol Physiol 2009;296:L3–11.
92. Singbartl K, Bishop JV, Wen X, et al. Differential effects of kidney-lung cross-talk during acute kidney injury and bacterial pneumonia. Kidney Int 2011;80:633–44.
93. Rossaint J, Spelten O, Kässens N, et al. Acute loss of renal function attenuates slow leukocyte rolling and transmigration by interfering with intracellular signaling. Kidney Int 2011;80:493–503.

Long-Term Follow-up of Acute Kidney Injury

James F. Doyle, MBChB, PGcertCU[a], Lui G. Forni, BSc, MB, PhD[a,b],*

KEYWORDS

- Acute kidney injury • Outcome • Follow-up • Critical illness • Critical care
- Intensive care

KEY POINTS

- Acute kidney injury (AKI) during critical illness has a high incidence. The standardized definitions of AKI have helped identify patients at risk and have highlighted worsening long-term outcomes in these patients.
- The development of a single episode of AKI during critical illness predisposes to chronic kidney disease (CKD).
- Active management with continuous renal replacement therapy (RRT), when indicated; appropriate fluid therapy; early nephrology referral; and on-going monitoring of renal parameters after the initial step down from an intensive care unit will hopefully improve long-term outcomes for AKI.
- Renal recovery may be more difficult to define than originally envisaged. Clinicians should be aware of the limitations of using creatinine as a marker of the glomerular filtration rate (GFR), particularly in those recovering from multiorgan failure where renal insufficiency may be overlooked.

INTRODUCTION

AKI confers an increased mortality risk owing to the interplay between the concomitant acidosis, volume overload, electrolyte disturbance, increased susceptibility to infection, and the impact on other organ functions that may ensue.[1] The sequelae of renal injury, however, are not limited to the acute episode, with growing evidence supporting the observation that an episode of AKI may increase the risk of both morbidity and mortality in the longer term.[2] This is of significance given that AKI is a

Disclosure statement: The authors have nothing to disclose.
[a] Intensive Care Unit, Department of Intensive Care Medicine, Surrey Peri-Operative Anaesthesia and Critical Care Collaborative Research Group, Royal Surrey County Hospital, NHS Foundation Trust, Egerton Road, Guildford, Surrey GU2 7XX, UK; [b] Faculty of Health and Medical Sciences, University of Surrey, Guildford, Surrey, UK
* Corresponding author. Intensive Care Unit, Department of Intensive Care Medicine, Surrey Peri-Operative Anaesthesia and Critical Care Collaborative Research Group, Royal Surrey County Hospital, NHS Foundation Trust, Egerton Road, Guildford, Surrey GU2 7XX, UK.
E-mail address: luiforni@nhs.net

Crit Care Clin 31 (2015) 763–772
http://dx.doi.org/10.1016/j.ccc.2015.06.017
0749-0704/15/$ – see front matter © 2015 Elsevier Inc. All rights reserved.
criticalcare.theclinics.com

common encounter in the general hospital setting where 15% of admitted patients sustain an episode of AKI, and in critical care this increases to over 25% whereas in pediatric practice the incidence varies depending on casemix.[3,4] The acute mortality of all critically ill patients has improved over the past 16 years but patients whose critical illness is complicated by AKI have a significantly higher risk of mortality, with this risk continuing for at least 2 years after the index ICU admission.[5] Furthermore, despite a temporal trend demonstrating a reduced risk of dialysis dependence after an episode of AKI, there are potentially more patients surviving, thereby increasing the burden on the health economy further.[6] This is reflected in the total annual cost of AKI-related inpatient care, which has been estimated at £1.02 billion, or just over 1% of the National Health Service budget, in the United Kingdom.[7] As a consequence, it is no surprise that the long-term outcome for patients with AKI, examining mortality, morbidity, and quality of life, is now receiving appropriate attention.[8,9] This article discusses some of the limitations in defining renal recovery using conventional methods and considers how the acute management of patients with AKI may influence long-term outcomes. The issue of identification of patients who may benefit from enhanced follow-up is addressed and long-term management principles for patients who have had an episode of AKI is considered.

DEFINING RECOVERY
What Is Meant by Recovery?

Since the first description of the Risk, Injury, Failure, Loss of Kidney Function, and End-stage Kidney Disease (RIFLE) criteria, the definition of AKI has undergone several reincarnations. More recently the Kidney Disease: Improving Global Outcomes (KDIGO) guidelines define AKI according to changes in serum creatinine and urine output and classify AKI by stages 1, 2, and 3.[10] Similarly, CKD is also defined by KDIGO and reflects both chronic structural change to the kidneys and functional change, for example, in terms of creatinine clearance.[11] The definition of CKD requires at least 2 creatinine estimations at least 90 days apart, which has led to the concept of acute kidney disease (AKD), which describes the transition between the acute and chronic states.[12] This in itself, however, is not straightforward. **Fig. 1** outlines the potential course of patients recovering from an episode of AKI. They may recover function (the definition of which is discussed) or progress to AKD. Further insult may lead,

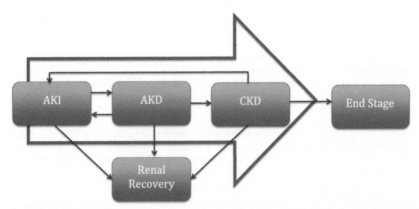

Fig. 1. Schematic describing the potential course of a patient surviving an episode of AKI.

however, to another episode of AKI and, thereafter, progress to CKD, or patients may suffer a further episode of AKI or may recover function. Hence, the recovery from an index episode of AKI does not then confer a steady transition from injury to recovery. So what defines recovery? Despite the efforts in defining AKI, the definition of renal recovery has not received as much attention; yet, a standardized definition of renal recovery is necessary to inform with regard to post-AKI epidemiology. This was first considered within the RIFLE criteria, where loss and end-stage kidney disease were described, which used both estimated GFR (eGFR) and time components within their metrics. Since then, a few studies have attempted to define recovery from AKI but often with regard to the necessity for RRT. Although it may be convenient to describe recovery as the cessation of RRT, the criteria for stopping are far from uniform, although some studies have addressed this[13]; also, recovery to a GFR of 20% of premorbid function, for example, cannot be considered recovery. Therefore, defining recovery needs to consider both the degree of recovery, which may be return to baseline, and the timing. To date no such consensus prevails.

Limitations of Conventional Markers of Acute Kidney Injury

Creatinine provides the mainstay for the outpatient management of chronic renal disease as a biomarker for the GFR, performing best under clinically stable conditions.[14] Despite this, creatinine is used as a surrogate for GFR during AKI in critically ill unstable patients because the GFR is rarely measured in clinical practice. Even in an outpatient setting, serum creatinine may be misleading and, therefore, various equations have been developed for eGFR from the serum creatinine where differences in age, gender, and race are considered. These include the Modification of Diet in Renal Disease and the Chronic Kidney Disease Epidemiology Collaboration equations.[15–17] AKI presents different challenges and creatinine performs less well in the intensive care environment. This is due in part to the reduction observed in muscle bulk in the critically ill coupled with reduced creatinine generation in sepsis that is encountered in approximately 50% of patients with AKI.[18–21] It follows that the application of those equations may lead to a significant overestimation of the GFR. Therefore, defining renal recovery where the eGFR is used is inherently flawed, and this has been observed in several studies where formal measurement of the GFR has been compared with the eGFR and considerable disparity observed.[22] So, this must be considered when defining renal recovery using eGFR, particularly in long-stay ICU patients. Similarly, creatinine by definition determines AKI but, given that there is a considerable delay between renal injury and any observed rise in creatinine, this again highlights the inadequacies of creatinine estimation in the critically ill.

A Role for Alternative Markers of Acute Kidney Injury

Given the inadequacies of currently readily available markers of renal function, attention has turned to newer biomarkers, which may provide more timely information regarding renal status. Several candidates have been championed almost exclusively as markers of renal injury with varying degrees of success,[23] although recently, a combination of biomarkers Tissue Inhibitor of Metalloproteinase-2/Insulin-Like Growth Factor-7 (TIMP-2/IGFBP7) with urine output and serum creatinine has been validated as superior to predicting dialysis at 9 months in patients with AKI.[24–27] Also, a residual effect from an episode of AKI on biomarkers of acute injury has been observed remaining elevated years after an episode of AKI after cardiac surgery in children.[28] Given the current research landscape, most efforts have addressed the need for early identification of AKI rather than evidence for renal repair. To date most efforts have been applied to predicting renal recovery or transition to CKD based on available clinical and laboratory variables.[29] There is limited knowledge regarding repair or progression-specific biomarkers. Recent evidence from animal studies suggest, however, upregulation of genes that code for biomarkers associated with renal injury may be surrogates for progressive renal injury following ischemic insult.[30] Further studies have shown that renal recovery was slower in patients who had increased concentrations of plasma interleukin (IL)-8, IL-18, and tumor necrosis factor receptor 1.[31] Potential processes involved in the transition between AKI, AKD, and CKD are outlined in **Fig. 2**. These early observations suggest that markers of kidney repair as well as disease progression may help untangle the complexities of renal repair and recovery after AKI and may eventually lead to a better description of AKD.[32]

ACUTE KIDNEY INJURY: WHAT ARE THE LONG-TERM RISKS?

There have been several studies supporting the observation that AKI and CKD may be associated but demonstration of a clear association does not necessarily confer causation.[33–35] Studies are often hindered by a lack of high-quality data, particularly regarding premorbid and post-AKI renal function; however, the evidence does support long-term follow-up of patients who have suffered an episode of AKI.[36] For example, data from Canada examined the effect of renal recovery after AKI in a population-based cohort study of 190,714 individuals. In those who did not recover kidney function, a higher risk for mortality and adverse renal outcomes was observed compared with those who recovered to within 25% of baseline creatinine.[37] Evidence for an increase in the long-term risk of coronary events after AKI is provided by data from Taiwan, which again showed an increase in mortality.[38] In individuals who required RRT for AKI, a higher risk of coronary events was observed compared with non-AKI controls (hazard ratio [HR] 1.67; 95% [95% CI], 1.36–2.04) and all-cause mortality (HR 1.67; 95% CI, 1.57–1.79). The same group also reported a significant increase in the risk of stroke events.[39] There are several ongoing prospective studies focusing on the link between AKI and CKD with detailed data collection, including biomarkers, which may well inform future practice.[40]

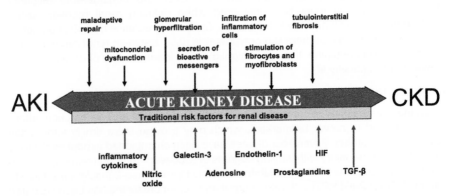

Fig. 2. Potential pathophysiologic processes involved in AKI/AKD/CKD pathway. HIF, hypoxia-inducible factor; TGF, transforming growth factor. (*Adapted from* Varrier M, Forni LG, Ostermann M. Long-term sequelae from acute kidney injury: potential mechanisms for the observed poor renal outcomes. Crit Care 2015;19(1):102; with permission.)

ETIOLOGY OF ACUTE KIDNEY INJURY AFFECTING OUTCOME

Although classically the etiology of AKI can be considered prerenal, renal, or postrenal, over the past few decades the incidence of AKI as a consequence of multiorgan dysfunction in ICUs has steadily risen. As a consequence, single organ failure is less commonly encountered in ICUs. Moreover, there has been a decrease in trauma-induced AKI and obstetric-related AKI[41] whereas severe sepsis is associated with AKI in 50% of critical care patients and has been shown to increase 2-year mortality.[42] AKI developing postoperatively is again thought to be multifactorial, and recent evidence demonstrated a recurrent kidney injury (RKI) rate of 31% and in the event of RKI an increase in 12-month mortality and long-term worsening of renal function.[43] A recent study suggests that outcome is related to etiology with sepsis-associated AKI having the worst outlook.[44]

CURRENT MANAGEMENT OF ACUTE KIDNEY INJURY AND AFFECT ON OUTCOME

The management of AKI remains supportive in nature. Guidelines exist as to the prevention and treatment of AKI, particularly in the ICU, but most of these are lacking in substantial robust evidence base. There is no evidence supporting any pharmaceutical interventions to date to treat AKI and as such it is unlikely that these will affect renal recovery and hence follow-up. What is clear is that overzealous use of intravascular fluid therapy resulting in volume overload is associated with worse renal outcomes and should be avoided.[45] Ideally, volume resuscitation in AKI should be targeted to defined endpoints to avoid unnecessary volume overload. There is also growing evidence that the mainstay of treatment of severe AKI, namely RRT, may play a role in long-term outcomes with continuous therapies providing a potential survival benefit, as suggested by a recent meta-analysis.[46] Although the mechanisms behind this remain unclear, it does not seem related to the dose of treatment delivered. An extended 4-year follow-up of the randomised evaluation of normal versus augmented level of renal replacement therapy in intensive care (RENAL) study confirmed that both short (90-day) and long (4-year) mortality or the subsequent need for chronic dialysis was not affected by the dosing of RRT.[5]

IDENTIFICATION OF THE PATIENT AT ENHANCED LONG-TERM RISK

AKI is, unfortunately, a common event in both primary and secondary care settings and, therefore, robust local pathways should be in place regarding follow-up and nephrology referral. Evidence suggesting that this does occur, however, is scarce. For example, a recent observational study from the United Kingdom identified 219 patients from an ICU cohort who had undergone RRT for severe AKI. Of these, only 57% had appropriate postdischarge investigations and only 12% of survivors received specialist nephrology follow-up.[47] These results are in keeping with an earlier study from the United States, which demonstrated a similarly depressing figure of less than 10%.[48] This is despite compelling evidence suggesting that nephrology follow-up reduces all-cause mortality in patients with severe AKI who undergo RRT as well as evidence that early referral to nephrology services in patients with CKD also demonstrates a survival benefit.[49,50] The transition from AKI to CKD provides a potential opportunity to influence patient outcome in those individuals who fulfill the AKD criteria. These criteria have been described by KDIGO as GFR less than 60 mL/min/1.73 m^2 for less than 3 months or decrease in GFR by greater than 35% or increase in serum creatinine by greater than 50% for less than 3 months.[10] Individuals at highest risk may also be identified by the application of risk prediction models; for

Table 1
Proposed patient pathway for monitoring of acute kidney disease

eGFR (mL/min/1.73 m²)		ACR Categories (mg/mmol)		
		<3 A1	3–30 A2	>30 A3
>90	G1	No features of significant renal disease Measure eGFR at 90 d	No features of significant renal disease Measure eGFR at 90 d	No features of significant renal disease Measure eGFR at 90 d Measure eGFR 2–4 wk postdischarge Nephrology referral
60–89	G2			
45–59	G3a			
30–44	G3b		Nephrology referral	
15–29	G4	Nephrology referral		
<15	G5			

Features of significant renal disease include persistent proteinuria and hematuria, suspected glomerulonephritis, known structural renal disease (eg, acute polycystic kidney disease), suspected urologic disease, and hypertension refractory to treatment.

Abbreviations: A1–A3, ACR categories; G1–G5, GFR categories.

example, in survivors of dialysis-requiring AKI who initially become dialysis independent, the subsequent need for chronic RRT is predicted by preexisting CKD, hypertension, and global comorbidities.[51] Although several such models have been described, they still require validation in larger study groups.[52] If patients with AKD who have survived severe AKI (KDIGO stage 2 at least) are considered, then timing of follow-up is determined by several features. The presence of chronic intrinsic renal diseases (eg, glomerulonephritis and vasculitis) requires specialist nephrologist intervention to manage therapies and their side effects that require close observation. A majority of patients, however, do not fall under this remit, so how is follow-up approached? Fortunately the management of CKD has robust recommendations regarding CKD follow-up, which rely on eGFR and the presence of proteinuria expressed as an albumin:creatinine ratio (ACR) in mg/mmol. A model can be envisaged whereby these parameters are incorporated into a proposed patient pathway, which should ensure appropriate referral. **Table 1** outlines such a proposed model and although this cannot possibly describe every potential clinical scenario, it provides a framework for referral and follows the CKD pathway described by KDIGO. Although this proposed model relies on the use of the eGFR with its inherent flaws, as highlighted previously, it remains the methodology used to classify and monitor CKD. Specific clinical evaluation is necessary for all patients with AKD, or AKI, although the diagnostic approach usually begins with assessment of the GFR and the serum creatinine assessment is not complete unless other markers of kidney damage have been performed. These markers include urinalysis, examination of the urinary sediment, and imaging studies as well as specific tests as appropriate. Identification of patients at risk should then allow referral to appropriate services.

LONG-TERM MANAGEMENT AFTER ACUTE KIDNEY INJURY

The long-term management of patients who have survived an episode of severe AKI should follow the aims of that described for management of patients with CKD.[11] Prevention of progression of CKD includes general measures, which have been shown to address cardiovascular health and include general lifestyle measures, control of hypertension following national guidelines, and interruption of the renin-angiotensin-aldosterone system. With regard to blood pressure control, these should be individualized to age, coexistent cardiovascular disease, and other comorbidities, with particular regard to the elderly. In patients with proteinuria (ACR <30 mg/24 h) and CKD, the blood pressure target should be consistently less than 140 mm Hg systolic and less than 90 mm Hg diastolic whereas in heavy proteinuric states the target should be consistently less than 130 mm Hg systolic and less than 80 mm Hg diastolic. Furthermore, in diabetic patients with CKD in the presence of microalbuminuria, renin-angiotensin-aldosterone system antagonism should be used. Given that CKD is a risk factor for AKI, patients with AKD or CKD should be considered high risk for further episodes of AKI, particularly during intercurrent illness or when undergoing investigation and procedures that are likely to increase the risk of AKI. In addition, patients with AKD/CKD should be offered dietary and lifestyle advice. Specific targeted therapy for the complications of CKD within this patient group may well have considerable repercussions with regard to long-term improvement in patient outcomes as well as considerable cost savings.

SUMMARY

The long-term sequelae of AKI are now more apparent and an episode of AKI, particularly when necessitating RRT, confers considerable future risks. This is reflected in an increase incidence of CKD, cardiovascular events, and stroke as well as significant effect on the quality of life of survivors. Unsurprisingly this is also associated with considerable health costs. Early identification of patients at risk of CKD and targeted referral where appropriate may go some way to improving patient outcomes and offering considerable cost savings to the local health economy.

REFERENCES

1. Srisawat N, Sileanu FE, Murugan R, et al. Variation in risk and mortality of acute kidney injury in critically ill patients: a multicenter study. Am J Nephrol 2015;41(1):81–8.
2. Heung M, Chawla LS. Acute kidney injury: gateway to chronic kidney disease. Nephron Clin Pract 2014;127(1–4):30–4.
3. Bedford M, Stevens PE, Wheeler TW, et al. What is the real impact of acute kidney injury? BMC Nephrol 2014;15:95.
4. Gulati S. Acute kidney injury in children. Clinical Queries: Nephrology 2012;1(1): 103–8.
5. Gallagher M, Cass A, Bellomo R, et al. Long-term survival and dialysis dependency following acute kidney injury in intensive care: extended follow-up of a randomized controlled trial. PLoS Med 2014;11(2):e1001601.
6. Schiffl H, Lang SM, Fischer R. Long-term outcomes of survivors of ICU acute kidney injury requiring renal replacement therapy: a 10-year prospective cohort study. Clin Kidney J 2012;5(4):297–302.
7. Kerr M, Bedford M, Matthews B, et al. The economic impact of acute kidney injury in England. Nephrol Dial Transplant 2014;29(7):1362–8.
8. Bell M. Acute kidney injury: new concepts, renal recovery. Nephron Clin Pract 2008;109(4):c224–8.
9. Fertmann J, Wolf H, Kuchenhoff H, et al. Prognostic factors in critically ill surgical patients requiring continuous renal replacement therapy. J Nephrol 2008;21(6):909–18.
10. Kidney Disease: Improving Global Outcomes (KDIGO) Acute Kidney Injury Work Group. KDIGO clinical practice guideline for acute kidney injury. Kidney Int 2012; 2(Suppl 1):1–138.
11. Kidney Disease: Improving Global Outcomes (KDIGO) Acute Kidney Injury Work Group. KDIGO clinical practice guideline for acute kidney injury. Kidney Int 2012; 2(Suppl 1):1–133.
12. Goldstein SL, Jaber BL, Faubel S, et al. AKI transition of care: a potential opportunity to detect and prevent CKD. Clin J Am Soc Nephrol 2013;8(3):476–83.
13. Palevsky PM, Zhang JH, O'Connor TZ, et al, The VA/NIH Acute Renal Failure Trial Network. Intensity of renal support in critically ill patients with acute kidney injury. N Engl J Med 2008;359(1):7–20.
14. Perrone RD, Madias NE, Levey AS. Serum creatinine as an index of renal function: new insights into old concepts. Clin Chem 1992;38(10):1933–53.
15. Stevens LA, Coresh J, Greene T, et al. Assessing kidney function–measured and estimated glomerular filtration rate. N Engl J Med 2006;354(23):2473–83.
16. Lai CF, Wu VC, Huang TM, et al. Kidney function decline after a non-dialysis-requiring acute kidney injury is associated with higher long-term mortality in critically ill survivors. Crit Care 2012;16(4):R123.
17. Carlier M, Dumoulin A, Janssen A, et al. Comparison of different equations to assess glomerular filtration in critically ill patients. Intensive Care Med 2015; 41(3):427–35.
18. Heimburger O, Stenvinkel P, Barany P. The enigma of decreased creatinine generation in acute kidney injury. Nephrol Dial Transplant 2012;27(11):3973–4.

19. Beddhu S, Samore MH, Roberts MS, et al. Creatinine production, nutrition, and glomerular filtration rate estimation. J Am Soc Nephrol 2003;14(4):1000–5.

20. Doi K, Yuen PS, Eisner C, et al. Reduced production of creatinine limits its use as marker of kidney injury in sepsis. J Am Soc Nephrol 2009;20(6):1217–21.

21. Wilson FP, Sheehan JM, Mariani LH, et al. Creatinine generation is reduced in patients requiring continuous venovenous hemodialysis and independently predicts mortality. Nephrol Dial Transplant 2012;27(11):4088–94.

22. Schetz M, Gunst J, Van den Berghe G. The impact of using estimated GFR versus creatinine clearance on the evaluation of recovery from acute kidney injury in the ICU. Intensive Care Med 2014;40(11):1709–17.

23. Ostermann M, Philips BJ, Forni LG. Clinical review: biomarkers of acute kidney injury: where are we now? Crit Care 2012;16:233.

24. Kashani K, Al-Khafaji A, Ardiles T, et al. Discovery and validation of cell cycle arrest biomarkers in human acute kidney injury. Crit Care 2013;17(1):R25.

25. Gocze I, Koch M, Renner P, et al. Urinary Biomarkers TIMP-2 and IGFBP7 early predict acute kidney injury after major surgery. PLoS One 2015;10(3):e0120863.

26. Meersch M, Schmidt C, Van Aken H, et al. Urinary TIMP-2 and IGFBP7 as early biomarkers of acute kidney injury and renal recovery following cardiac surgery. PLoS One 2014;9(3):e93460.

27. Koyner JL, Shaw AD, Chawla LS, et al. Tissue inhibitor Metalloproteinase-2 (TIMP-2)-IGF-Binding Protein-7 (IGFBP7) levels are associated with adverse long-term outcomes in patients with AKI. J Am Soc Nephrol 2014;26:1747–54.

28. Cooper DS, Claes DC, Goldstein SG, et al. Novel urinary biomarkers remain elevated years after acute kidney injury following cardiac surgery in children. Pediatr Crit Care Med 2014;15(4 Suppl):25.

29. Chawla LS, Eggers PW, Star RA, et al. Acute kidney injury and chronic kidney disease as interconnected syndromes. N Engl J Med 2014;371(1):58–66.

30. Ko GJ, Grigoryev DN, Linfert D, et al. Transcriptional analysis of kidneys during repair from AKI reveals possible roles for NGAL and KIM-1 as biomarkers of AKI-to-CKD transition. Am J Physiol Renal Physiol 2010;298:F1472–83.

31. Murugan R, Wen X, Shah N, et al. Plasma inflammatory and apoptosis markers are associated with dialysis dependence and death among critically ill patients receiving renal replacement therapy. Nephrol Dial Transplant 2014;29(10):1854–64.

32. Kashani K, Kellum JA. Novel biomarkers indicating repair or progression after acute kidney injury. Curr Opin Nephrol Hypertens 2015;24(1):21–7.

33. Leung KC, Tonelli M, James MT. Chronic kidney disease following acute kidney injury-risk and outcomes. Nat Rev Nephrol 2012;9(2):77–85.

34. Venkatachalam MA, Griffin KA, Lan R, et al. Acute kidney injury: a springboard for progression in chronic kidney disease. Am J Physiol Renal Physiol 2010;298:F1078–94.

35. Bucaloiu ID, Kirchner HL, Norfolk ER, et al. Increased risk of death and de novo chronic kidney disease following reversible acute kidney injury. Kidney Int 2012;81:477–85.

36. Bagshaw SM, Laupland KB, Doig CJ, et al. Prognosis for long-term survival and renal recovery in critically ill patients with severe acute renal failure: a population-based study. Crit Care 2005;9(6):R700–9.

37. Pannu N, James M, Hemmelgarn B, et al. Association between AKI, recovery of renal function, and long-term outcomes after hospital discharge. Clin J Am Soc Nephrol 2013;8(2):194.

38. Wu V-C, Wu CH, Huang TM, et al. Long-term risk of coronary events after AKI. J Am Soc Nephrol 2014;25(3):595.

39. Wu V-C, Wu PC, Wu CH, et al. The impact of acute kidney injury on the long-term risk of stroke. J Am Heart Assoc 2014;3(4):595–605.

40. Varrier M, Forni LG, Ostermann M. Long-term sequelae from acute kidney injury: potential mechanisms for the observed poor renal outcomes. Crit Care 2015; 19(1):102.

41. Shah SH, Mehta RL. Acute kidney injury in critical care: time for a paradigm shift? Curr Opin Nephrol Hypertens 2006;15(6):561–5.

42. Lopes JA, Fernandes P, Jorge S, et al. Long-term risk of mortality after acute kidney injury in patients with sepsis: a contemporary analysis. BMC Nephrol 2010; 11:9.

43. Harris DG, Koo G, McCrone MP, et al. Recurrent kidney injury in critically ill surgical patients is common and associated with worse outcomes. J Trauma Acute Care Surg 2014;76(6):1397–401.

44. Waikar SS, Liu KD, Chertow GM. Diagnosis, epidemiology and outcomes of acute kidney injury. Clin J Am Soc Nephrol 2008;3(3):844–61.

45. Bouchard J, Soroko SB, Chertow GM, et al. Fluid accumulation, survival and recovery of kidney function in critically ill patients with acute kidney injury. Kidney Int 2009;76:422–7.

46. Schneider AG, Bellomo R, Bagshaw SM, et al. Choice of renal replacement therapy modality and dialysis dependence after acute kidney injury: a systematic review and meta-analysis. Intensive Care Med 2013;39(6):987–97.

47. Kirwan CJ, Blunden MJ, Dobbie H, et al. Critically ill patients requiring acute renal replacement therapy are at an increased risk of long-term renal dysfunction, but rarely receive specialist nephrology follow-up. Nephron 2015;129(3):164–70.

48. Siew ED, Peterson JF, Eden SK, et al. Outpatient nephrology referral rates after acute kidney injury. J Am Soc Nephrol 2012;23(2):305–12.

49. Harel Z, Wald R, Bargman JM, et al. Nephrologist follow-up improves all-cause mortality of severe acute kidney injury survivors. Kidney Int 2013;83(5):901–8.

50. Smart NA, Dieberg G, Ladhani M, et al. Early referral to specialist nephrology services for preventing the progression to end-stage kidney disease. Cochrane Database Syst Rev 2014;(6):CD007333.

51. Harel Z, Bell CM, Dixon SN, et al. Predictors of progression to chronic dialysis in survivors of severe acute kidney injury: a competing risk study. BMC Nephrol 2014;15:114.

52. Heung M, Chawla LS. Predicting progression to chronic kidney disease after recovery from acute kidney injury. Curr Opin Nephrol Hypertens 2012;21(6): 628–34.

Preventing Acute Kidney Injury

Etienne Macedo, MD, PhD[a,b], Ravindra L. Mehta, MD[a,*]

KEYWORDS

- Acute kidney injury • Prevention • Epidemiology

KEY POINTS

- The International Society of Nephrology 0by25 initiative's main goal is to reduce avoidable acute kidney injury (AKI)–related deaths around the world by 2025.
- The 0by25 initiative proposed the use of the 5R (risk assessment, recognition, response, renal support, and rehabilitation) framework.
- Awareness of the factors that affect AKI outcomes is a key step for implementing initiatives and reducing AKI-related mortality and morbidity.
- A general risk score for AKI can help select patients for closer follow-up and early nephrology referral.

INTRODUCTION

The worldwide application of the RIFLE/AKIN, and most recently KDIGO, acute kidney injury (AKI) classification systems has confirmed the increasing incidence of AKI in different settings. The efforts of nephrology and critical care societies and groups to unify a classification system have enabled comparisons of AKI incidence and outcomes across diverse populations. The resultant epidemiologic studies have shown increasing severity of AKI and higher risk of death associated with AKI in both hospital and community settings.[1–3] In addition, AKI is now a recognized important risk factor for new-onset chronic kidney disease (CKD), determining acceleration in progression to end-stage renal disease (ESRD), and leading to poor quality of life, disability, and long-term costs.[4–6]

Although the effects of these efforts to spread the use of a standardized AKI classification system are unquestionable, clinical application can still be improved. Most studies on AKI are derived from developed countries and mainly focus on intensive

Disclosures: None.
[a] Department of Medicine, University of California San Diego, 200 West Arbor Drive, San Diego, CA 92103, USA; [b] Nephrology Division, University of Sao Paulo, Brazil
* Corresponding author.
E-mail address: rmehta@ucsd.edu

Crit Care Clin 31 (2015) 773–784
http://dx.doi.org/10.1016/j.ccc.2015.06.011
0749-0704/15/$ – see front matter © 2015 Elsevier Inc. All rights reserved.

care unit (ICU) populations. In developed countries, the easy access to patients' data, laboratory tests, and computerized systems improves the quantity and the quality of AKI information. Information on the increasing associated mortality of even mild AKI and the effects of an AKI episode on long-term outcomes has driven more investment into early detection and treatment of AKI. The focus in more developed areas, especially in ICU patients, is to learn how to apply new biomarkers of AKI to determine risk, avoid progression, and treat AKI earlier.

However, in less developed areas of the globe, especially in low-income countries (LIC) and low-middle–income countries (LMIC), where 85% of the world's population lives, the epidemiology of AKI is diverse and access to care is limited. In LMIC, the lack of infrastructure and resources are key problems. Limited availability of health workers, diagnostic equipment, and limited hospital resources are among the reasons why AKI is poorly recognized and treated in LMIC. Scattered data from these regions show a high incidence of avoidable deaths from AKI. With identification of risk, routines for screening, provision of simpler tests, and basic treatment, most of these AKI cases would be treatable and often reversible.[7] In more severe cases, availability of dialysis could avoid deaths. However, dialysis is unavailable for large parts of the population in LMIC because most national health systems in the poorest nations do not provide dialysis facilities.

The lack of knowledge and recognition that the kidney is essential to maintain life is another barrier to increasing the awareness of AKI. Because AKI is not associated with any specific symptoms and the diagnosis is largely based on measurement of laboratory parameters, AKI is often not recognized. Caregivers may not be equipped with the knowledge for early recognition, timely intervention, and effective follow-up. Thus, key opportunities to prevent and treat AKI are lost and this results in disability and a significant loss of life.[8]

INITIATIVE GOALS

The main goal of the International Society of Nephrology (ISN) 0by25 initiative is to eliminate, or at least reduce, avoidable AKI-related deaths around the world by 2025 (www.0by25.org). Two key points are fundamental in order to implement the initiative: defining preventable death from AKI and promoting local recommendations for AKI care considering the health care infrastructure and socioeconomic conditions. Preventable deaths from AKI occur as a result of 3 different situations[8]: (1) secondary to public health problems such as unclean water, diarrhea, and endemic infections; (2) because of delay or lack of recognition, lack of access to laboratory studies, or inadequate response or iatrogenic factors resulting in additional insults to a failing kidney; (3) because of lack of dialysis support to treat life-threatening hyperkalemia, fluid overload, and acidosis. Knowledge of the factors that affect AKI outcomes is a key step for implementing initiatives and reducing AKI-related mortality and morbidity. The strategies to reduce the burden of AKI need to be based on the identification of patients at risk, implementation of preventive actions, application of diagnostic methods, and timely referral for specialist care.[9–11] Development of educational and training tools for increasing awareness and standardizing care of patients with AKI is also essential.

STRATEGIES

The initiative proposed a 3-step strategy to address these issues. First, analyze existing data to determine how AKI contributes to the global burden of health loss. Second, increase awareness of AKI in the worldwide community and reduce variations in management of AKI. Third, develop a sustainable infrastructure to enable need-based approaches for education, training, and care delivery and pilot studies of appropriate, well-thought-out interventions and measurable outcomes.

Increasing Awareness of Acute Kidney Injury

To generate the database supporting the need for this initiative, a meta-analysis of epidemiology of AKI around the world was conducted. In addition, the ISN launched a prospective cohort global snapshot of AKI over a 10-week period and a subsequent longitudinal AKI cohort study in selected centers in LMIC.

In the meta-analysis, involving a systematic search of the literature from January 2012 to August 2014, 499 articles for all definitions and 266 articles for KDIGO or equivalent AKI definitions were included.[8] Analysis of the pooled incidence rate by KDIGO stage in 266 studies (4,502,158 subjects) shows an overall incidence of 20.9% of hospital admissions, which is in agreement with current estimates of incidence around the world. The overall incidence of dialysis-requiring AKI in KDIGO-defined studies is small, at 2.3% of hospital admissions (11% of all AKI), whereas KDIGO stage 1 had an incidence of 11.5% of hospital admissions (79.7% of all AKI).[8] In this analysis the pooled incidence rate in LMIC seems increasingly close to that of developed countries, in contrast with previous reports.[12–14] The results also indicate that the use of comparable definitions (KDIGO or KDIGO equivalent) is already making the understanding of AKI in those regions more reliable.[3] In addition, the estimates for AKI incidence in LMIC are becoming more accurate and problems with underreporting may be decreasing.[8] Nevertheless, mortalities continue to be high in all regions and there is continued association of nonrenal recovery following AKI.

Acute Kidney Injury and the Global Burden of Disease Study

The Global Burden of Disease (GBD) study is an effort of the World Health Organization (WHO) to quantify leading causes of health loss secondary to illness or injury throughout the world.[15] The GBD study categorizes causes of health loss by age, sex, and geography for specific time points. This time-based measure combines years of life lost because of premature mortality and years of life lost because of time lived in states of less than full health. The DALY metric was developed in the original GBD 1990 study to assess the burden of disease consistently across diseases, risk factors, and regions. As a part of the 0by25 initiative, the ISN has partnered with the Institute of Health Metrics and Evaluation, which coordinates the GBD study to include AKI in the 2015 GBD report. Incorporating AKI into the GBD will involve determining the relationship between AKI as an intermediate event associated with disability or death. It will be possible to follow the leading causes of AKI, and the segments of the population most susceptible to AKI-related health loss.

In order to enable the inclusion of AKI in GBD, the ISN 0by25 initiative helped to generate AKI epidemiologic data at the population level. The 0by25 initiative enabled the AKI Global Snapshot, a prospective observational cohort study to compare risk factors, causes, diagnosis, management, and outcomes of AKI. The study was conducted from 29 September to 7 December 2014, with more than 600 participating centers in more than 93 countries. One of the most important aims of the study was to understand the resources available for the nondialytic and dialytic management of AKI in different settings around the globe. Following the AKI Global Snapshot, additional longitudinal studies are planned to include centers across the globe to capture sequential data on AKI and its long-term outcomes. This study will use an open source platform, developed from the need for simple but robust data collection in settings with poor resources. The platform can be reached via smartphone, tablets, and other informatics tools that are easily available, even in poor countries and keep.isn.org).

The Global Snapshot and the AKI Cohort Study will provide update information on the growing burden of AKI as well as how it is identified, managed, and treated in these different settings. Furthermore, the inclusion of AKI in GBD will be the first attempt to characterize AKI burden across worldwide geography, time, and lifespan. The effort will allow the characterization of specific causes of AKI in different regions and help governments in the challenge of health care resource allocation.

Strategies for Increasing Awareness and Reducing Variations in Acute Kidney Injury Management

A comprehensive approach for education and training of health care personnel is fundamental to achieving increase awareness and better care delivery in AKI. The heterogeneity in cause, setting, and course of AKI demands an integrative approach. The 0by25 initiative proposed the use of the 5R framework (risk assessment, recognition, response, renal support and rehabilitation) for critically ill patients (**Fig. 1**).[7,8]

Key points in the management of AKI:

- Identification of high-risk patients for developing AKI
- Diagnostic testing to confirm AKI
- Implementation of initial maneuvers to correct reversible factors
- Recognition of need for renal support
- Referral for nephrology care

It is fundamental to recognize that the approach to increase awareness and improve quality of care differs across ICUs around the globe. Educational campaigns on the importance of AKI must occur in cooperation with the public health administration, private health insurance companies, and medical societies. In ICU settings, development

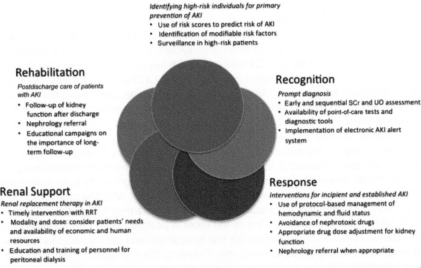

Risk
Identifying high-risk individuals for primary prevention of AKI
- Use of risk scores to predict risk of AKI
- Identification of modifiable risk factors
- Surveillance in high-risk patients

Rehabilitation
Postdischarge care of patients with AKI
- Follow-up of kidney function after discharge
- Nephrology referral
- Educational campaigns on the importance of long-term follow-up

Recognition
Prompt diagnosis
- Early and sequential SCr and UO assessment
- Availability of point-of-care tests and diagnostic tools
- Implementation of electronic AKI alert system

Renal Support
Renal replacement therapy in AKI
- Timely intervention with RRT
- Modality and dose: consider patients' needs and availability of economic and human resources
- Education and training of personnel for peritoneal dialysis

Response
Interventions for incipient and established AKI
- Use of protocol-based management of hemodynamic and fluid status
- Avoidance of nephrotoxic drugs
- Appropriate drug dose adjustment for kidney function
- Nephrology referral when appropriate

Fig. 1. ISN AKI 0by25. Key elements for a sustainable infrastructure to support AKI care in critically ill patients. RRT, renal replacement therapy; SCr, serum creatinine; UO, urine output. (*Adapted from* Mehta RL, Cerdá J, Burdmann EA, et al. International Society of Nephrology's 0by25 initiative for acute kidney injury (zero preventable deaths by 2025): a human rights case for nephrology. Lancet 2015;385:2628; with permission.)

of protocols for prevention, recognition, treatment, and follow-up of AKI can help standardize care delivery. We believe that the AKI KDIGO guidelines are already helping to improve the development of more homogeneous approaches in management of AKI.[16] In addition, we expect that the 5R framework approach will streamline efforts to establish a formal program for the prevention and treatment of AKI.

Risk: identifying high-risk individuals for primary prevention of acute kidney injury
Early identification of patients at increased risk for AKI is the first step for implementing preventive strategies. Most of the known risk factors associated with AKI have been identified in hospitalized patients in developed countries. In these settings, efforts toward potentially modifiable factors are the main approach to prevention.[17–19] However, several different exposures contributing to AKI in different settings are unknown or difficult to access, challenging the development of a unified tool for risk assessment (**Table 1**).[12,20–26] Nevertheless, individuals exposed to these insults must have a careful determination of overall risk of AKI, and, when possible, the exposure should be avoided.

Risk scores to estimate the probability of AKI are still underdeveloped tools. Several risk scores for AKI have already been proposed.[27,28] Malhotra and colleagues[28] developed a risk classification system for ICU patients based on chronic comorbidities and acute events to estimate the risk of developing AKI and adverse outcomes within 48 hours of ICU admission. The presence of chronic liver disease, congestive heart failure, hypertension, atherosclerotic coronary vascular disease, pH less than or equal to 7.30, nephrotoxic exposure, sepsis, mechanical ventilation, and anemia were identified as independent predictors of AKI. This risk assessment tool could help clinicians to stratify patients for surveillance, prevention, and early therapeutic intervention in the ICU. However, most of the available scores are specific for a particular risk setting (eg, ICU, post-operative setting), and were developed based on data from hospitalized patients in developed countries. In addition to patient risk factors, environmental and infrastructure particularities, such as inadequate sanitation, limited clean water availability, inadequate control of parasites and infection-carrying vectors, and poor transportation, can increase the risk of AKI (see **Table 1**).[8] There is a need to develop a general risk score for AKI that could be assessed in the general population globally. This risk score would greatly enhance identification of high-risk patients and facilitate preventive strategies.

Recognition: prompt diagnosis
Understanding the dynamic nature of AKI is key to avoiding further injury and progression of the disease.[29,30] Hence, timely diagnosis should be the focus in secondary prevention. Delays in AKI are common and occur frequently, even in tertiary centers in developed countries. Without team integration and protocols to maintain surveillance, delay in recognition is an important factor contributing to adverse outcomes. Intensivists and emergency department physicians must emphasize early and sequential serum creatinine (SCr) and urinary output assessment for screening of high-risk patients. This approach is possible for most LIC and for high-income countries.

The lack of infrastructure or the inaccessibility of diagnostic tools, often caused by financial constraints, coupled with limited access to health care and physician referral, contribute to the high morbidity and mortality of AKI in LMIC. In addition to increasing awareness and implementing protocols, making point-of-care tests available for physicians and other health care professionals could affect the course of AKI.

In settings in which laboratory examinations are part of an electronic patient file, the implementation of an electronic AKI alert system can help early AKI detection. In a Belgian ICU, Electronic AKI alerting covering all beds was associated with a shorter

Table 1
Main risk factors for developing AKI

	Patient		Exposures		Environmental and
Nonmodifiable	Modifiable	Developed areas	LMIC and less Developed Areas		Infrastructure
Comorbid medical conditions	Dehydration	Sepsis	Diarrhea		Inadequate sanitation
CKD	Intravascular volume depletion	Circulatory shock	Obstetric complications (including septic absorption)		Limited clean water availability
Diabetes mellitus	Hypotension	Trauma	Infectious diseases (malaria, leptospirosis, dengue, cholera, yellow fever, tetanus, Hantavirus)		Inadequate control of parasites
Cancer	Anemia	Cardiac surgery (especially with cardiopulmonary bypass)			Inadequate control of infection-carrying vectors
Chronic heart disease	Hypoxia	Major noncardiac surgery	Animal venoms (snakes, bees and wasps, *Loxosceles* spiders, *Lonomia* caterpillars)		Poor transportation
Chronic lung disease	Use of nephrotoxic agents (antibiotics, iodinated contrast, nonsteroidal antiinflammatory drugs, anticancer drugs, antiretrovirals, calcineurin blockers)	Nephrotoxic drugs and agents	Natural medicines		Inadequate health budget
Chronic gastrointestinal disease		Burns	Prolonged physically overwhelming work in an unhealthy environment		Insufficient health care human resources
Demographic factors					Insufficient health services and hospitals
Gender	—	—	Natural dyes		—
Older age	—	—			—

Adapted from Mehta RL, Cerdá J, Burdmann EA, et al. International Society of Nephrology's 0by25 initiative for acute kidney injury (zero preventable deaths by 2025): a human rights case for nephrology. Lancet 2015;385:2637; with permission time to therapeutic intervention and a higher frequency of normalization of SCr levels.[31] Whether the use of an electronic alert system for AKI will improve clinical outcomes among patients in hospital is still debatable. In a recent study in Philadelphia, Pennsylvania, there was no difference in the composite outcome of relative maximum change in creatinine, dialysis, and death between the alert group and the usual-care groups.[32] In the United Kingdom, the implementation of a real-time alert for the detection of in-hospital AKI (SCr changes) showed that early detection allowed an early treatment of AKI, potentially reversing a proportion of stage 1 AKI, and minimizing progression to more severe stages.

Response: interventions for incipient and established acute kidney injury

Of the known modifiable factors associated with AKI development and progression, extracellular volume depletion is likely the most frequent. Assessment of the patient's volume status should be the first priority for preventing AKI secondary to multiple kidney-injuring situations. However, attempts to correct volume depletion must be individualized and based on frequent monitoring of physiologic parameters. Avoiding fluid overload should also be a main concern, because fluid accumulation has been associated with higher mortality in patients with AKI.[33] Monitoring of urine output and body weight is a simple and inexpensive way to prevent fluid overload and can be implemented in all ICUs. The KDIGO AKI guidelines using protocol-based methods for optimization of hemodynamics and oxygenation should be interpreted with flexibility, according to particular aspects of the patient, the medical staff, and the health care infrastructure, and should be monitored for efficacy and changed as necessary.[17,34–39]

The avoidance of drugs and nephrotoxins that cause AKI, and the appropriate dose adjustment for kidney function medications, are important for AKI management.[40] In children, the implementation of a systematic electronic health record screening and decision support process (trigger) was associated with a 42% reduction in AKI intensity.[41] Although a large proportion of nephrotoxic AKIs are not able to be predicted or avoided, a systematic screening for nephrotoxic medication exposure and AKI detection can decrease AKI progression.

Despite efforts to implement protocols and the emphasis on educational strategies as a pivotal basis for the 0by25 AKI initiative, the importance of nephrology referral should be mentioned. Recent evidence has strengthened the importance of early nephrology referral.[42–45] However, the number of trained nephrologists available is insufficient to care for the growing number of cases of AKI around the globe. In many African countries, the density of physicians is 0.02 to 0.29 per 1000 population, considerably less than the rate of 2.28 professionals per 1000 population recommended by the WHO.[46] The training of primary care physicians and other health care givers to increase awareness and provide easy-to-use tools for knowledge and practical management of AKI is imperative, but is particularly important in LMIC.[8]

Renal support: renal replacement therapy in acute kidney injury

Despite the efforts to increase knowledge regarding renal replacement therapy (RRT), timing of initiation, type, and dose, are still topics of debate. At present, the available data suggest that early initiation of RRT favors better outcomes.[17] It is clear that RRT should be started when life-threatening alterations in fluid status, serum electrolyte levels, and/or acid-base balance occur. More subtle indications for RRT, such as increasing fluid overload, must be evaluated on a case-by-case and moment-by-moment basis.[17] Large variations in availability of, access to, and procedures for RRT occur in LMIC compared with developed countries.[8,47–51] Availability of and access to RRT strongly depend on the level of socioeconomic development and health system organization, not only of the country but also of particular areas of the same country. It is common that equipment and medical supplies resources and trained personnel are sparse or insufficient.

Choosing RRT modality has to include consideration not only of the patients' needs but also of the context of availability of economic and human resources. An option that has been more frequently reported in the last several years is the use of peritoneal dialysis (PD) for AKI. Recent studies have showed that PD has similar efficacy to extracorporeal blood purification techniques in specific populations with AKI.[52–55] In centers with experience in the technique, PD is a safe and less expensive RRT method, particularly useful in areas with less developed health infrastructure.[56–58] Intraperitoneal flexible catheters should be preferentially used for acute PD.[59] Trained nephrologists, intensivists, or emergency care physicians can perform the insertion procedure. Programs launched in Africa in countries where RRT availability is severely restricted were lifesaving for dialysis-dependent patients with AKI.[60–63]

In LIC, a structured referral and follow-up structure is crucial in order to optimize RRT to patients with AKI. Decisions regarding initiation, method, and frequency have to consider the limited availability of trained personnel and RRT equipment. Mild to moderate cases could be treated in secondary level hospitals; if RRT is indicated, consideration should be given to PD. In the context of multiorgan dysfunction, patients with AKI should be transferred to a tertiary center. The geographic distribution of the reference centers and corresponding catchment areas should be based on the local epidemiology and demographic variables.[8]

Rehabilitation: postdischarge care of patients with acute kidney injury

Frequently, patients surviving an AKI episode are not follow by a nephrologist and do not have long-term assessment of kidney function.[64] Inadequate follow-up of kidney function is an even greater problem in LMIC, affecting patients' chances of recovery and progression to CKD. Ideally, patients should be followed for more than 3 months after discharge, and have their SCr levels routinely measured to assess for recovery of renal function and/or progression of renal injury. In developed countries, it is increasingly recognized that a substantial proportion of the total AKI burden is caused by incomplete renal recovery with subsequent CKD.

With the increasing number of patients recovering from AKI, it will be necessary to direct efforts into education and training of health providers to follow kidney function recovery. Appropriate management of patients with incomplete kidney recovery may delay the progressive loss of kidney function, ultimately preventing the incremental increase in the need for chronic dialysis. Educational campaigns on the importance of long-term follow-up of patients with AKI must be planned accordingly to the level of health organization and must involve the whole health care team, including physicians, nurses, and allied medical personnel.

SUMMARY

The ISN 0by25 initiative's aim is to reduce avoidable AKI-related deaths. Progress in the last decade has made this goal achievable. The application of a standardized classification system has made epidemiologic studies possible and increased awareness of the burden of AKI. The importance of risk assessment and early diagnosis has been emphasized since the recognition that minimal changes of kidney function affect outcomes. Studies have shown that the application of risk prediction tools and electronic alerts have the potential to decrease the incidence and progression of AKI in different settings. New biomarkers of early AKI detection will enable the development of new strategies and possible new drugs for prevention and treatment of AKI. However, although progress in AKI management is a reality at ICUs in developed countries, basic conditions need to be achieved before progress can be reflected elsewhere, especially in LIC and LMIC. Key elements include improvement in health care and diagnostics tools availability, and provision of acute RRT for patients in need. The ISN Oby25 initiative offers a critical opportunity to help improve education, training, care delivery, and the implementation of diagnostic and intervention studies in AKI.

REFERENCES

1. Coca SG, Yusuf B, Shlipak MG, et al. Long-term risk of mortality and other adverse outcomes after acute kidney injury: a systematic review and meta-analysis. Am J Kidney Dis 2009;53(6):961–73.
2. Daher EF, Silva Junior GB, Santos SQ, et al. Differences in community, hospital and intensive care unit-acquired acute kidney injury: observational study in a nephrology service of a developing country. Clin Nephrol 2012;78(6):449–55.
3. Susantitaphong P, Cruz DN, Cerda J, et al, Acute Kidney Injury Advisory Group of the American Society of Nephrology. World incidence of AKI: a meta-analysis. Clin J Am Soc Nephrol 2013;8(9):1482–93.
4. Chawla LS, Kimmel PL. Acute kidney injury and chronic kidney disease: an integrated clinical syndrome. Kidney Int 2012;82(5):516–24.
5. Coca SG. Long-term outcomes of acute kidney injury. Curr Opin Nephrol Hypertens 2010;19(3):266–72.
6. Coca SG, Singanamala S, Parikh CR. Chronic kidney disease after acute kidney injury: a systematic review and meta-analysis. Kidney Int 2012;81(5):442–8.
7. Lewington AJ, Cerda J, Mehta RL. Raising awareness of acute kidney injury: a global perspective of a silent killer. Kidney Int 2013;84(3):457–67.
8. Mehta RL, Cerdá J, Burdmann EA, et al. International Society of Nephrology's Oby25 initiative for acute kidney injury (zero preventable deaths by 2025): a human rights case for nephrology. Lancet 2015;385:2616–43.
9. Chawla LS, Amdur RL, Shaw AD, et al. Association between AKI and long-term renal and cardiovascular outcomes in United States veterans. Clin J Am Soc Nephrol 2014;9(3):448–56.
10. Leung KC, Tonelli M, James MT. Chronic kidney disease following acute kidney injury-risk and outcomes. Nat Rev Nephrol 2013;9(2):77–85.
11. Li PK, Burdmann EA, Mehta RL. Acute kidney injury: global health alert. Kidney Int 2013;83(3):372–6.
12. Cerda J, Bagga A, Kher V, et al. The contrasting characteristics of acute kidney injury in developed and developing countries. Nat Clin Pract Nephrol 2008;4(3): 138–53.
13. Jha V, Parameswaran S. Community-acquired acute kidney injury in tropical countries. Nat Rev Nephrol 2013;9(5):278–90.
14. Naicker S, Aboud O, Gharbi MB. Epidemiology of acute kidney injury in Africa. Semin Nephrol 2008;28(4):348–53.
15. Murray CJ, Ezzati M, Flaxman AD, et al. GBD 2010: design, definitions, and metrics. Lancet 2012;380(9859):2063–6.
16. Thomas ME, Blaine C, Dawnay A, et al. The definition of acute kidney injury and its use in practice. Kidney Int 2015;87:62–73.
17. Group KAW. KDIGO clinical practice guideline for acute kidney injury. Kidney Int 2012;2(Supplement):1–138.

18. Finlay S, Bray B, Lewington AJ, et al. Identification of risk factors associated with acute kidney injury in patients admitted to acute medical units. Clin Med 2013; 13(3):233–8.

19. Huang TM, Wu VC, Young GH, et al. Preoperative proteinuria predicts adverse renal outcomes after coronary artery bypass grafting. J Am Soc Nephrol 2011; 22(1):156–63.

20. Lombardi R, Yu L, Younes-Ibrahim M, et al. Epidemiology of acute kidney injury in Latin America. Semin Nephrol 2008;28(4):320–9.

21. Daher Ede F, Junior Silva GB, Vieira AP, et al. Acute kidney injury in a tropical country: a cohort study of 253 patients in an infectious diseases intensive care unit. Rev Soc Bras Med Trop 2014;47(1):86–9.

22. Saravu K, Rishikesh K, Parikh CR. Risk factors and outcomes stratified by severity of acute kidney injury in malaria. PLoS One 2014;9(3):e90419.

23. Esezobor CI, Ladapo TA, Osinaike B, et al. Paediatric acute kidney injury in a tertiary hospital in Nigeria: prevalence, causes and mortality rate. PLoS One 2012; 7(12):e51229.

24. Mathew AJ, George J. Acute kidney injury in the tropics. Ann Saudi Med 2011; 31(5):451–6.

25. Lombardi R, Rosa-Diez G, Ferreiro A, et al. Acute kidney injury in Latin America: a view on renal replacement therapy resources. Nephrol Dial Transplant 2014; 29(7):1369–76.

26. Paula Santos U, Zanetta DM, Terra-Filho M, et al. Burnt sugarcane harvesting is associated with acute renal dysfunction. Kidney Int 2015;87(4):792–9.

27. McMahon GM, Zeng X, Waikar SS. A risk prediction score for kidney failure or mortality in rhabdomyolysis. JAMA Intern Med 2013;173(19):1821–8.

28. Malhotra R, Macedo E, Bouchard J, et al. Development and validation of a risk score for predicting acute kidney injury in intensive care unit patients. J Am Soc Nephrol 2014;25:81A.

29. Palmieri T, Lavrentieva A, Greenhalgh DG. Acute kidney injury in critically ill burn patients. Risk factors, progression and impact on mortality. Burns 2010;36(2):205–11.

30. Porter CJ, Juurlink I, Bisset LH, et al. A real-time electronic alert to improve detection of acute kidney injury in a large teaching hospital. Nephrol Dial Transplant 2014;29(10):1888–93.

31. Colpaert K, Hoste EA, Steurbaut K, et al. Impact of real-time electronic alerting of acute kidney injury on therapeutic intervention and progression of RIFLE class. Crit Care Med 2012;40:1164–70.

32. Wilson FP, Shashaty M, Testani J, et al. Automated, electronic alerts for acute kidney injury: a single-blind, parallel-group, randomised controlled trial. Lancet 2015;385(9981):1966–74.

33. Bouchard J, Soroko SB, Chertow GM, et al. Fluid accumulation, survival and recovery of kidney function in critically ill patients with acute kidney injury. Kidney Int 2009;76(4):422–7.

34. Brienza N, Giglio MT, Marucci M, et al. Does perioperative hemodynamic optimization protect renal function in surgical patients? A meta-analytic study. Crit Care Med 2009;37(6):2079–90.

35. Lin SM, Huang CD, Lin HC, et al. A modified goal-directed protocol improves clinical outcomes in intensive care unit patients with septic shock: a randomized controlled trial. Shock 2006;26:551–7.

36. Ng RR, Chew ST, Liu W, et al. Identification of modifiable risk factors for acute kidney injury after coronary artery bypass graft surgery in an Asian population. J Thorac Cardiovasc Surg 2014;147:1356–61.

37. Murakami R, Kumita S, Hayashi H, et al. Anemia and the risk of contrast-induced nephropathy in patients with renal insufficiency undergoing contrast-enhanced MDCT. Eur J Radiol 2013;82:e521–4.
38. Karkouti K, Wijeysundera DN, Yau TM, et al. Influence of erythrocyte transfusion on the risk of acute kidney injury after cardiac surgery differs in anemic and non-anemic patients. Anesthesiology 2011;115:523–30.
39. Khan UA, Coca SG, Hong K, et al. Blood transfusions are associated with urinary biomarkers of kidney injury in cardiac surgery. J Thorac Cardiovasc Surg 2014; 148:726–32.
40. Philips BJ, Lane K, Dixon J, et al. The effects of acute renal failure on drug metabolism. Expert Opin Drug Metab Toxicol 2014;10:11–23.
41. Goldstein SL, Kirkendall E, Nguyen H, et al. Electronic health record identification of nephrotoxin exposure and associated acute kidney injury. Pediatrics 2013; 132(3):e756–67.
42. Mehta RL, McDonald B, Gabbai F, et al. Nephrology consultation in acute renal failure: does timing matter? Am J Med Sci 2002;113:456–61.
43. Costa e Silva VT, Liaño F, Muriel A, et al. Nephrology referral and outcomes in critically ill acute kidney injury patients. PLoS One 2013;8:e70482.
44. Ponce D, Zorzenon Cde P, dos Santos NY, et al. Early nephrology consultation can have an impact on outcome of acute kidney injury patients. Nephrol Dial Transplant 2011;26:3202–6.
45. Meier P, Bonfils RM, Vogt B, et al. Referral patterns and outcomes in noncritically ill patients with hospital-acquired acute kidney injury. Clin J Am Soc Nephrol 2011;6:2215–25.
46. Kinfu Y, Dal Poz MR, Mercer H, et al. The health worker shortage in Africa: are enough physicians and nurses being trained? Bull World Health Organ 2009; 87:225–30.
47. Overberger P, Pesacreta M, Palevsky PM, VA/NIH Acute Renal Failure Trial Network. Management of renal replacement therapy in acute kidney injury: a survey of practitioner prescribing practices. Clin J Am Soc Nephrol 2007;2: 623–30.
48. Investigators RS. Renal replacement therapy for acute kidney injury in Australian and New Zealand intensive care units: a practice survey. Crit Care Resusc 2008; 10:225–30.
49. Basso F, Ricci Z, Cruz D, et al. International survey on the management of acute kidney injury in critically ill patients: year 2007. Blood Purif 2010;30:214–20.
50. Legrand M, Darmon M, Joannidis M, et al. Management of renal replacement therapy in ICU patients: an international survey. Intensive Care Med 2013;39: 101–8.
51. Jamal JA, Mat-Nor MB, Mohamad-Nor FS, et al. A national survey of renal replacement therapy prescribing practice for acute kidney injury in Malaysian intensive care units. Nephrology (Carlton) 2014;19:507–12.
52. Gabriel DP, Caramori JT, Martim LC, et al. High volume peritoneal dialysis vs daily hemodialysis: a randomized, controlled trial in patients with acute kidney injury. Kidney Int Suppl 2008;108:S87–93.
53. Ponce D, Berbel MN, Regina de Goes C, et al. High-volume peritoneal dialysis in acute kidney injury: indications and limitations. Clin J Am Soc Nephrol 2012;7: 887–94.
54. Ponce D, Berbel MN, Abrão JM, et al. A randomized clinical trial of high volume peritoneal dialysis versus extended daily hemodialysis for acute kidney injury patients. Int Urol Nephrol 2013;45:869–78.

55. Bonilla-Félix M. Peritoneal dialysis in the pediatric intensive care unit setting: techniques, quantitations and outcomes. Blood Purif 2013;35:77–80.
56. Burdmann EA, Chakravarthi R. Peritoneal dialysis in acute kidney injury: lessons learned and applied. Semin Dial 2011;24:149–56.
57. Chionh CY, Soni SS, Finkelstein FO, et al. Use of peritoneal dialysis in AKI: a systematic review. Clin J Am Soc Nephrol 2013;8:1649–60.
58. Obiagwu PN, Abdu A. Peritoneal dialysis vs. haemodialysis in the management of paediatric acute kidney injury in Kano, Nigeria: a cost analysis. Trop Med Int Health 2015;20(1):2–7.
59. Cullis B, Abdelraheem M, Abrahams G, et al. Peritoneal dialysis for acute kidney injury. Perit Dial Int 2014;34(5):494–517.
60. Kilonzo KG, Ghosh S, Temu SA, et al. Outcome of acute peritoneal dialysis in northern Tanzania. Perit Dial Int 2012;32:261–6.
61. Kilonzo K, Mathew A, Croome A. Establishment of an acute peritoneal dialysis program in Tanzania. Kidney Int Suppl 2013;3:186–9.
62. Ademola AD, Asinobi AO, Ogunkunle OO, et al. Peritoneal dialysis in childhood acute kidney injury: experience in southwest Nigeria. Perit Dial Int 2012;32: 267–72.
63. Callegari J, Antwi S, Wystrychowski G, et al. Peritoneal dialysis as a mode of treatment for acute kidney injury in sub-Saharan Africa. Blood Purif 2013;36: 226–30.
64. USRDS Annual Report 2007 Department of Health and Human Services, NIDDK, United States Renal Data System (USRDS). 2007. vol. 1. p. 240–1. NIH publication no 07-3176.

Principles of Fluid Management

Oleksa Rewa, MD, FRCPC, Sean M. Bagshaw, MD, MSc, FRCPC*

KEYWORDS

- Crystalloid • Colloid • Resuscitation • Intravenous • Fluid balance • Toxicity

KEY POINTS

- Intravenous (IV) fluids should be recognized and prescribed as drugs.
- Fluid therapy is a dynamic intervention. Its prescription can be viewed as occurring across distinct but interrelated phases of resuscitation (rescue, optimization, stabilization, and de-escalation) whereby the goals of fluid therapy naturally vary.
- Natural colloids, such as albumin, have similar effectiveness as resuscitation fluid in critical illness and have a role in prevention of hepatorenal syndrome; however, their use in traumatic brain injury is associated with higher mortality.
- The issue of fluid toxicity is important and associated with increased mortality. Accumulated fluid should be mobilized and removed aggressively as patients recover from their critical illness.

INTRODUCTION

IV fluid therapy remains the most ubiquitous intervention administered in acutely ill hospitalized patients.[1] Fluid therapy is routinely prescribed across a broad range of clinical settings, including in the management of critically ill patients with infections, hypovolemia, and in those with hemodynamic deterioration deemed to be volume responsive, and for the perioperative replacement of significant fluid deficits and losses. In these contexts, fluid therapy is generally perceived to have benefit for patients. However, there is wide variation in practice.[2,3] Fluid therapy prescription varies considerably depending on where care is provided (ie, country, region, hospital, care unit) and by provider specialty (ie, surgical, medical, anesthesia, emergency).[4] This variation stems from several factors such as the physiologic complexity of bedside determination of

Dr S.M. Bagshaw is supported by a Canada Research Chair in Critical Care Nephrology and Clinical Investigator Award from Alberta Innovates - Health Solutions.
Division of Critical Care Medicine, Faculty of Medicine and Dentistry, University of Alberta, 8440-112 Street Northwest, Edmonton, Alberta T6G 2B7, Canada
* Corresponding author. Division of Critical Care Medicine, Faculty of Medicine and Dentistry, University of Alberta, 2-124E Clinical Sciences Building, 8440-112 Street Northwest, Edmonton, Alberta T6G 2B7, Canada.
E-mail address: bagshaw@ualberta.ca

Crit Care Clin 31 (2015) 785–801
http://dx.doi.org/10.1016/j.ccc.2015.06.012
0749-0704/15/$ – see front matter © 2015 Elsevier Inc. All rights reserved.

the optimal type, volume and rate of fluid administration, the mechanisms for assessing the response to fluid loading, and due to many prescribing clinicians having limited expertise and underappreciation for the potential for harm.[5–7] This variation has also historically stemmed from a general lack of clarity in the literature on the principles of optimal fluid prescription (ie, efficacy and safety), the idea of prescribing fluid therapy for "the right patient, at the right time, and in the right context."[1]

In the last few years, several large high-quality randomized trials have reported on the efficacy and safety of IV fluid therapy for acute resuscitation in the critically ill.[8–12] These data provide greater clarity to long-standing debates regarding fluid type and dose, during and after acute resuscitation, and better inform best clinical practice to improve patient outcomes. In addition, several organizations have published consensus statements, performed quality assurance audits, and implemented evidenced-based recommendations regarding fluid therapy for acutely ill patients.[5,7,13] More commonly, there has been a recommendation for clinicians to give the same attention to prescribing IV fluid therapy as they would any other drug **(Table 1)**. IV fluids should be prescribed for specific indications; should have the type, dose, and rate specified; and should have recognized contraindications. Fluid therapy should be prescribed with an appreciation for the potential for adverse effects; this is particularly relevant when considering that the vast majority of acutely ill hospitalized patients, including children, receive IV fluid therapy in some form or another, usually as some combination of crystalloids, colloids, and blood products. This review provides an overview of recent relevant evidence related to the management of fluid therapy used in acutely ill and hospitalized patients.

HISTORICAL CONTEXT

We owe the origins of the salt solution for IV resuscitation to the Scottish physician William O'Shaughnessy, who in 1831 recommended the use of a dilute salt solution as a novel therapy to counteract the profound hypovolemia associated with cholera.[13]

Table 1
Overview of the analogy of prescribing fluid therapy and prescribing a drug

Steps for Prescribing a Drug	Prescribing an Oral Hypoglycemic Medication	Prescribing Fluid Therapy
Define the clinical problem	Diabetes mellitus	Hypovolemia or other fluid responsive state
Specify the therapeutic objective	Lower blood glucose	Restore absolute/relative fluid deficit
Verify the suitability of the drug	Class of oral hypoglycemic agent	Crystalloid, colloid, or blood product
Write a prescription to start the use of drug	Order written by MD, verified and dispensed by pharmacy	Order written by MD; verified by pharmacy, blood bank, or RN; administered by RN
Monitor therapeutic response of the drug	Blood glucose or hemoglobin A1C, evidence of adverse effect/toxicity	Monitor hemodynamic profile and end-organ perfusion, evidence of dose-response toxicity
Write an order to discontinue	Order written by MD, verified by pharmacy	Order written by MD, administered by RN

Adapted from Raghunathan K, Shaw AD, Bagshaw SM. Fluids are drugs. Curr Opin Crit Care 2013;19(4):290–8; with permission.

The first clinical use of IV fluids for resuscitation followed shortly thereafter, when Dr Thomas A. Latta administered a warmed IV solution of "two drachms of muriate, two scruples of carbonate of soda to sixty ounces of water" to combat the refractory hypovolemia attributable to cholera in 6 patients hospitalized at the Leith Infirmary in Scotland.[14] The clinical and physiologic response was described by Latta as immediate and profound and seemingly able to "reanimate the dead."[14] Latta described significant volumes of fluid being given to patients (more than 12 L in some cases) to restore hemodynamics, and he later described "...an immediate return of the pulse, and improvement in the respiration...[and in] the appearance of the patient [were] the immediate effects." Yet, even in 1832, an editorial subsequently published in the *Lancet* commented that "...the mass of the profession is unable to decide; and thus, instead of any uniform mode of treatment, every town and village has its different system or systems..." and that "...a suitable clinical investigation is required to resolve between such conflicting authorities...."[14] It would seem ironic that after nearly 2 centuries of advancements in modern medicine, including impressive growth of the types of fluid therapy available for patient care, this editorial seems to be remarkably familiar in many respects to the current state of knowledge regarding the optimal prescription of fluid therapy for acutely ill patients. Accordingly, despite medicine's deeply anchored confidence in fluid therapy, numerous fundamental questions about its efficacy and safety remain that are increasingly being challenged in modern clinical contexts.

PHASES OF FLUID THERAPY

Despite the wide variety of IV fluid types available for use in clinical practice, the general principles behind IV fluid therapy remain similar today as they did in the nineteenth century, to restore cardiac output, blood pressure, and organ and microcirculatory tissue perfusion and ensure adequate tissue oxygen delivery.[15]

The fluid needs for critically ill patients are not static and evolve in accordance with their phase of acute illness.[1] A conceptual framework outlining 4 distinct yet interrelated phases of resuscitation has been proposed. These phases have been described as rescue (or salvage), optimization, stabilization, and de-escalation and are intended to span initial acute resuscitation to illness resolution (**Fig. 1**).[6,16] Logically, fluid therapy follows similar phases during resuscitation.

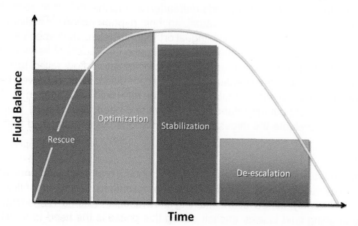

Fig. 1. Patient volume status at different phases of resuscitation. (Copyright © 2013 ADQI.)

Rescue

This phase, also referred to as salvage, is characterized by life-threatening shock characterized by hypotension and impaired organ perfusion. In this phase, patients are given rapid fluid bolus therapy as the mainstay of treatment to rapidly reverse volume-responsive shock states and improve organ perfusion while concomitantly identifying and treating the underlying precipitate (ie, major trauma, sepsis, or gastrointestinal bleeding). These patients are best transferred to settings with enhanced invasive (ie, arterial catheter, central venous pressure, central venous oxygen saturation) and noninvasive (ie, echocardiography, pulse pressure, stroke volume variation) monitoring capabilities to guide ongoing resuscitation and organ support (ie, vasoactive therapy, mechanical ventilation).

Optimization

In this phase, the patient is no longer at imminent risk of life-threatening shock but often requires fluid therapy to optimize cardiac function, sustain tissue perfusion, mitigate organ dysfunction, and achieve physiologic end points.[17] The optimal end points for resuscitation remain uncertain; however, consensus generally supports restoration of central venous oxygen saturation and clearance of arterial lactate as dynamic goals of resuscitation that correlate with improved patient outcome.[18,19] Although multicenter randomized trials have challenged the specific bundled elements of protocolized early goal-directed therapy in sepsis, the overarching philosophy of early and aggressive resuscitation targeting improvements in bedside hemodynamics and physiology generally remains uncontested.[20–22] During optimization, fluid challenge therapy using fluid volumes of 250 to 500 mL over 15 to 20 minutes is often used to evaluate the effect of additional fluid therapy on targeted end points of resuscitation. Clinicians must recognize there may be significant heterogeneity in the response to fluid therapy during this early phase of resuscitation that may relate to differences in patient susceptibilities and case mix. As an example, a randomized trial of fluid bolus therapy in hypoperfused African children with severe infection, contrary to the study central hypothesis, found a striking increase in mortality within 48 hours after intervention, attributable to cardiovascular collapse, in settings where modern intensive care was largely unavailable.[23,24]

There may be biphasic and/or variable responses to normalization of resuscitation variables (eg, rapid initial improvement in Scvo$_2$, capillary refill time, and lactate clearance may be followed by slower trends thereafter) and further delays to normalization due to confounding by impaired hepatosplanchnic hypoperfusion.[25,26] Microcirculatory capillary blood flow (ie, use of sublingual orthogonal polarization spectral imaging) is commonly found abnormal among critically ill patients. Recent observational data have shown that disturbance in sublingual microcirculatory flow failed to correlate with patient survival, possibly because of a significant dissociation observed between sublingual and intestinal microcirculatory perfusion after fluid resuscitation.[27,28] These data reinforce the critical importance of the constant need for clinicians to monitor, reassess, and reevaluate the necessity for and response to ongoing fluid therapy.

Stabilization

During this phase, the main goals are to provide ongoing organ support, prevent worsening organ dysfunction, and avoid iatrogenic complications. The need for fluid during this phase is largely aimed at maintaining intravascular volume homeostasis and replacing ongoing fluid losses. Implicit during this phase is the need to monitor and assess volume status and fluid balance. In particular, patients are susceptible to progressive, excessive, and, in many circumstances, unnecessary fluid accumulation and overload termed fluid creep.[29] This condition was first described in patients with major burn injury; however, it can essentially be applied to any patient who has been subject to overly judicious fluid administration. Although iatrogenic fluid accumulation is important to monitor and unnecessary fluid overload important to avoid whenever possible, the optimal method to mitigate or even actively remove accumulated fluid remains uncertain.[30–32] The excessive removal or too conservative use of fluid early during convalescence can precipitate hypotension or organ hypoperfusion and may contribute to long-term risk of neuropsychological impairment and delayed recovery.[33]

De-escalation

The final phase is characterized by ongoing recovery whereby patients are weaned from ventilatory and vasoactive support and accumulated fluid is mobilized and removed. This deresuscitation is aimed to achieve a negative fluid balance and relieve or avert the quantitative toxicity of fluid therapy. Late conservative fluid management strategies and achievement of a negative fluid balance have been associated with improved patient outcome, including reduced duration of mechanical ventilation, earlier discharge from the intensive care unit (ICU), and survival.[30,34] Unfortunately, there is a paucity of evidence on measures to effectively and safely remove resuscitation fluid. In addition, as mentioned earlier, the ideal mechanisms to remove accumulated fluid (ie, diuretic therapy, ultrafiltration) and optimal rate at which fluid can be safely removed remain to be determined.

MONITORING AND REASSESSMENT

Owing to large differences in baseline susceptibility and case mix, patients may rapidly transition from a phase in which active resuscitation is ongoing to one in which the complications attributable to fluid overload manifest. Although patients may perceive to progress through these phases of resuscitation, they do not necessarily all start at the same point. Some patients do not present in life-threatening shock and, accordingly, may present at the optimization phase. Similarly, patients may develop new disease processes or suffer acute deterioration while having fluid mobilized, necessitating a recurrent episode of resuscitation. This patient variability in fluid needs is a dynamic process and does not necessarily follow a fixed temporal pattern or time scale.[35] This dynamism creates challenges for determining optimal or protocolized practices for fluid management.[36] Accordingly, an integrated and targeted evaluation of volume status, fluid balance, and ongoing fluid requirements centers on several parameters, including routine vital signs, hemodynamic profile, physical examination, biochemical parameters, and diagnostic imaging for evidence of complications of fluid therapy that are potentially actionable (see **Fig. 3**; **Table 2**). The critical pearl for clinicians is constant evaluation and reevaluation of the volume status, fluid balance, and ongoing fluid needs of the patient.

TYPE OF FLUID THERAPY

There are now innumerable types of fluids available for patient care. For a given dose of a given type of fluid administered, clinical efficacy is for the most part similar (with the exception of blood in hemorrhagic shock); however, the attributable toxicity may vary depending on the type, composition, and dose of fluid being administered, coupled with patient susceptibilities, physiologic reserve, and clinical context.

Table 2
Measures of fluid status and end points of resuscitation

Physical Examination		Biochemical Parameters		Echocardiography & Ultrasonography	Radiography
Static Variables	Dynamic Variables	Static Variables	Dynamic Variables		
Vital signs (HR, BP)	Pulse pressure variation	Scvo$_2$	Lactate clearance	Stroke volume variation	Chest radiograph
Physical examination (skin turgor, capillary refill, skin perfusion)	Passive leg raises	Blood lactate		IVC/SVC diameter	Chest computed tomography
		Urinary biochemistry (FeNa, urea)		Ejection fraction	
Central venous pressure				Fractional shortening	
Serial weight				Lung ultrasonography	
Cumulative fluid balance (ins and outs)		Bioelectrical impedance and vector analysis			
Urinary output					
Historical information (recent fluid losses, oral intake, medications)					

Abbreviations: BP, blood pressure; HR, heart rate; IVC, inferior vena cava; SVC, superior vena cava.

The controversy weighing the relative merits and risks of selection of colloid over crystalloid solutions and vice versa remains unsettled. Although various iterations of crystalloid solutions have been used for resuscitation in humans since the 1830s, it was approximately 100 years later when the technology was available to isolate albumin from serum. Synthetic colloids such as dextrans, hydroxyethyl starches (HES), and gelatins have, until recently, been considered reasonable alternatives to albumin, because of a misguided perception of increased mortality with use of albumin and various theoretic advantages such as avoiding the infectious risks associated with human blood products, improving blood rheology and microvascular flow, and modulating neutrophil aggregation.[37] Indeed, an international study of 391 ICUs across 25 countries found a 6-fold difference between countries in the primary fluid type used for acute resuscitation and that colloid therapy was the most common fluid type used for fluid bolus therapy in acute resuscitation (48% of instances), whereas crystalloid solutions and blood products represented 33% and 28% of encounters, respectively.[4] Although both patient-specific and context-specific factors need to be considered when selecting the type of fluid therapy to be administered, the choice of fluid used in clinical practice has largely been dictated by regional or local institutional practice and individual provider preferences rather than guided by high-quality evidence from randomized trials.[38]

CRYSTALLOID SOLUTIONS

The ideal electrolyte solution is yet undiscovered; however, for acute resuscitation, one that near parallels the plasma chloride concentration and has a strong ion difference (SID) that is greater than zero (unlike 0.9% saline) but less than plasma during resuscitation should be used. Although 0.9% saline remains the most commonly prescribed crystalloid solution, recent data have suggested clinically important outcomes differ when comparing it to physiologically balanced crystalloid solutions.

In the last few years, several studies have described reduced complications and improved patient outcomes based on the relative chloride concentration load of fluid therapy.[39–45] Consistent with experimental and small human clinical studies, use of crystalloid solutions with lower chloride content were found to be beneficial.[46–48] Saline (0.9%) solution is nonphysiologic, and the high chloride concentration and lower SID compared with plasma (0.9% saline, SID 0 mmol/L vs Plasma, SID 40 mmol/L) directly incites an iatrogenic hyperchloremic metabolic acidosis, which may mask, simulate, and/or precipitate to occurrence of significant adverse effects. This effect can often be exaggerated among patients with impaired kidney function because of diminished capacity to excrete excess chloride. In a controlled experimental model of resuscitation after uncontrolled hemorrhagic shock, resuscitation with the more balanced crystalloid Lactated Ringers compared with 0.9% saline required significantly less fluid to maintain mean arterial pressure and was associated with less hyperchloremia, less acidemia, higher plasma fibrinogen levels, and lower plasma [lactate] at the end of the study.[48] The higher total fluid requirements associated with 0.9% saline are believed attributable to untoward effects of the hyperchloremic acidosis, including depressed myocardial performance, diminished peripheral vascular resistance, reduced inotropic response to catecholamines and arrhythmias.[49] In addition, 0.9% saline has been associated with platelet dysfunction, disruption of the coagulation cascade, greater relative blood loss, and significantly higher need for transfused blood products when compared with resuscitation with balanced crystalloid solutions.[39,50] The use of balanced crystalloid solutions for initial resuscitation in patients with diabetic ketoacidosis, despite the theoretic concern that the added [potassium] content ([K$^+$] 5.0 mmol/L) may exacerbate hyperkalemia, was found to be associated with more rapid correction of base deficit when compared with 0.9% saline.[41] In a cohort of adult patients undergoing major open abdominal surgery, the use of balanced crystalloid solutions when compared with 0.9% saline was associated with less electrolyte disturbances, fewer blood transfusions, decreased number of acidosis investigations, fewer complications including acute renal replacement therapy (RRT), and an overall trend toward lower hospital mortality.[39] These observations were likewise found in a cohort of critically ill patients with systemic inflammatory response and sepsis.[51] In a randomized crossover trial of healthy volunteers, renal blood flow and renal cortical perfusion were found to decrease significantly after the bolus administration of 2 L of 0.9% saline compared with the balanced crystalloid solution Plasma-Lyte 148. These observations of the direct negative effects of high chloride load on kidney function have been corroborated.[46] Recent data have also clearly shown that high chloride concentration solutions contribute to renal vasoconstriction, decreased glomerular filtration, and greater interstitial fluid accumulation, along with increased risk of acute kidney injury (AKI) and utilization of RRT.[39,40,42,44,51,52] Although much of these data are derived from observational studies and not randomized trials, the weight of evidence would imply that balanced crystalloid solutions are a safe and reasonable default choice for initial resuscitation fluid in acutely ill patients.[38] In the meantime, randomized comparisons of balanced versus 0.9% saline solutions as primary resuscitation fluid in critically ill patients are ongoing.[53]

COLLOIDS

Several studies have consistently shown a physiologic rationale for the preferential use of a colloid (with an emphasis on HES) over crystalloid therapy for resuscitation in septic shock and in other states of acute stress such as perioperatively. Selected colloids, such as HES solutions have been suggested to attenuate inflammation, mitigate endothelial barrier dysfunction and vascular leak, and preserve intestinal barrier function. Small clinical trials have suggested superiority of colloid solutions for resuscitation of the microcirculation in sepsis.[54] Small randomized trials have suggested early fluid resuscitation with colloid solutions, in particular HES, to result in more rapid hemodynamic stabilization and shock reversal when compared with crystalloid solutions and to require less resuscitation fluid to restore and maintain intravascular volume homeostasis.[55,56] Accordingly, accumulated evidence had suggested improved efficacy on various physiologic outcomes for colloid solutions compared with crystalloids; however, few of these earlier trials had focused on patient-centered outcomes.

Several high-quality multicenter randomized controlled trials have specifically evaluated the colloid/crystalloid hypothesis for fluid resuscitation across a range in case mix of critically ill patients. The saline versus albumin fluid evaluation (SAFE) study SAFE (4% albumin in 0.9% saline vs 0.9% saline), CHEST (6% HES in 0.9% saline vs 0.9% saline), 6S (6% HES in Ringer acetate vs Ringer acetate); ALBIOS (20% albumen plus crystalloid to target serum albumin 30 g/L vs crystalloid); and CRISTAL (any colloid vs any crystalloid) trials were specifically designed to evaluate the safety, efficacy, and effectiveness of colloids compared with crystalloids.

First, these trials have confirmed that the efficacy of volume expansion of colloids over crystalloids (ie, the ability to increase plasma volume) is modestly greater for colloids (ratio 1.2–1.4:1 for crystalloid:colloid); however, it is far less than traditional teachings and evidence from animal models.[8] This finding may be due to failure of the classical Starling model understanding of fluid movement across capillary membranes in critically ill states, whereby the vascular endothelium is damaged (ie, loss of the endothelial glycocalyx) and hydrostatic (ie, systemic venous hypertension due to fluid overload) and oncotic (ie, hypoproteinemia) forces are disrupted[1]; this implies that capillary leak and fluid extravasation into the interstitium in critically ill states can occur with similar propensity for crystalloids and colloids.[15]

Second, these trials have largely supported the view that colloids generally show no greater effectiveness for patient-centered outcomes than crystalloids, with few exceptions, for acute resuscitation in critical illness.[57] The SAFE trial, comparing 4% albumin to 0.9% saline for resuscitation in critically ill patients was the first large high-quality randomized controlled trial to establish no difference in mortality or resource utilization between colloids and crystalloids. In the SAFE study, a preplanned analysis of the septic subgroup suggested lower mortality in those receiving 4% albumin compared with 0.9% saline. The ALBIOS trial, however, failed to show that albumin replacement in addition to crystalloids, as compared with crystalloids alone, improved survival.[12]

Third, these trials have also confirmed concerns about colloid use in selected subgroups of patients and specific types of colloids showing evidence of harm. In the SAFE study, preplanned subgroup analyses suggested higher mortality in patients with trauma, predominantly with head injury. Further post hoc long-term follow-up of patients with traumatic brain injury in the SAFE study confirmed a higher mortality in those receiving 4% albumin.[58]

Several randomized trials have concluded increased concern for adverse effects related to the use of HES solutions. Although there has been suggestion of an improved safety profile for HES solutions with a lower molecular weight and lower degree of molar substitution, with respect to coagulopathy, bleeding, and AKI, these findings have been inconsistent. Before the efficacy of volume substitution and insulin therapy in severe sepsis (VISEP) study 6S, and CHEST trials, the literature comprised small lower-quality trials that failed to adequately inform the full extent of toxicity risk.[59–61] Moreover, wide-scale retractions due to fraudulent reporting on the efficacy and safety of HES have further undermined provider confidence.[60] More recent data from higher-quality randomized trials have described serious safety concerns about the dose-associated kidney toxic effects of HES.[9,11,62] Additional data have shown that newer low-molecular-weight HES solutions still accumulate in tissues shortly after administration, including in the liver, kidney, lung, spleen, and lymph nodes.[63,64] A most recent Cochrane review concluded that there is no evidence from randomized controlled trials that resuscitation with colloids reduces the risk of death compared with resuscitation with crystalloids and that the use of HES may increase mortality.[65] The VISEP trial, comparing 10% HES (200/0.5) to lactated Ringer for fluid resuscitation in septic shock, was terminated prematurely because of the higher incidence of AKI and a trend toward mortality associated with 10% HES. These findings were confirmed in 2 recent large randomized trials. The CHEST trial compared 6% HES (130/0.4) in 0.9% saline to 0.9% saline for acute resuscitation in critically ill patients. No difference in mortality was evident; however, utilization of RRT in those receiving HES was significantly higher. Similarly, the 6S trial compared 6% HES (130/0.42) Ringers acetate with Ringers acetate for resuscitation in severe sepsis. Rates of AKI, RRT, and mortality were higher among those allocated to receive HES. These data imply a clear increased risk for harm associated with HES solutions and has lead the European Society of Intensive Care Medicine to recommend against the use of HES in patients with severe sepsis or those at risk for AKI.[66] In the United States, the US Food and Drug Administration issued a black boxed warning against HES use in critically ill patients because of the increased risk of AKI and death.[67]

Finally, colloid solutions are vastly more expensive than crystalloids and not likely to be cost-effective given the preponderance of evidence of equivalence and/or harm. In the absence of compelling evidence to the contrary with respect to patient-centered outcomes, colloid use should be minimized to indications for which robust evidence may exist (ie, albumin) or be avoided altogether (ie, HES).

QUANTITATIVE TOXICITY OF FLUID THERAPY

As mentioned earlier, a central theme in dosing fluid therapy for acutely ill patients is the need to actively evaluate existing need and losses along with iterative reassessment for additional fluid therapy; this reinforces the need to recognize that patients are heterogeneous, vary considerably with respect to baseline susceptibilities and case mix, and are bound to respond variably to fluid loading during resuscitation and de-escalation. Fluid therapy must be individualized for patient-specific resuscitation goals that ideally integrate functional hemodynamic measures in addition to generic resuscitation end points. Numerous studies in perioperative and critical care settings support this concept of ebb and flow in fluid loading and fluid accumulation and removal. The long-standing practice of providing a baseline maintenance prescription or the routine replacement of unmeasured fluid deficits such as third space losses for many patients should be challenged and unchecked may simply contribute to preventable fluid accumulation. Fluid therapy is an important modifiable aspect of the care of acutely ill patients and if managed poorly can contribute to iatrogenic harm. Inappropriate fluid therapy, regardless of fluid type, may disrupt compensatory mechanisms and worsen outcome.[23,24]

After the rescue and optimization phases of resuscitation, excessive fluid accumulation and fluid overload portend worse clinical outcome, across a range in clinical settings and particularly in AKI whereby clearance of salt and water are further impaired. Among critically ill patients with septic AKI, sustained fluid therapy in the setting of a stabilized systemic hemodynamic profile has been shown to not only not improve kidney function but also worsen lung function and oxygenation.[68,69] Fluid accumulation in critically ill adults with septic AKI predicts 60-day mortality (hazard ratio, 1.21 per L/24 h; 95% confidence interval, 1.13–1.28; $P<.001$).[31] In addition, although the fluid and catheter treatment trial (FACCT) trial did not demonstrate a mortality difference between a liberal and a more conservative fluid management strategy in the setting of acute lung injury, the conservative strategy was associated with improved lung function, reduced length of stay in ICU, and a trend for lower utilization of RRT.[34] A greater degree of fluid overload when RRT is started is associated with higher mortality and lower likelihood of kidney recovery. For each 1% increase in percentage fluid overload (%FO, calculated by the following formula) at RRT initiation, risk of death increased by 3%.[70]

$$\%FO = [(\text{total fluid in} - \text{total fluid out})/\text{admission body weight} \times 100]$$

These observations highlight the importance of monitoring fluid balance and evaluating for the degree of fluid accumulation in acutely ill patients, in particular after rescue and optimization, whereby the obligatory daily fluid administered (ie, due to need for vital medications and nutrition) can exceed the daily spontaneous output (ie, due to relative oliguria or AKI), contributing to rapid fluid accumulation. In these circumstances, there should be concerted effort to minimize or avoid all nonessential fluid therapy. However, data on fluid accumulation in critically ill patients are almost entirely post hoc, associative, and not causal. Very few prospective interventional studies, with the exception of the FACCT trial and selected studies of conservative perioperative fluid regimens, have informed on the optimal fluid management strategies, in particular with respect to fluid mobilization in the stabilization and de-escalation phases, and evaluated their association with organ function, adverse events, and survival.[34,71]

MITIGATION OF FLUID ACCUMULATION

The optimal timing for when to begin fluid mobilization and the ideal rate at which fluid can be mobilized to avoid iatrogenic complications in acute ill patients who have significant fluid accumulation remain uncertain (**Fig. 2**; see **Table 2**). Although there has been little investigation on the process of deresuscitation in critically ill patients with respect to fluid accumulation to guide practice, studies are ongoing.[72] Accordingly, there is likely wide practice variation on this issue. In general, the process of removal of fluid should be patient- and context-specific and guided by clinical, physiologic, biochemical, and radiographic parameters, with the aim of maintaining euvolemia and avoiding iatrogenic complications such as hemodynamic instability. In patients with significant fluid accumulation or overload, there are really only 3 strategies to mitigate additional fluid accumulation and stimulate fluid removal. Patients can either passively remove fluid spontaneously or have active assistance with pharmacologic diuresis/natriuresis (ie, diuretics) or mechanical fluid removal (ie, ultrafiltration) (**Fig. 3**).

Ideally, when patients transition to the stabilization and de-escalation phases concomitant with recovery, excess accumulated fluid should be mobilized. However, patients are generally unable to spontaneously achieve fluid mobilization due several factors such as persistent AKI or hypoalbuminemia. Accordingly, based on the clinical context, an initial trial of pharmacologic management to promote fluid removal is appropriate.[36] Diuretic drugs, such as the loop diuretic furosemide, are most commonly used and have been shown to achieve a negative fluid balance and recently have shown trends for improve outcomes, after adjustment for fluid balance.[31,73] These findings contradict earlier data and the long-held paradigm that diuretics are associated with increased risk for death and nonrecovery of kidney function.[74] In these studies, the delayed referral for RRT among patients with severe diuretic-unresponsive AKI was likely an important source of bias in the association between diuretic therapy and mortality.[74–76]

Although an initial trial of pharmacologic management may be a temporizing measure, patients with symptomatic and resistant fluid overload refractory to diuretic therapy (ie, inadequate diuresis or development of worsening AKI or metabolic complications such as hypernatremia), those with relative oliguria in the setting of large obligatory fluid requirements, or those with an imminent life-threatening complication attributable to fluid overload (ie, pulmonary edema) should have RRT organized,

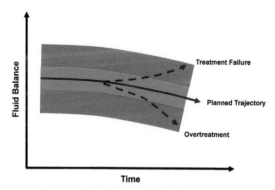

Fig. 2. Fluid balance and removal trajectory. Clinical care encompasses adherence to an intended fluid balance trajectory. Deviation from the trajectory (either above or below the intended pathway) should prompt adjustments in fluid management strategy. (Copyright © 2013 ADQI.)

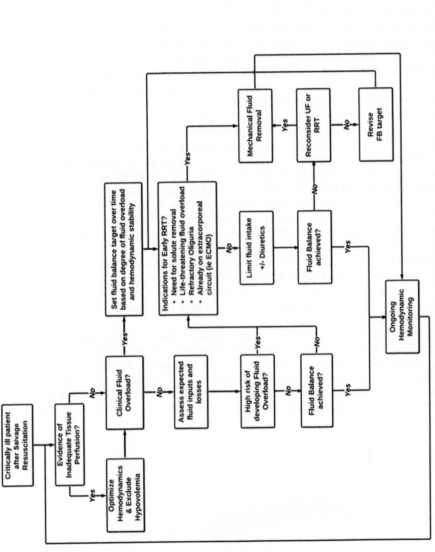

Fig. 3. Fluid management strategies in acutely ill patients. Once intravascular fluid deficits and hypovolemia have been corrected, unnecessary fluid accumulation and overload should be avoided. If clinically significant fluid overload occurs or is anticipated, early use of diuretic therapy or extracorporeal fluid removal should be considered. During therapy, hemodynamic and intravascular volume status should be monitored and fluid removal rate and fluid balance targets regularly reassessed to avoid iatrogenic clinical stability. Within this pathway, RRT should be considered at any time point if additional solute/volume removal is necessary that is refractory to diuretic therapy. (Copyright © 2013 ADQI.)

in particular when concomitant indications for RRT are present (ie, hyperkalemia, azotemia, acidosis). There are several forms of mechanical fluid removal that can be used, but the most common are isolated intermittent ultrafiltration/dialysis or continuous ultrafiltration/RRT in acutely ill patients.[77] During the initial phases of recovery, slower and sustained fluid removal by continuous RRT (CRRT) techniques may better achieve negative fluid balance and enable vascular refilling while minimizing the risk of iatrogenic hemodynamic instability.[78,79] This technique represents a plausible mechanism whereby initial therapy with CRRT may be associated with greater likelihood of kidney recovery among those with severe AKI and decreased risk of long-term RRT dependence.[80,81]

SUMMARY

IV fluid therapy remains one of the most common interventions received by acutely ill hospitalized patients. It is prescribed across a broad range of clinical settings, for several differing indications and by providers with a large range in experience. There are wide variations in practice. Increasingly, the prescription for fluid therapy is being recognized as being similar to the prescription of any drug, whereby it must be prescribed for clear indications and the type, dose, and rate must be specified. The fluid needs of patients are dynamic, differ according to the phase of resuscitation, and must be iteratively evaluated and reevaluated. Physiologically balanced crystalloid solutions have been shown to be equally efficacious as 0.9% saline with fewer complications and potentially improved outcomes for patients. Pending contrary data, balanced crystalloids solutions should be considered the default resuscitation fluid for most acute ill patients. Colloid therapy, with few exceptions, is only marginally more efficacious for hemodynamic stabilization compared with crystalloids; however, it is no more effective in terms of patient outcomes, is not likely cost-effective, and in selected patients has shown evidence of harm (ie, HES in sepsis, albumin in traumatic brain injury). Excessive and unnecessary fluid accumulation, in particular when patients transition to more convalescent phases of resuscitation, should be avoided, including active efforts to prevent complications of overt fluid overload. Minimization of nonessential fluid and active fluid removal with diuretic therapy or RRT may be necessary.

REFERENCES

1. McDermid RC, Radhunathan K, Romanosvsky A, et al. Controversies in fluid therapy: type, dose and toxicity. World J Crit Care Med 2014;3(1):24.
2. Chong PC, Greco EF, Stothart D, et al. Substantial variation of both opinions and practice regarding perioperative fluid resuscitation. Can J Surg 2009;52(3):207.
3. McIntyre LA, Hebert PC, Fergusson D, et al. A survey of Canadian intensivists' resuscitation practices in early septic shock. Crit Care 2007;11(4):R74.
4. Finfer S, Liu B, Taylor C, et al. Resuscitation fluid use in critically ill adults: an international cross-sectional study in 391 intensive care units. Crit Care 2010;14(5):R185.
5. NICE Clinical Guidelines, no. 174. Intravenous fluid therapy in adults. 2013. Available at: http://www.ncbi.nlm.nih.gov/pubmedhealth/PMH0068965/. Accessed May 14, 2015.
6. Hoste EA, Maitland K, Brudney CS, et al. Four phases of intravenous fluid therapy: a conceptual model. Br J Anaesth 2014;113(5):740-7.
7. 2011 NCEPOD report [Internet]. 2015. p. 1–18. Available at: http://www.ncepod. org.uk/2011report2/downloads/POC_summary.pdf. Accessed May 14, 2015.

8. Finfer S, Bellomo R, Boyce N, et al. A comparison of albumin and saline for fluid resuscitation in the intensive care unit. N Engl J Med 2004;350(22):2247–56.

9. Myburgh JA, Finfer S, Bellomo R, et al. Hydroxyethyl starch or saline for fluid resuscitation in intensive care. N Engl J Med 2012;367(20):1901–11.

10. Annane D. Effects of fluid resuscitation with colloids vs crystalloids on mortality in critically ill patients presenting with hypovolemic shock. JAMA 2013;310(17):1809.

11. Perner A, Haase N, Guttormsen AB. Hydroxyethyl starch 130/0.42 versus Ringer's acetate in severe sepsis. N Engl J Med 2012;367:124–34.

12. Caironi P, Tognoni G, Masson S, et al. Albumin replacement in patients with severe sepsis or septic shock. N Engl J Med 2014;370(15):1412–21.

13. Kellum JA, Mythen MG, Shaw AD, et al. The 12th consensus conference of the Acute Dialysis Quality Initiative (ADQI XII). Br J Anaesth 2014;113(5):729–31.

14. Awad S, Allison SP, Lobo DN. The history of 0.9% saline. Clin Nutr 2008;27(2):179–88.

15. Payen D. Back to basic physiological questions and consideration of fluids as drugs. Br J Anaesth 2014;113(5):732–3.

16. Finfer SR, Vincent J-L, De Backer D. Circulatory shock. N Engl J Med 2013;369(18):1726–34.

17. Goldstein SL. Fluid management in acute kidney injury. J Intensive Care Med 2014;29(4):183–9.

18. Jones AE, Shapiro NI, Trzeciak S, et al. Lactate clearance vs central venous oxygen saturation as goals of early sepsis therapy: a randomized clinical trial. JAMA 2010;303(8):739–46.

19. Jansen TC, van Bommel J, Schoonderbeek FJ, et al. Early lactate-guided therapy in intensive care unit patients. Am J Respir Crit Care Med 2010;182(6):752–61.

20. ARISE Investigators, ANZICS Clinical Trials Group, Peake SL, et al. Goal-directed resuscitation for patients with early septic shock. N Engl J Med 2014;371(16):1496–506.

21. The ProCESS Investigators. A randomized trial of protocol-based care for early septic shock. N Engl J Med 2014;370(18):1683–93.

22. Mouncey PR, Osborn TM, Power GS, et al. Trial of early, goal-directed resuscitation for septic shock. N Engl J Med 2015;372(14):1301–11.

23. Maitland K, Kiguli S, Opoka RO, et al. Mortality after fluid bolus in African children with severe infection. N Engl J Med 2011;364(26):2483–95.

24. Maitland K, George EC, Evans JA, et al. Exploring mechanisms of excess mortality with early fluid resuscitation: insights from the FEAST trial. BMC Med 2013;11(1):68.

25. Hernandez G, Regueira T, Bruhn A, et al. Relationship of systemic, hepatosplanchnic, and microcirculatory perfusion parameters with 6-hour lactate clearance in hyperdynamic septic shock patients: an acute, clinical-physiological, pilot study. Ann Intensive Care 2012;2:44.

26. Hernandez G, Luengo C, Bruhn A, et al. When to stop septic shock resuscitation: clues from a dynamic perfusion monitoring. Ann Intensive Care 2014;4:30.

27. Vellinga NAR, Boerma EC, Koopmans M, et al. International study on microcirculatory shock occurrence in acutely ill patients. Crit Care Med 2015;43(1):48–56.

28. Edul VSK, Ince C, Navarro N, et al. Dissociation between sublingual and gut microcirculation in the response to a fluid challenge in postoperative patients with abdominal sepsis. Ann Intensive Care 2014;4(1):39.

29. Saffle JR. The phenomenon of "fluid creep" in acute burn resuscitation. J Burn Care Res 2007;28(3):382–95.

30. Murphy CV, Schramm GE, Doherty JA, et al. The importance of fluid management in acute lung injury secondary to septic shock. Chest 2009;136(1):102–9.
31. Grams ME, Estrella MM, Coresh J, et al. Fluid balance, diuretic use, and mortality in acute kidney injury. Clin J Am Soc Nephrol 2011;6:966–73.
32. Bellomo R. Issue and challenges of fluid removal in the critically ill. Br J Anaesth 2014;113(5):734–5.
33. Mikkelsen ME, Christie JD, Lanken PN, et al. The adult respiratory distress syndrome cognitive outcomes study. Am J Respir Crit Care Med 2012;185(12):1307–15.
34. Wiedermann HP, Wheeler AP, Bernard GR, et al. Comparison of two fluid-management strategies in acute lung injury. N Engl J Med 2006;354(24):2564–75.
35. Raghunathan K, Shaw AD, Bagshaw SM. Fluids are drugs. Curr Opin Crit Care 2013;19(4):290–8.
36. Goldstein S, Bagshaw S, Cecconi M, et al. Pharmacological management of fluid overload. Br J Anaesth 2014;113(5):756–63.
37. Cochrane Injuries Group Albumin Reviewers. Human albumin administration in critically ill patients: systematic review of randomized controlled trials. BMJ 1998;317(7153):235–40.
38. Raghunathan K, Murray PT, Beattie WS, et al. Choice of fluid in acute illness: what should be given? An international consensus. Br J Anaesth 2014;113(5):772–83.
39. Shaw AD, Bagshaw SM, Goldstein SL, et al. Major complications, mortality, and resource utilization after open abdominal surgery. Ann Surg 2012;255(5):821–9.
40. Yunos NM, Bellomo R, Hegarty C, et al. Association between a chloride-liberal vs chloride-restrictive intravenous fluid administration strategy and kidney injury in critically ill adults. JAMA 2012;308(15):1566–72.
41. Chua H-R, Venkatesh B, Stachowski E, et al. Plasma-Lyte 148 vs 0.9% saline for fluid resuscitation in diabetic ketoacidosis. J Crit Care 2012;27(2):138–45.
42. Krajewski ML, Raghunathan K, Paluszkiewicz SM, et al. Meta-analysis of high-versus low-chloride content in perioperative and critical care fluid resuscitation. Br J Surg 2015;102(1):24–36.
43. Shaw AD, Raghunathan K, Peyerl FW, et al. Association between intravenous chloride load during resuscitation and in-hospital mortality among patients with SIRS. Intensive Care Med 2014;40(12):1897–905.
44. McCluskey SA, Karkouti K, Wijeysundera D, et al. Hyperchloremia after noncardiac surgery is independently associated with increased morbidity and mortality. Anesth Analg 2013;117(2):412–21.
45. Young JB, Utter GH, Schermer CR, et al. Saline versus Plasma-Lyte A in initial resuscitation of trauma patients. Ann Surg 2014;259(2):255–62.
46. Chowdhury AH, Cox EF, Francis ST, et al. A randomized, controlled, double-blind crossover study on the effects of 2-l infusions of 0.9% saline and Plasma-Lyte® 148 on renal blood flow velocity and renal cortical tissue perfusion in healthy volunteers. Ann Surg 2012;256(1):18–24.
47. Wilcox CS. Regulation of renal blood flow by plasma chloride. J Clin Invest 1983;71(3):726–35.
48. Todd SR, Malinoski D, Muller PJ, et al. Lactated Ringer's is superior to normal saline in the resuscitation of uncontrolled hemorrhagic shock. J Trauma 2007;62(3):636–9.
49. Burch JM, Ortiz VB, Richardson RJ, et al. Abbreviated laparotomy and planned reoperation for critically injured patients. Ann Surg 1992;215(5):476–83.
50. Orbegozo Cortés D, Rayo Bonor A, Vincent JL. Isotonic crystalloid solutions: a structured review of the literature. Br J Anaesth 2014;112(6):968–81.

51. Raghunathan K, Shaw A, Nathanson B, et al. Association between the choice of IV crystalloid and in-hospital mortality among critically ill adults with sepsis. Crit Care Med 2014;42(7):1585–91.

52. Yunos NM, Kim IB, Bellomo R, et al. The biochemical effects of restricting chloride-rich fluids in intensive care. Crit Care Med 2011;39(11):2419–24.

53. Reddy SK, Bailey MJ, Beasley RW, et al. A protocol for the 0.9% saline versus Plasma-Lyte 148 for intensive care fluid therapy (SPLIT) study. Crit Care Resusc 2014;16(4):274–9.

54. Marx G, Pedder S, Smith L, et al. Resuscitation from septic shock with capillary leakage: hydroxyethyl starch (30KD), but not Ringer's solution maintains plasma volume and systemic oxygenation. Shock 2004;21(4):336–41.

55. Guidet B, Soni N, Rocca Della G, et al. A balanced view of balanced solutions. Crit Care 2010;14(5):325.

56. Magder S, Potter BJ, Varennes BD, et al. Fluids after cardiac surgery: a pilot study of the use of colloids versus crystalloids. Crit Care Med 2010;38(11):2117–24.

57. Sort P, Navasa M, Arroyo V, et al. Effect of intravenous albumin on renal impairment and mortality in patients with cirrhosis and spontaneous bacterial peritonitis. N Engl J Med 1999;341(6):403–9.

58. Myburgh J, Cooper DJ, Finfer S, et al. Saline or albumin for fluid resuscitation in patients with traumatic brain injury. N Engl J Med 2007;357:874–84.

59. Gattas DJ, Dan A, Myburgh J, et al. Fluid resuscitation with 6% hydroxyethyl starch (130/0.4 and 130/0.42) in acutely ill patients: systematic review of effects on mortality and treatment with renal replacement therapy. Intensive Care Med 2013;39(4):558–68.

60. Hartog CS, Skupin H, Natanson C, et al. Systematic analysis of hydroxyethyl starch (HES) reviews: proliferation of low-quality reviews overwhelms the results of well-performed meta-analyses. Intensive Care Med 2012;38(8):1258–71.

61. Antonelli M, Sandroni C. Hydroxyethyl starch for intravenous volume replacement: more harm than benefit. JAMA 2013;309(7):723–4.

62. Brunkhorst FM, Engel C, Bloos F, et al. Intensive insulin therapy and pentastarch resuscitation in severe sepsis. N Engl J Med 2008;358(2):125–39.

63. Wilkes MM, Navickis RJ, Sibbald WJ. Albumin versus hydroxyethyl starch in cardiopulmonary bypass surgery: a meta-analysis of postoperative bleeding. Ann Thorac Surg 2001;72(2):527–33.

64. O'Malley CMN, Frumento RJ, Hardy MA, et al. A randomized, double-blind comparison of lactated Ringer's solution and 0.9% NaCl during renal transplantation. Anesth Analg 2005;100(5):1518–24.

65. Perel P, Roberts I, Ker K. Colloids versus crystalloids for fluid resuscitation in critically ill patients. Cochrane Database Syst Rev 2013;(2):CD000567.

66. Reinhart K, Perner A, Sprung CL, et al. Consensus statement of the ESICM task force on colloid volume therapy in critically ill patients. Intensive Care Med 2012;38(3):368–83.

67. Hydroxyethyl starch solutions: FDA safety communication - Boxed warning on increased mortality and severe renal injury and risk of bleeding [Internet]. 2015. p. 1–2. Available at: http://www.fda.gov/safety/medwatch/safetyinformation/safetyalertsforhumanmedicalproducts/ucm358349.htm. Accessed May 14, 2015.

68. Biesen V, Yegenaga I, Vanholder R, et al. Relationship between fluid status and its management on acute renal failure (ARF) in intensive care unit (ICU) patients with sepsis: a prospective analysis. J Nephrol 2005;18(1):54–60.

69. Arikan AA, Zappitelli M, Goldstein SL, et al. Fluid overload is associated with impaired oxygenation and morbidity in critically ill children. Pediatr Crit Care Med 2012;13(3):253–8.

70. Sutherland SM, Zappitelli M, Alexander SR, et al. Fluid overload and mortality in children receiving continuous renal replacement therapy: the prospective pediatric continuous renal replacement therapy registry. Am J Kidney Dis 2010;55(2): 316–25.

71. Brandstrup B, Tønnesen H, Beier-Holgersen R, et al. Effects of intravenous fluid restriction on postoperative complications: comparison of two perioperative fluid regimens. Ann Surg 2003;238(5):641–8.

72. Oczkowski SJW, Mazzetti I, Meade MO, et al. Furosemide and albumin for diuresis of edema (FADE): a study protocol for a randomized controlled trial. Trials 2014;15(1):222.

73. Teixeira C, Garzotto F, Piccinni P, et al. Fluid balance and urine volume are independent predictors of mortality in acute kidney injury. Crit Care 2013;17(1):R14.

74. Mehta RL, Pascual MT, Soroko S, et al. Diuretics, mortality, and nonrecovery of renal function in acute renal failure. JAMA 2002;288(20):2547–53.

75. Chawla LS, Davison DL, Brasha-Mitchell E, et al. Development and standardization of afurosemide stress test to predict the severity of acute kidney injury. Crit Care 2013;17(5):R207.

76. Shilliday IR, Quinn KJ, Allison ME. Loop diuretics in the management of acute renal failure: a prospective, double-blind, placebo-controlled, randomized study. Nephrol Dial Transplant 1997;12(12):2592–6.

77. Rosner MH, Ostermann M, Murugan R, et al. Indications and management of mechanical fluid removal in critical illness. Br J Anaesth 2014;113(5):764–71.

78. Bouchard J, Mehta RL. Volume management in continuous renal replacement therapy. Semin Dial 2009;22(2):146–50.

79. Bouchard J, Soroko SB, Chertow GM, et al. Fluid accumulation, survival and recovery of kidney function in critically ill patients with acute kidney injury. Kidney Int 2009;76(4):422–7.

80. Wald R, Shariff SZ, Adhikari NKJ, et al. The association between renal replacement therapy modality and long-term outcomes among critically ill adults with acute kidney injury. Crit Care Med 2014;42(4):868–77.

81. Schneider AG, Bellomo R, Bagshaw SM, et al. Choice of renal replacement therapy modality and dialysis dependence after acute kidney injury: a systematic review and meta-analysis. Intensive Care Med 2013;39(6):987–97.

Fluid Overload

Michael E. O'Connor, MBBS, BSc, MRCP, FRCA[a,b],
John R. Prowle, MA, MB BChir, MSc, MD, FRCP, FFICM[a,b,c],*

KEYWORDS

- Fluid overload • Edema • Critical illness • Diuretics • Ultrafiltration

KEY POINTS

- Fluid overload is an almost universal finding in the critically ill, despite little evidence to justify fluid therapy within the intensive care unit after initial resuscitation.
- Hemodynamic responses to fluid administration are unpredictable and short lived, which may contribute to recurrent fluid administration.
- Positive fluid balances have been consistently associated with adverse outcomes and organ dysfunction in critical illness.
- Structural and functional changes in the endothelium and extracellular matrix during systemic inflammation leads to sequestration of administered fluid outside the circulation, promoting fluid accumulation and impeding its removal.
- Strategies to manage fluid balances in the critically ill require close attention to true need for fluid administration and active prevention or management of fluid overload.

INTRODUCTION: ASSOCIATION BETWEEN FLUID OVERLOAD AND ADVERSE OUTCOMES IN CRITICAL ILLNESS

When delivered correctly for the right reasons and at the appropriate time, intravenous fluid can be lifesaving. However, in established critical illness, a combination of increased fluid intake and relatively reduced urine output frequently results in accumulation of excess fluid within the body (**Table 1**). In particular, critically ill patients with sepsis frequently receive very large volumes of fluid resulting in significantly positive fluid balances; for example, in a retrospective analysis of data from the Vasopressin in Septic Shock Trial (VASST), the mean fluid balance was on average +4.2 L at 12 hours after

Disclosures: Dr J.R. Prowle has received speakers and consultant's fees from Baxter and institutional funding from NIKKISO Europe GmbH, both manufactures of continuous renal replacement therapy technology.
[a] Adult Critical Care Unit, The Royal London Hospital, Barts Health NHS Trust, Whitechapel Road, London E1 1BB, UK; [b] Centre for Translational Medicine & Therapeutics, William Harvey Research Institute, Queen Mary University of London, Charterhouse Square, London EC1M 6BQ, UK; [c] Department of Renal and Transplant Medicine, The Royal London Hospital, Barts Health NHS Trust, Whitechapel Road, London E1 1BB, UK
* Corresponding author. Adult Critical Care Unit, The Royal London Hospital, Barts Health NHS Trust, Whitechapel Road, London E1 1BB, UK.
E-mail address: j.prowle@qmul.ac.uk

Crit Care Clin 31 (2015) 803–821
http://dx.doi.org/10.1016/j.ccc.2015.06.013
0749-0704/15/$ – see front matter © 2015 Elsevier Inc. All rights reserved.

Table 1		
Contributions to positive fluid balances in critical illness		
	Early in Admission to Intensive Care	Later in Admission to Intensive Care
Excessive intake of fluid	Need for blood products Intravenous fluid resuscitation	Obligate daily fluid needs in terms of drug therapies and nutrition Intercurrent clinical events requiring fluid resuscitation
Inadequate fluid elimination	Acute or chronic kidney disease Acute hemodynamic instability Fluid losses from circulation to interstitial space	Ongoing renal impairment Cardiac and liver dysfunction Sequestration of fluid in the interstitium and body cavities

presentation with severe sepsis and +11.0 L by day 4 after enrollment.[1] Crucially, in this analysis, the upper 2 quartiles of fluid balance were associated with progressively worse survival than patients with less positive fluid balance, even after adjustment for baseline illness severity and demographics. It is pertinent to consider the magnitude of fluid excess we are dealing with here. The fluid balance in the mid upper quartile of the VASST analysis at 4 days was +20.5 L; that is about *50% of the normal total body water*, clearly far in excess of any plausible volume deficit at baseline. Despite clinicians' apparent willingness to administer very large volumes of fluid over several days to the sickest critically ill patients, when the relationship between fluid balance and outcome has been examined a consistent association has been demonstrated between positive fluid balance and prolonged intensive care unit (ICU) stay, development or worsening of organ dysfunction and excess mortality.[2–11] A recent systematic review considered 17 observational studies reporting fluid balances in relation to clinical outcomes including data from more than 5000 ICU patients; in these results, nonsurvivors (48% mortality) had a more positive cumulative fluid balance by day 7 of their ICU stay than survivors by, on average, 4.35 L.[12] In parallel to the adverse effects of fluid overload, patients instead achieving a negative fluid balance in the ICU have an increased survival from septic shock[13] and in acute kidney injury (AKI) treated with continuous renal replacement therapy[8] and have a shorter duration of mechanical ventilation and ICU stay.[6,14] Of course, demonstration of an association between positive fluid balance and adverse outcomes does not prove a causative role of fluid overload in mediating adverse outcomes; undoubtedly, positive fluid balances are a marker of severity critical illness both as a reflection of the degree of physiologic instability and physician response to it.[15] However, the authors think there are strong biological arguments, supported by a wealth of observational evidence, that fluid overload does worsen organ function; therefore, excessive fluid accumulation is an avoidable source of iatrogenic morbidity and mortality in at least a proportion of patients. Many causative mechanisms could mediate a direct association between the development of interstitial edema and the development of progressive organ dysfunction; these include impaired oxygen and metabolite diffusion, distorted tissue architecture, obstruction of organ perfusion, venous outflow and lymphatic drainage, and disturbed cell-cell interaction.

Evidence of the adverse effects of fluid overload can be found in almost all organ systems (**Fig. 1**), including the gastrointestinal tract,[16] the liver,[17,18] the cardiovascular system,[19–22] the central nervous system,[23,24] and skin and soft tissues.[25–28] In particular, fluid overload and the resultant visceral edema is a risk factor for intra-abdominal hypertension (IAH). In an ICU population, positive fluid balances have been associated with an increased risk of IAH,[29–31] which in turn is strongly associated with the development of other organ dysfunction, particularly the development of AKI.[12,29,31–34] The

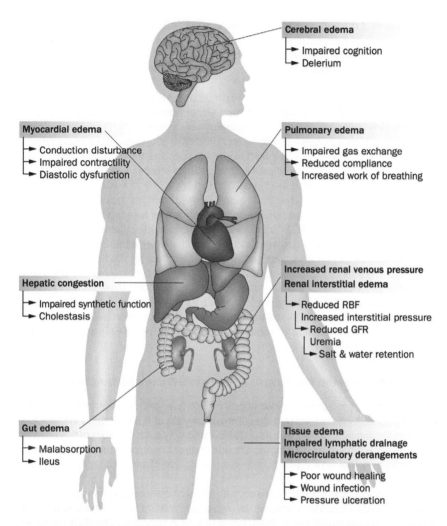

Fig. 1. Pathologic sequelae of fluid overload in organ systems. GFR, glomerular filtration rate; RBF, renal blood flow. (*From* Prowle JR, Echeverri JE, Ligabo EV, et al. Fluid balance and acute kidney injury. Nat Rev Nephrol 2010;6(2):110; with permission.)

effects of fluid overload are perhaps most well recognized in the respiratory system where the development or worsening of pulmonary edema can lead to impaired gas exchange, reduced lung compliance, and increased work of breathing.[35] Positive fluid balances and liberal fluid strategies have been associated with decreased survival, greater duration of mechanical ventilation, and an increased ICU length of stay in retrospective analyses of patient outcomes in acute lung injury[7,36] and prospective studies.[37] Importantly, the only multicenter prospective randomized controlled study examining fluid management strategies in the ICU focused on a group with severe lung injury, the Fluid And Catheter Treatment Trial (FACTT).[6] FACTT compared a liberal versus conservative fluid management strategy in patients with acute respiratory distress syndrome. Fluid restriction and diuretics were used to maintain lower central venous or pulmonary capillary wedge pressure in patients in the conservative arm of the study; over 7 days, this strategy achieved a neutral fluid balance in the conservative arm compared with, on average, a positive fluid balance of +7 L in the liberal arm. The conservative fluid management strategy led to fewer ventilator days,[6] and a post hoc analysis indicated that achieving a negative fluid balance with diuretics was associated with improved survival.[14]

Finally, the relationship between fluid overload and AKI is of particular interest given the role of the kidney in maintaining salt and water homeostasis. Traditional teaching has emphasized the need for fluid resuscitation aiming to maintain renal perfusion and maintain urine output in patients with or at risk of AKI. However, the clinical literature has consistently demonstrated the fluid overload is particularly harmful in AKI; in a previous review,[38] the authors identified 17 observational studies examining fluid balance and outcomes in patients with AKI from 2008 to 13,[8,9,11,14,39–50] and all demonstrated evidence of harm from fluid overload and/or benefit from its resolution. Prospective evidence supporting improved renal outcome with active avoidance of fluid overload is also available from the FACTT study whereby conservative fluid management was associated with a strong trend toward a lower need for renal replacement therapy[6] and a lower incidence of AKI in a post hoc analysis adjusted for fluid balance.[51] Strong physiologic arguments support a causative role for fluid overload in the persistence of AKI whereby increased venous pressure, extrarenal compression, and intrarenal interstitial pressure all potentially act to oppose renal blood flow and reduce glomerular ultrafiltration gradient,[38] in-line with an observed association between more positive fluid balance at initiation of renal replacement therapy (RRT) and poorer renal outcomes in severe AKI.[39]

DEVELOPMENT OF FLUID OVERLOAD: A PATIENT-PHYSICIAN INTERACTION

Given very significant adverse associations of fluid overload, the authors think there is a clinical imperative to minimize the extent and impact of fluid overload in the ICU. To achieve this, clinicians need to appreciate how and why such degrees of fluid overload occur. Because almost all fluid inputs are under direct control of the clinical team, we first have to consider how and why we give fluid therapy in the ICU and the evidence underlying this practice.

Conventional management of patients with signs of inadequate tissue perfusion is to ensure adequate circulating volume by rapid administration of intravenous fluids. Although the administration of an initial bolus of fluid in shocked patients is considered an essential feature of emergency management, continued or repeated fluid therapy beyond the very initial phase of management may not be beneficial. Three large randomized controlled trials[52–54] have now demonstrated that, in the first 6 hours after presentation with sepsis, management strategies including administration of intravenous fluids targeting the restoration of surrogate end points for tissue perfusion (central venous oxygen saturation) and volume status (central venous pressure [CVP]) are not associated with improved outcomes. Thus, even during the earliest phase of critical illness, the rationale and indications for fluid therapy, beyond an initial bolus, are not well established. In light of these findings, the Surviving Sepsis Campaign has, in March 2015, revised their 2012 guidelines[55] to remove the use of CVP and central venous oxygen saturation as targets for hemodynamic therapy, including intravenous fluids.[56]

Once in the ICU, bolus fluid therapy is frequently continued provided with the intention of improving systemic hemodynamics and tissue perfusion. The rationale of bolus fluid is to augment cardiac output in the context of presumed inadequate ventricular preload. However, routine hemodynamic targets of resuscitation (blood pressure, heart rate, CVP) are poorly predictive of cardiac output and much less indicative of adequate tissue perfusion; the effects of acute illness, chronic disease, and drug therapy can unpredictably alter the response of the cardiovascular system to fluid administration. In particular, there are no clinical data to support a link between CVP and circulating volume or hemodynamic response to fluid therapy,[57] as the relationship between CVP, cardiac performance, and fluid responsiveness is highly variable depending on the clinical context.[58] Generally in critical illness, the cardiovascular response to fluid is modified by diverse factors, including myocardial function,[19,59,60] arterial resistance, regional perfusion,[61,62] venous reservoir capacity, and capillary permeability,[63] making the clinical assessment of the response to fluid therapy very challenging resulting in considerable clinical practice variation. Importantly, although fluid therapy will only effectively treat hypovolemic shock,[64–66] it is frequently used in the context of cardiogenic and vasodilatory shock to rule out a hypovolemic component, with little regard to the substantial risks of fluid accumulation in these conditions. Measurements of cardiac output do provide information on global tissue perfusion and allow fluid and other inotropic therapies to be titrated against cardiac response and should be considered if there is any uncertainty about the potential response to fluid therapy; however, in practice, these are not routinely used in contemporary ICUs.[67] However, indiscriminate use of intravenous fluid to *maximize* cardiac output in established critical illness might not be beneficial if the effects are short lived or do not correlate with improvement in tissue oxygenation. For instance, in a large animal model, intravenous fluid boluses caused short-lived increases in cardiac output and blood pressure[68] but no change in renal oxygen delivery. Similarly, in a rat model of hemorrhagic shock, fluid resuscitation with crystalloids could restore systemic blood pressure but had no effect on renal microvascular oxygenation.[69]

The natural consequence of exploratory fluid therapy and persistent boluses given to achieve short-lived hemodynamic responses is fluid accumulation.[68,70] This fluid accumulation is particularly pronounced in systematic inflammatory states. In sepsis, rapid fluid redistribution from damaged and leaky capillaries means only 5% of the volume of fluid infused is estimated to remain in the intravascular compartment after 90 minutes[71]; even in an intact circulation, only around 20% of infused crystalloid remains in the vascular compartment after redistribution.[72] These effects, combined with obligate fluid input, are from a multitude of sources[73]; the relative inability of the kidney to manage salt and water homeostasis in the context of critical illness means that almost all critically ill patients are at risk of fluid overload.[17] As the adverse effects of fluid overload and limited clinical effects of fluid therapy are increasingly recognized,[74] clinical fluid administration is likely to shift from ensuring adequacy of fluid resuscitation to focus much more on the prevention and treatment of fluid overload. However, in order to confidently make this paradigm shift from a deeply engrained culture of repeated fluid boluses, a sound understanding of the pathophysiology of the development of fluid overload, its adverse effects on organ systems, and the therapeutic strategies for its resolution are required.

PATHOGENESIS OF FLUID OVERLOAD

Fluid overload can be defined as a pathologic accumulation of water and dissolved electrolytes in the body beyond that seen in healthy individuals. In general, this excess fluid accumulates as extracellular fluid in expandable interstitial compartments as interstitial edema and as macroscopic fluid collections in the thorax (pleural effusions) or abdomen (ascites). Thus, fluid overload is predominantly a syndrome of interstitial edema and total of body sodium excess (the predominant extracellular cation). As discussed, interstitial edema is likely to mediate many of the adverse effects of fluid overload.[17] At an organ level, tissue edema impedes capillary blood flow and lymphatic drainage, especially in encapsulated organs, such as the kidneys and liver, where additional volume cannot be accommodated without an increase in interstitial pressure,[75] causing further impairment of organ perfusion and function.

The dynamic role of vascular integrity in maintaining vascular volume means that it is crucial to consider key structures, such as the endothelial glycocalyx, when considering the development and treatment of fluid overload.[76,77] In recent years, our understanding of the vascular biology of edema formation in the capillary bed has progressed from a balance of pressure-driven plasma ultrafiltration across the capillary wall and colloid-osmotic pressure–mediated plasma reabsorption, in the classic Starling model, to a revised model incorporating our knowledge of the structure and function of the glycocalyx.[78,79] The glycocalyx is a complex network of cell-bound proteoglycans, glycosaminoglycan side chains, and sialo-proteins that envelop the luminal side of intact endothelium including the intercellular endothelial cleft where intercellular transcapillary water fluxes occur.[80] The glycocalyx participates in numerous physiologic functions from regulating vascular permeability to storing a large proportion of noncirculating plasma volume and modulating inflammation and hemostasis. An important functional role of the glycocalyx is to bind plasma proteins; this effectively excludes proteins from the subendothelial cleft (ETC) resulting in a local oncotic gradient between the plasma and cleft opposing transcapillary water efflux.[78,79] An understanding of the glycocalyx function has, thus, led to a revised Starling model whereby a local oncotic gradient that remains fairly constant along the capillary and opposes and attenuates pressure-mediated plasma water efflux without ever causing reabsorption of fluid from the interstitium, except in specialized vascular beds in the renal tubules and the intestines.[78] This model has several important physiologic implications. Firstly, the primary pathology resulting in increased capillary permeability in inflammatory states is the disruption of the glycocalyx, which is a physical process that will not be rapidly reversible once established. Secondly, rates of fluid loss from capillaries will be determined by capillary pressure (increased by increased venous pressure and the extent of precapillary arteriolar vasodilation, which transmits systemic pressure to the capillary bed) but relatively little by plasma oncotic pressure, as the oncotic gradient in the small ETC is chiefly determined by glycocalyx integrity. Finally, as transcapillary fluxes are smaller than previously predicted and unidirectional, almost all vascular refilling from the interstitium occurs via lymphatic channels.[78,79] These observations have corresponding clinical implications: Firstly, once the glycocalyx is disrupted, patients will be at ongoing risk of fluid interstitial accumulation. Secondly, manipulation of the colloid concentration in plasma is not likely to provide much more effective vascular filling and certainly will not encourage vascular refilling form the capillary bed findings consistent with the limited hemodynamic benefit of colloids over crystalloids in resuscitation[72] and absence of any fluid sparing effect in patients with severe sepsis.[81] Finally, vascular refilling during fluid removal is likely to be slow and relatively fixed; therefore, tolerance of rapid rates of fluid removal in critically ill patients will be poor and a little offset by elevating colloid-osmotic pressure. Evidence of widespread alteration and breakdown of the endothelial glycocalyx has been demonstrated in disease states, such as sepsis,[82–85] major surgery,[85] trauma,[86] and postischemic states[87]; this process occurs both because of the direct effect of ischemia, oxidative stress, and pathogen-host response–mediated injury or because of the effect of circulating toxins, such as lipopolysaccharide and inflammatory mediators, particularly tumor necrosis factor (TNF) α.[82,84,88] Acute hyperglycemia, a common finding in critical illness, has also been associated with loss of glycocalyx integrity.[89] As well as leading to plasma water and protein extravasation, loss of glycocalyx potentiates ongoing inflammatory responses by of exposure of endothelial cell adhesion molecules.[76,90] Such mechanisms may mediate important pathologic events associated with interstitial edema, such as acute lung injury.[84]

In combination, loss of fluid from the vascular space and loss of glycocalyx volume itself, which causes an increase vascular fluid capacitance, create a potential need for fluid replacement, but in a context whereby further interstitial edema may rapidly arise. This circumstance presents a clinical dilemma of providing enough fluid to avoid overt hypovolemia while avoiding a vicious cycle whereby volume expansion leads to worsening tissue edema impairing further organ function. Although squaring this circle may by impossible in many patients, an awareness of these mechanisms should prompt fluid therapy to be regarded not as an obligation but as a powerful drug therapy to be carefully titrated.

In addition to a clear role in the development of edema in systemic inflammation, glycocalyx dysfunction seems to play a central role in edematous states more generally, emphasizing the key importance of this mechanism. For instance, in nephrotic syndrome, the primary processes driving edema are now thought to be primary renal salt and water retention and systemic inflammation involving TNF α[91] rather than hypoalbuminemia, which, in isolation, does not cause edema. Similarly, atrial natriuretic peptide release, stimulated by mechanical wall stress cardiac atria, has been shown to cause acute deterioration of the glycocalyx and is associated with increased vascular permeability and intestinal fluid shift.[92,93] Perioperatively, volume expansion has been shown to mediate atrial natriuretic peptide (ANP) release and shedding of glycocalyx,[94] raising the possibility that fluid therapy can indirectly compromise vascular integrity and worsen fluid shifts to the interstitium. These mechanisms suggest that there may be an unappreciated, long-lasting effect of strategies to elevate CVP or maximize cardiac output with volume expansion in the critically ill if this triggers ANP release.

Another underappreciated mechanism of edema formation is alteration of structure and function of the extracellular matrix (ECM) in systemic inflammation and critical illness.[95] Normally, fluid loss from capillaries leads to increased interstitial pressure opposing transcapillary ultrafiltration and promoting lymphatic filling, which is the initial process in lymphatic drainage. However, after local tissue injury or exposure to inflammatory mediators, interstitial pressure has been noted to decrease, despite rapid efflux of fluid to the interstitium. Decreased interstitial pressure is thought to arise because of the release of cellular tension exerted on the collagen and microfibril networks in the ECM by mechanisms including release of collagen-binding β1-integrins.[96] In addition to the loss of ECM mechanical integrity, the resultant exposure of glycosaminoglycan ground substance, which is normally compressed and underhydrated, expands and takes up fluid.[95] Local injury[97] and a wide range of local and systemic inflammatory mediators[98] and toxins, including lipopolysaccharide,[99] have been shown to mediate such ECM changes with a decrease in interstitial pressure, which promotes the development and retention of tissue edema. Finally, low interstitial pressure in combination with disruption of local lymphatic architecture and the direct effect of inflammatory mediators and immobility on lymphatic function will result in impaired lymphatic drainage of accumulated tissue fluid, further contributing to interstitial fluid accumulation.[100]

Overall, the current understanding of the vascular biology of interstitial edema emphasizes the structural changes in the capillaries and endothelium that predispose to interstitial fluid accumulation, which are mechanisms that are not directly related to plasma protein loss or colloid osmotic pressure (**Fig. 2**). These changes may actually be worsened by excessive volume loading through direct and endocrine mechanisms.

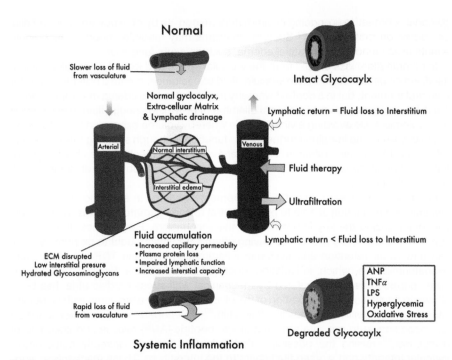

Fig. 2. Systemic inflammation results in disruption of endothelial glycocalyx and changes in the ECM and lymphatic drainage that promote loss of plasma fluid to the extracellular space and its retention in the interstitial compartment. These processes have implications for the magnitude and duration of response to fluid therapy and ability to resolve fluid overload once it has arisen. LPS, lipopolysaccharide.

An important consequence of the modified Starling model incorporating understanding of the role of the glycocalyx is that as return of fluid to the circulation is predominantly by lymphatic drainage, the ability to rapidly resolve fluid accumulation by diuresis or ultrafiltration will be limited. Thus, although the prevention of fluid overload in critical illness will be very challenging, every fluid administration should be carefully considered, as resolution of the resultant interstitial edema is likely to be very difficult.

MANAGEMENT OF FLUID OVERLOAD
Controlling Fluid Intake

Equipped with an appreciation of the causes and consequences of fluid overload, clinicians can adopt a more systematic approach to fluid management in the ICU. Thus, the process has to commence with the rationale management of fluid resuscitation to minimization initial fluid accumulation. In brief, recent conceptual models of resuscitation of the critically ill have emphasized sequential phases of fluid resuscitation.[101] In this approach, fluid therapy is provided emergently during very acute clinical instability (*rescue* phase) but is rapidly tempered to judicious use of intravenous fluid to *optimize* the hemodynamic status and thence to a *stabilization* phase whereby clinicians aim for an even or slightly negative fluid balance. Finally, in the *de-escalation* phase, the clinician aims to mobilize accumulated fluid during the initial resuscitation. This approach places the consideration of fluid overload at the center of the hemodynamic management of shock rather than as an after thought and emphasizes the need to consider the need for fluid therapy in the context of clinical response and fluid balance at all stages of critical illness. In line with this concept, the authors have suggested an approach whereby, beyond the initial first few hours of acute critical illness, evidence of inadequate organ function should prompt the assessment of the cardiac output and bolus fluid therapy should be considered only in the context of inadequate cardiac output and evidence of volume responsiveness, with an end point of an acceptable level of cardiac output and system perfusion and not with the intention to maximize stroke volume.[38] This strategy sets several hurdles to justify fluid therapy, reflecting the complexity of the assessment of volume status in critical illness, the short-lived effect of fluid therapy, the longer-term adverse effects of fluid overload, and the great difficulty of removing fluid once it has been lost to the interstitium.

Fluid Removal: Diuretics, Ultrafiltration, and Monitoring

The more rigorous approach to the assessment of need for fluid therapy described earlier is then accompanied by a process of continued assessment and management of fluid balance, with the intention of preventing or resolving fluid overload once stability has been achieved. A schematic approach to this process has been suggested[38,73]; if signs of fluid overload are present, then steps to resolve this should be undertaken, whereas if a patient is perceived to be euvolemic, then fluid balance should be actively managed to prevent the acquisition of fluid overload, particularly if prescribed fluid inputs is high (**Fig. 3**). Choice of diuretic therapy over mechanical fluid removal will depend on renal function, baseline urine output, and severity of fluid overload; however, the response to therapy should be regularly reassessed. Although evidence suggests that the use of diuretics to treat established AKI is ineffective[102] and may delay definitive AKI management with RRT,[103] their use in a large population of patients with AKI in the ICU has not been associated with increased mortality[104]; thus the use of diuretics to manage fluid balance, paying close attention to clinical response, is logical and clinically supportable.[105] A diuretic challenge at an adequate dose of 1.0 to 1.5 mg/kg furosemide may be useful in making an early assessment of patients likely to respond and those that may require RRT to avoid definite fluid management in those likely to require it.[106,107]

When using an active fluid management strategy with diuretics or mechanical ultrafiltration, it is important to distinguish between the overall level of fluid overload (the eventual target) and the ability to remove fluid from the circulation without inducing hemodynamic instability. In the sickest patients, these two factors may be disassociated necessitating a slow transition from prevention of further accumulation of fluid to slow fluid removal. Different forms of monitoring inform clinicians on these differing aspects of therapy; static assessments of fluid status inform on the extent of fluid accumulation, whereas dynamic assessments of cardiac output and tissue perfusion provide information on tolerance of rate of removal (**Table 2**).

Determining the total quantity of fluid overload and the goal of therapy is challenging, as charted fluid balances are often inaccurate and do not account for unmeasured fluid losses or change in flesh weight during prolonged critical illness. However, charted daily fluid balance do seem to be a more useful guide in determining the risk of fluid overload than daily weights in the ICU, which can be inaccurate in guiding fluid management in the critical care setting.[108] Bioelectrical impedance body-composition analysis (BIA), a noninvasive method of fluid assessment, can provide estimates of total-body, extracellular, and intracellular water to allow the quantification of fluid overload and setting of dry weight[109,110]; BIA is used widely in determining the fluid status in patients with end-stage renal failure on hemodialysis or peritoneal dialysis. However, this technology has not been extensively validated in critical care; its benefit over use of a well-kept fluid balance has not yet been established.

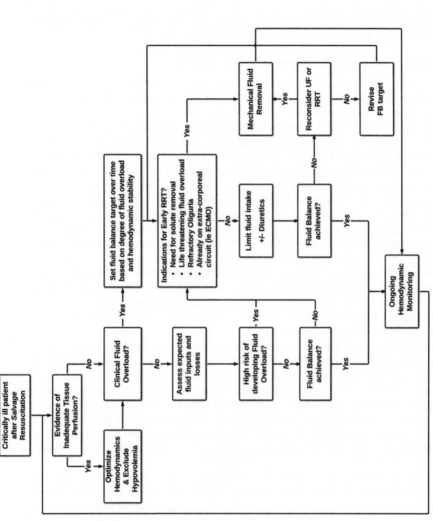

Fig. 3. A clinical approach to prevention and treatment of fluid overload after the initial phase of critical illness. Many different technologies for hemodynamic and fluid balance assessment can be applied within this philosophy. ECMO, extracorporeal membrane oxygenation; FB, fluid balance; UF, ultrafiltration. (*Adapted from* Rosner MH, Ostermann M, Murugan R, et al. Indications and management of mechanical fluid removal in critical illness. Br J Anaesth 2014;113(5):764–71; with permission.)

Table 2
Methodology for assessment of response to changes in circulating volume and quantification fluid overload in critically ill patients

Measure	Characteristics
Measures of fluid responsiveness and tolerance of fluid removal	
Stroke volume variation Pulse pressure variation	Requires mandatory mechanical ventilation Indicates position on Frank-Starling curve not extent of tissue fluid overload
Echocardiography	Subjective impression of right ventricular filling and inferior vena cava collapse Requires technical expertise Poor windows in critically ill
Passive straight leg raise	Provides impression of fluid responsiveness without requirement for fluid challenge Difficult or impossible in some patients
Stroke volume or other hemodynamic response to fluid challenge	Require administration of fluid Positive response does not imply fluid is clinically indicated or that response will be sustained Fluid responsiveness is normal physiologic state
Central venous or pulmonary artery wedge pressure	No evidence that absolute values or relative changes correlate with cardiac output or fluid responsiveness Very low values may imply right ventricular preload could be increased with fluid therapy
Blood volume monitoring (continuous hematocrit)	A monitor of reverse fluid responsiveness, the hemodynamic effect of fluid removal Currently available during hemodialysis only May be too imprecise to preempt hypotension during ultrafiltration in the critically ill
Measures of fluid overload	
Clinical examination (peripheral and pulmonary edema)	Significant volume overload can occur without edema Edema and intravascular volume depletion may coexist Wide range of addition contributing causes
Serial weight	Quantifies extent of fluid overload Difficult to perform in critically ill Loss of muscle and fat mass may mask fluid gain
Cumulative fluid balance	Quantifies extent of fluid overload Often imprecisely recorded Difficult to account for insensible losses
Chest radiograph	Gives impression of pulmonary edema only Wide differential diagnosis
Oxygenation indices Ventilatory requirements	Nonspecific for fluid overload depending on clinical context
Lung ultrasound	More sensitive for early pulmonary congestion before chest radiograph, oxygenation, and symptomatic changes[116] Requires technical expertise May be confounded by other pulmonary pathology
Echocardiography	Subjective impression of right ventricular or inferior vena cava distension Requires technical expertise Poor windows in critically ill

(continued on next page)

Table 2
(continued)

Measure	Characteristics
Intra-abdominal pressure	Only significant if abnormal
	Cause may be primary or secondary (fluid overload)
Bioimpedance analysis of body composition	Noninvasive
	Enables separate estimate of extracellular volume over hydration and intracellular (muscle) volume
	Quantifies extent of fluid overload
	Methodology not validated in critically ill
	May be difficult to perform good-quality measurements at bedside in ICU
	Requires accurate weight measurement
	Range of algorithms to calculate volume measurements, which are device specific and may not be applicable to critically ill

Adapted from Prowle JR, Kirwan CJ, Bellomo R. Fluid management for the prevention and attenuation of acute kidney injury. Nat Rev Nephrol 2014;10(1):42; with permission.

Given the difficulty in determining the true extent of fluid overload and the uncertain tolerance of fluid removal even when significant overload is present, dynamic monitoring of fluid removal should not be neglected. The commencement of fluid removal could be considered a reverse fluid challenge using the same clinical and hemodynamic monitoring that would be used to assess the response to fluid administration. These considerations are important in assessing the outcomes of fluid removal strategies. A follow-up of a sample of patients from the FACCT study demonstrated that patients in the conservatively managed group tended to have poorer cognitive function after recovery from critical illness; hypothetically, this could be linked to transient episodes of hypoperfusion during fluid management.[111] In line with this, although patients in FACCT only received fluid removal when strict criteria for hemodynamic stability were present, there was a higher incidence of new shock in the conservative arm. A recent follow-up nonrandomized study examined a FACCT-Lite conservative fluid strategy,[112] which resulted in an approximately 2-L positive fluid balance over 7 days (compared with even and +7-L balances, respectively, with conservative and liberal strategies in FACCT); this approach demonstrated similar respiratory and renal outcomes to the conservative group in FACCT but with a new shock incidence similar to the liberal arm, suggesting this may be a safer approach. Further evidence for the importance of hemodynamic stability during fluid removal is found in the large body of observation evidence suggesting that the use of continuous renal replacement therapy for the treatment of AKI in the ICU is associated with improved long-term renal outcomes compared with intermittent dialysis.[113,114] This observation is potentially related to lower rates of hemodynamic instability and recurrent renal ischemia associated with slower fluid removal that allows for the slow vascular refilling during continuous or extended ultrafiltration.[115] Related to improved tolerance of fluid removal, continuous therapy has been shown to better allow negative fluid balances to be achieved in the ICU compared with intermittent therapy, which was associated with progressive fluid accumulation.[11] Thus, continuous use of extended RRT modalities may be beneficial to long-term organ function both by avoiding recurrent hemodynamic instability and by achieving better resolution of fluid overload. Collectively, this evidence suggests that fluid removal strategies do need to be carefully titrated and monitored and that futures trials considering such approaches will have to consider measures on longer-term organ functions as well as short-term ICU outcomes.

SUMMARY

In the critically ill, fluid overload is widely prevalent and has been consistently associated with adverse outcomes and organ dysfunction. Although some degree of fluid accumulation is an almost inevitable consequence of early resuscitation requirements and obligate fluid intakes, many patients receive multiple fluid boluses to ill-defined indications and with, at best, very short-term hemodynamic effects. Once accrued, fluid overload is challenging to resolve, as structural changes in the vascular bed and the ECM promote fluid sequestration in the interstitial compartment. Thus, any approach to fluid management requires careful attention to the true requirement for fluid therapies; fluids should be regarded as powerful drugs with serious potential adverse effects rather than a default low-risk response to clinical changes.

Critical care should involve the regular assessment, management, and prevention of fluid overload. When fluid removal is attempted, careful and continued monitoring is essential, as vascular refilling is likely to be slow and the extent of total fluid accumulation and tolerance of fluid removal may be poorly correlated. As yet there is little prospective evidence to guide clinicians in this area, and therapy should be tailored to individual patient requirements.

REFERENCES

1. Boyd JH, Forbes J, Nakada TA, et al. Fluid resuscitation in septic shock: a positive fluid balance and elevated central venous pressure are associated with increased mortality. Crit Care Med 2011;39:259–65.
2. Pan SW, Kao HK, Lien TC, et al. Acute kidney injury on ventilator initiation day independently predicts prolonged mechanical ventilation in intensive care unit patients. J Crit Care 2011;26:586–92.
3. Vieira JM Jr, Castro I, Curvello-Neto A, et al. Effect of acute kidney injury on weaning from mechanical ventilation in critically ill patients. Crit Care Med 2007;35:184–91.
4. Stein A, de Souza LV, Belettini CR, et al. Fluid overload and changes in serum creatinine after cardiac surgery: predictors of mortality and longer intensive care stay. A prospective cohort study. Crit Care 2012;16:R99.
5. Toraman F, Evrenkaya S, Yuce M, et al. Highly positive intraoperative fluid balance during cardiac surgery is associated with adverse outcome. Perfusion 2004;19:85–91.
6. National Heart Lung Blood Institute Acute Respiratory Distress Syndrome Clinical Trials Network, Wiedemann HP, Wheeler AP, et al. Comparison of two fluid-management strategies in acute lung injury. N Engl J Med 2006; 354:2564–75.
7. Murphy CV, Schramm GE, Doherty JA, et al. The importance of fluid management in acute lung injury secondary to septic shock. Chest 2009;136:102–9.
8. RENAL Replacement Therapy Study Investigators, Bellomo R, Cass A, et al. An observational study fluid balance and patient outcomes in the Randomized Evaluation of Normal vs. Augmented Level of Replacement Therapy trial. Crit Care Med 2012;40:1753–60.
9. Payen D, de Pont AC, Sakr Y, et al. A positive fluid balance is associated with a worse outcome in patients with acute renal failure. Crit Care 2008;12:R74.

10. Vincent JL, Sakr Y, Sprung CL, et al. Sepsis in European intensive care units: results of the SOAP study. Crit Care Med 2006;34:344–53.

11. Bouchard J, Soroko SB, Chertow GM, et al. Fluid accumulation, survival and recovery of kidney function in critically ill patients with acute kidney injury. Kidney Int 2009;76:422–7.

12. Malbrain ML, Marik PE, Witters I, et al. Fluid overload, de-resuscitation, and outcomes in critically ill or injured patients: a systematic review with suggestions for clinical practice. Anaesthesiol Intensive Ther 2014;46:361–80.

13. Alsous F, Khamiees M, DeGirolamo A, et al. Negative fluid balance predicts survival in patients with septic shock: a retrospective pilot study. Chest 2000; 117:1749–54.

14. Grams ME, Estrella MM, Coresh J, et al. Fluid balance, diuretic use, and mortality in acute kidney injury. Clin J Am Soc Nephrol 2011;6:966–73.

15. Bagshaw SM, Brophy PD, Cruz D, et al. Fluid balance as a biomarker: impact of fluid overload on outcome in critically ill patients with acute kidney injury. Crit Care 2008;12(4):169.

16. Lobo DN. Fluid, electrolytes and nutrition: physiological and clinical aspects. Proc Nutr Soc 2004;63:453–66.

17. Marik PE. Iatrogenic salt water drowning and the hazards of a high central venous pressure. Ann Intensive Care 2014;4:21.

18. Gieling RG, Ruijter JM, Maas AA, et al. Hepatic response to right ventricular pressure overload. Gastroenterology 2004;127:1210–21.

19. Bouhemad B, Nicolas-Robin A, Arbelot C, et al. Acute left ventricular dilatation and shock-induced myocardial dysfunction. Crit Care Med 2009;37: 441–7.

20. Desai KV, Laine GA, Stewart RH, et al. Mechanics of the left ventricular myocardial interstitium: effects of acute and chronic myocardial edema. Am J Physiol Heart Circ Physiol 2008;294:H2428–34.

21. Madias JE. Apparent amelioration of bundle branch blocks and intraventricular conduction delays mediated by anasarca. J Electrocardiol 2005;38:160–5.

22. Boyle A, Maurer MS, Sobotka PA. Myocellular and interstitial edema and circulating volume expansion as a cause of morbidity and mortality in heart failure. J Card Fail 2007;13:133–6.

23. El-Sharkawy AM, Sahota O, Maughan RJ, et al. The pathophysiology of fluid and electrolyte balance in the older adult surgical patient. Clin Nutr 2014;33:6–13.

24. Veiga D, Luis C, Parente D, et al. Postoperative delirium in intensive care patients: risk factors and outcome. Rev Bras Anestesiol 2012;62:469–83.

25. Nisanevich V, Felsenstein I, Almogy G, et al. Effect of intraoperative fluid management on outcome after intra-abdominal surgery. Anesthesiology 2005;103:25–32.

26. Brandstrup B, Tønnesen H, Beier-Holgersen R, et al. Effects of intravenous fluid restriction on postoperative complications: comparison of two perioperative fluid regimens: a randomized assessor-blinded multicenter trial. Ann Surg 2003;238: 641–8.

27. Rahbari NN, Zimmermann JB, Schmidt T, et al. Meta-analysis of standard, restrictive and supplemental fluid administration in colorectal surgery. Br J Surg 2009;96:331–41.

28. Lobo DN, Dube MG, Neal KR, et al. Peri-operative fluid and electrolyte management: a survey of consultant surgeons in the UK. Ann R Coll Surg Engl 2002;84: 156–60.

29. Dalfino L, Tullo L, Donadio I, et al. Intra-abdominal hypertension and acute renal failure in critically ill patients. Intensive Care Med 2008;34:707–13.

30. Malbrain ML, Chiumello D, Pelosi P, et al. Incidence and prognosis of intra-abdominal hypertension in a mixed population of critically ill patients: a multiple-center epidemiological study. Crit Care Med 2005;33:315–22.

31. Vidal MG, Ruiz Weisser J, Gonzalez F, et al. Incidence and clinical effects of intra-abdominal hypertension in critically ill patients. Crit Care Med 2008;36:1823–31.

32. Malbrain ML, Cheatham ML, Kirkpatrick A, et al. Results from the International Conference of Experts on Intra-abdominal Hypertension and Abdominal Compartment Syndrome. I. Definitions. Intensive Care Med 2006;32:1722–32.

33. Firth JD, Raine AE, Ledingham JG. Raised venous pressure: a direct cause of renal sodium retention in oedema? Lancet 1988;1:1033–5.

34. Cordemans C, De Laet I, Van Regenmortel N, et al. Fluid management in critically ill patients: the role of extravascular lung water, abdominal hypertension, capillary leak, and fluid balance. Ann Intensive Care 2012;2:S1.

35. Schrier RW, Wang W. Acute renal failure and sepsis. N Engl J Med 2004;351: 159–69.

36. Rosenberg AL, Dechert RE, Park PK, et al. Review of a large clinical series: association of cumulative fluid balance on outcome in acute lung injury: a retrospective review of the ARDSnet tidal volume study cohort. J Intensive Care Med 2009;24:35–46.

37. Martin GS, Moss M, Wheeler AP, et al. A randomized, controlled trial of furosemide with or without albumin in hypoproteinemic patients with acute lung injury. Crit Care Med 2005;33:1681–7.

38. Prowle JR, Kirwan CJ, Bellomo R. Fluid management for the prevention and attenuation of acute kidney injury. Nat Rev Nephrol 2014;10:37–47.

39. Teixeira C, Garzotto F, Piccinni P, et al. Fluid balance and urine volume are independent predictors of mortality in acute kidney injury. Crit Care 2013;17:R14.

40. Askenazi DJ, Koralkar R, Hundley HE, et al. Fluid overload and mortality are associated with acute kidney injury in sick near-term/term neonate. Pediatr Nephrol 2013;28:661–6.

41. Basu RK, Andrews A, Krawczeski C, et al. Acute kidney injury based on corrected serum creatinine is associated with increased morbidity in children following the arterial switch operation. Pediatr Crit Care Med 2013;14:e218–24.

42. Hazle MA, Gajarski RJ, Yu S, et al. Fluid overload in infants following congenital heart surgery. Pediatr Crit Care Med 2013;14:44–9.

43. Vaara ST, Korhonen AM, Kaukonen KM, et al. Fluid overload is associated with an increased risk for 90-day mortality in critically ill patients with renal replacement therapy: data from the prospective FINNAKI study. Crit Care 2012;16:R197.

44. Prowle JR, Chua HR, Bagshaw SM, et al. Clinical review: volume of fluid resuscitation and the incidence of acute kidney injury - a systematic review. Crit Care 2012;16:230.

45. Selewski DT, Cornell TT, Blatt NB, et al. Fluid overload and fluid removal in pediatric patients on extracorporeal membrane oxygenation requiring continuous renal replacement therapy. Crit Care Med 2012;40:2694–9.

46. Dass B, Shimada M, Kambhampati G, et al. Fluid balance as an early indicator of acute kidney injury in CV surgery. Clin Nephrol 2012;77:438–44.

47. Kambhampati G, Ross EA, Alsabbagh MM, et al. Perioperative fluid balance and acute kidney injury. Clin Exp Nephrol 2012;16:730–8.

48. Selewski DT, Cornell TT, Lombel RM, et al. Weight-based determination of fluid overload status and mortality in pediatric intensive care unit patients requiring continuous renal replacement therapy. Intensive Care Med 2011; 37:1166–73.

49. Fulop T, Pathak MB, Schmidt DW, et al. Volume-related weight gain and subsequent mortality in acute renal failure patients treated with continuous renal replacement therapy. ASAIO J 2010;56:333–7.
50. Sutherland SM, Zappitelli M, Alexander SR, et al. Fluid overload and mortality in children receiving continuous renal replacement therapy: the prospective pediatric continuous renal replacement therapy registry. Am J Kidney Dis 2010;55:316–25.
51. Liu KD, Thompson BT, Ancukiewicz M, et al. Acute kidney injury in patients with acute lung injury: impact of fluid accumulation on classification of acute kidney injury and associated outcomes. Crit Care Med 2011;39:2665–71.
52. ARISE Investigators, ANZICS Clinical Trials Group, Peake SL, et al. Goal-directed resuscitation for patients with early septic shock. N Engl J Med 2014;371:1496–506.
53. Angus DC, Yealy DM, Kellum JA. Protocol-based care for early septic shock. N Engl J Med 2014;371:386.
54. Mouncey PR, Osborn TM, Power GS, et al. Trial of early, goal-directed resuscitation for septic shock. N Engl J Med 2015;372:1301–11.
55. Dellinger RP, Levy MM, Rhodes A, et al. Surviving Sepsis Campaign: international guidelines for management of severe sepsis and septic shock: 2012. Crit Care Med 2013;41:580–637.
56. Surviving Sepsis Campaign Guidelines Committee. Surviving Sepsis Campaign 6hr bundle. 2015. Available at: http://www.survivingsepsis.org/SiteCollection Documents/SSC_Bundle.pdf. Accessed April 1, 2015.
57. Marik PE, Cavallazzi R. Does the central venous pressure predict fluid responsiveness? An updated meta-analysis and a plea for some common sense. Crit Care Med 2013;41:1774–81.
58. Berlin DA, Bakker J. Starling curves and central venous pressure. Crit Care 2015;19:55.
59. Bouhemad B. Isolated and reversible impairment of ventricular relaxation in patients with septic shock. Crit Care Med 2008;36:766–74.
60. Rudiger A, Singer M. Mechanisms of sepsis-induced cardiac dysfunction. Crit Care Med 2007;35:1599–608.
61. Di Giantomasso D, May CN, Bellomo R. Vital organ blood flow during hyperdynamic sepsis. Chest 2003;124:1053–9.
62. Ruokonen E. Regional blood flow and oxygen transport in septic shock. Crit Care Med 1993;21:1296–303.
63. Fleck A. Increased vascular permeability: a major cause of hypoalbuminaemia in disease and injury. Lancet 1985;325:781–4.
64. LeDoux D, Astiz ME, Carpati CM, et al. Effects of perfusion pressure on tissue perfusion in septic shock. Crit Care Med 2000;28:2729–32.
65. Marik PE, Baram M, Vahid B. Does central venous pressure predict fluid responsiveness? A systematic review of the literature and the tale of seven mares. Chest 2008;134:172–8.
66. Michard F, Teboul JL. Predicting fluid responsiveness in ICU patients: a critical analysis of the evidence. Chest 2002;121:2000–8.
67. Boulain T, Boisrame-Helms J, Ehrmann S, et al. Volume expansion in the first 4 days of shock: a prospective multicentre study in 19 French intensive care units. Intensive Care Med 2015;41:248–56.
68. Wan L, Bellomo R, May CN. A comparison of 4% succinylated gelatin solution versus normal saline in stable normovolaemic sheep: global haemodynamic, regional blood flow and oxygen delivery effects. Anaesth Intensive Care 2007; 35:924–31.

69. Legrand M, Mik EG, Balestra GM, et al. Fluid resuscitation does not improve renal oxygenation during hemorrhagic shock in rats. Anesthesiology 2010; 112:119–27.
70. Wan L, Bellomo R, May CN. The effect of normal saline resuscitation on vital organ blood flow in septic sheep. Intensive Care Med 2006;32:1238–42.
71. Sanchez M, Jiménez-Lendínez M, Cidoncha M, et al. Comparison of fluid compartments and fluid responsiveness in septic and non-septic patients. Anaesth Intensive Care 2011;39:1022–9.
72. Jacob M, Chappell D, Hofmann-Kiefer K, et al. The intravascular volume effect of Ringer's lactate is below 20%: a prospective study in humans. Crit Care 2012; 16:R86.
73. Rosner MH, Ostermann M, Murugan R, et al. Indications and management of mechanical fluid removal in critical illness. Br J Anaesth 2014;113:764–71.
74. Goldstein SL. Fluid management in acute kidney injury. J Intensive Care Med 2012;29:183–9.
75. Prowle JR, Echeverri JE, Ligabo EV, et al. Fluid balance and acute kidney injury. Nat Rev Nephrol 2010;6:107–15.
76. Becker BF, Chappell D, Jacob M. Endothelial glycocalyx and coronary vascular permeability: the fringe benefit. Basic Res Cardiol 2010;105: 687–701.
77. Chawla LS, Ince C, Chappell D, et al. Vascular content, tone, integrity, and haemodynamics for guiding fluid therapy: a conceptual approach. Br J Anaesth 2014;113:748–55.
78. Levick JR, Michel CC. Microvascular fluid exchange and the revised Starling principle. Cardiovasc Res 2010;87:198–210.
79. Woodcock TE, Woodcock TM. Revised Starling equation and the glycocalyx model of transvascular fluid exchange: an improved paradigm for prescribing intravenous fluid therapy. Br J Anaesth 2012;108:384–94.
80. Reitsma S, Slaaf DW, Vink H, et al. The endothelial glycocalyx: composition, functions, and visualization. Pflugers Arch 2007;454:345–59.
81. Perner A, Haase N, Guttormsen AB, et al. Hydroxyethyl starch 130/0.42 versus Ringer's acetate in severe sepsis. N Engl J Med 2012;367:124–34.
82. Chelazzi C, Villa G, Mancinelli P, et al. Glycocalyx and sepsis-induced alterations in vascular permeability. Crit Care 2015;19:26.
83. Donati A, Damiani E, Domizi R, et al. Alteration of the sublingual microvascular glycocalyx in critically ill patients. Microvasc Res 2013;90:86–9.
84. Schmidt EP, Yang Y, Janssen WJ, et al. The pulmonary endothelial glycocalyx regulates neutrophil adhesion and lung injury during experimental sepsis. Nat Med 2012;18:1217–23.
85. Steppan J, Hofer S, Funke B, et al. Sepsis and major abdominal surgery lead to flaking of the endothelial glycocalix. J Surg Res 2011;165:136–41.
86. Johansson PI, Stensballe J, Rasmussen LS, et al. A high admission syndecan-1 level, a marker of endothelial glycocalyx degradation, is associated with inflammation, protein C depletion, fibrinolysis, and increased mortality in trauma patients. Ann Surg 2011;254:194–200.
87. Rehm M, Bruegger D, Christ F, et al. Shedding of the endothelial glycocalyx in patients undergoing major vascular surgery with global and regional ischemia. Circulation 2007;116:1896–906.
88. Kolarova H, Ambrůzová B, Svihálková Šindlerová L, et al. Modulation of endothelial glycocalyx structure under inflammatory conditions. Mediators Inflamm 2014;2014:694312.

89. Nieuwdorp M, van Haeften TW, Gouverneur MC, et al. Loss of endothelial glyco-calyx during acute hyperglycemia coincides with endothelial dysfunction and coagulation activation in vivo. Diabetes 2006;55:480–6.

90. Van Teeffelen JW, Brands J, Stroes ES, et al. Endothelial glycocalyx: sweet shield of blood vessels. Trends Cardiovasc Med 2007;17:101–5.

91. Doucet A, Favre G, Deschenes G. Molecular mechanism of edema formation in nephrotic syndrome: therapeutic implications. Pediatr Nephrol 2007;22: 1983–90.

92. Bruegger D, Jacob M, Rehm M, et al. Atrial natriuretic peptide induces shed-ding of endothelial glycocalyx in coronary vascular bed of guinea pig hearts. Am J Physiol Heart Circ Physiol 2005;289:H1993–9.

93. Bruegger D, Schwartz L, Chappell D, et al. Release of atrial natriuretic peptide precedes shedding of the endothelial glycocalyx equally in patients undergoing on- and off-pump coronary artery bypass surgery. Basic Res Cardiol 2011;106: 1111–21.

94. Chappell D, Bruegger D, Potzel J, et al. Hypervolemia increases release of atrial natriuretic peptide and shedding of the endothelial glycocalyx. Crit Care 2014; 18:538.

95. Reed RK, Rubin K. Transcapillary exchange: role and importance of the intersti-tial fluid pressure and the extracellular matrix. Cardiovasc Res 2010;87:211–7.

96. Reed RK, Rubin K, Wiig H, et al. Blockade of beta 1-integrins in skin causes edema through lowering of interstitial fluid pressure. Circ Res 1992;71:978–83.

97. Lund T, Onarheim H, Wiig H, et al. Mechanisms behind increased dermal imbi-bition pressure in acute burn edema. Am J Physiol 1989;256:H940–8.

98. Nedrebo T, Berg A, Reed RK. Effect of tumor necrosis factor-alpha, IL-1beta, and IL-6 on interstitial fluid pressure in rat skin. Am J Physiol 1999;277: H1857–62.

99. Nedrebo T, Reed RK. Different serotypes of endotoxin (lipopolysaccharide) cause different increases in albumin extravasation in rats. Shock 2002;18: 138–41.

100. Aukland K, Reed RK. Interstitial-lymphatic mechanisms in the control of extra-cellular fluid volume. Physiol Rev 1993;73:1–78.

101. Hoste EA, Maitland K, Brudney CS, et al. Four phases of intravenous fluid ther-apy: a conceptual model. Br J Anaesth 2014;113:740–7.

102. Ho KM, Sheridan DJ. Meta-analysis of frusemide to prevent or treat acute renal failure. BMJ 2006;333:420.

103. Mehta RL, Pascual MT, Soroko S, et al. Diuretics, mortality, and nonrecovery of renal function in acute renal failure. JAMA 2002;288:2547–53.

104. Uchino S, Doig GS, Bellomo R, et al. Diuretics and mortality in acute renal fail-ure. Crit Care Med 2004;32:1669–77.

105. Goldstein S, Bagshaw S, Cecconi M, et al. Pharmacological management of fluid overload. Br J Anaesth 2014;113:756–63.

106. Chawla LS, Davison DL, Brasha-Mitchell E, et al. Development and standardiza-tion of a furosemide stress test to predict the severity of acute kidney injury. Crit Care 2013;17:R207.

107. Koyner JL, Davison DL, Brasha-Mitchell E, et al. Furosemide stress test and bio-markers for the prediction of AKI severity. J Am Soc Nephrol 2015. http://dx.doi.org/10.1681/ASN.2014060535.

108. Schneider AG, Baldwin I, Freitag E, et al. Estimation of fluid status changes in critically ill patients: fluid balance chart or electronic bed weight? J Crit Care 2012;27:745.e7–12.

109. Uszko-Lencer NH, Bothmer F, van Pol PE, et al. Measuring body composition in chronic heart failure: a comparison of methods. Eur J Heart Fail 2006;8:208–14.
110. Parrinello G, Paterna S, Di Pasquale P, et al. The usefulness of bioelectrical impedance analysis in differentiating dyspnea due to decompensated heart failure. J Card Fail 2008;14:676–86.
111. Mikkelsen ME, Christie JD, Lanken PN, et al. The adult respiratory distress syndrome cognitive outcomes study: long-term neuropsychological function in survivors of acute lung injury. Am J Respir Crit Care Med 2012;185:1307–15.
112. Grissom CK, Hirshberg EL, Dickerson JB, et al. Fluid management with a simplified conservative protocol for the acute respiratory distress syndrome*. Crit Care Med 2015;43:288–95.
113. Schneider AG, Bellomo R, Bagshaw SM, et al. Choice of renal replacement therapy modality and dialysis dependence after acute kidney injury: a systematic review and meta-analysis. Intensive Care Med 2013;39:987–97.
114. Wald R, Shariff SZ, Adhikari NK, et al. The association between renal replacement therapy modality and long-term outcomes among critically ill adults with acute kidney injury: a retrospective cohort study*. Crit Care Med 2014;42:868–77.
115. Ronco C, Brendolan A, Bellomo R. Online monitoring in continuous renal replacement therapies. Kidney Int Suppl 1999;(72):S8–14.
116. Zoccali C, Torino C, Tripepi R, et al. Pulmonary congestion predicts cardiac events and mortality in ESRD. J Am Soc Nephrol 2013;24:639–46.

Fluid Composition and Clinical Effects

Matt Varrier, MBBS, MRCP, Marlies Ostermann, PhD, MD, FRCP, EDIC*

KEYWORDS

- Crystalloid • Colloid • Fluid therapy • Critical illness • Balanced solutions
- Unbalanced solutions

KEY POINTS

- Crystalloids differ in electrolyte composition, pH, osmolarity, effect on acid base status, and strong ion difference and can be divided into balanced and unbalanced solutions based on their similarity with plasma.
- Colloids are crystalloid solutions containing oncotic macromolecules, which are protein or carbohydrate based. They differ in the type of macromolecule, electrolyte composition, and carrier fluid.
- The degree of volume expansion following fluid administration depends on the molecular weight and half-life of the components, function of the endothelial glycocalyx layer, endothelial integrity, and hydrostatic and osmotic pressure gradient between the intravascular and extravascular compartment.
- The adverse effects of different crystalloid and colloid fluids vary and include nephrotoxicity, anticoagulation, acid base disturbance, and anaphylactoid reactions.
- Knowledge of the characteristics of the different types of fluids and their potential effects following administration is essential to prescribe the most appropriate fluid according to the physiologic needs of patients.

INTRODUCTION

Fluids and oxygen are the most ubiquitous therapeutic interventions in critically ill patients. Typical indications for fluid administration range from simple replacement of insensible volume loss in patients unable to take fluids orally to correction of intravascular hypovolemia, augmentation of cardiac output, and administration of injectable medications and electrolytes.

Fluids exert their therapeutic effects by expansion of the intravascular, interstitial, and intracellular compartments.[1] There is evidence that their electrolyte composition

Disclosures: The authors have nothing to declare.
King's College London, Guy's and St Thomas Hospital, Department of Critical Care, London, UK
* Corresponding author.
E-mail address: Marlies.Ostermann@gstt.nhs.uk

Crit Care Clin 31 (2015) 823–837
http://dx.doi.org/10.1016/j.ccc.2015.06.014 **criticalcare.theclinics.com**

and the particle size of components have an effect on the acid base status, renal function, and coagulation and may also affect patient outcome. The choice of fluid and the rate of administration should be guided by the physiologic needs of individual patients.[2–4] Knowledge of the composition of different types of fluids and their physiochemical characteristics is important to ensure that the right fluid is administered at the right dose and the right time for the right duration and tailored to the pathophysiologic phase of critical illness.[3–6]

The following review describes the characteristics of individual types of fluids, their effects on different organ systems, and potential indications in clinical practice.

TYPES OF FLUIDS
Crystalloids

Crystalloids are aqueous solutions containing minerals and/or salts of organic acids. They differ in electrolyte composition, pH, osmolarity, effect on acid base status, and strong ion difference and can be divided into balanced and unbalanced solutions based on their similarity with plasma[7] (**Table 1**).

Unbalanced crystalloids

Dextrose solutions Dextrose solutions contain glucose dissolved in either water (dextrose 5%, 10%, or 20%) or 0.9% sodium chloride (NaCl) (D5NS = 5% dextrose in 0.9% NaCl; D5 1/2 NS = dextrose 5% in 0.45% NaCl). They are hypotonic and can be used to provide glucose and free water in conditions associated with hypoglycemia or loss of water.

0.9% Sodium chloride Saline 0.9% is the most commonly used fluid worldwide. After infusion, it is rapidly distributed between the compartments of the extracellular space. In health, approximately 60% of the infused volume diffuses from the intravascular space into the interstitial compartment within 20 minutes of administration.[8] These fluid shifts are even faster in conditions associated with endothelial dysfunction.

NaCl 0.9% has a nonphysiologic ion content and supraphysiologic concentration of chloride (see **Table 1**). As a result, administration of 0.9% NaCl can lead to hyperchloremia and metabolic acidosis.

Sodium bicarbonate solutions Intravenous sodium bicarbonate ($NaHCO_3$) is available in different concentrations (1.26%, 1.4%, 4.2%, and 8.4%). In vivo, it dissociates to provide Na^+ and HCO_3^- anions and buffers excess hydrogen ions. Carbonic acid quickly dissolves to water and carbon dioxide (CO_2). The CO_2 is excreted via the lungs.

Balanced crystalloids

Balanced crystalloids are solutions with an ionic composition more similar to plasma than 0.9% NaCl. Several types are commercially available. They differ in their ionic makeup, osmolarity, tonicity, and type of metabolizable anion, such as acetate, lactate, and malate (see **Table 1**).

Ringer lactate solution has an osmolarity of 273 mosmol/L and can cause a small reduction in plasma osmolality.

Hartmann's solution is a slightly modified form of Ringer lactate.

Plasma-Lyte and Sterofundin contain electrolytes in concentrations that are more similar to plasma compared with Hartmann and Ringer lactate (see **Table 1**).

Colloids

Colloids are crystalloid solutions containing oncotic macromolecules that largely remain in the intravascular space and, thereby, generate an oncotic pressure

(**Table 2**). The macromolecules may be protein or carbohydrate based. All available colloids are synthetically produced with the exception of albumin (and other fluids derived from donated blood, which are not discussed in this review). The synthetic processes create heterogeneity in the weight of molecules present called polydispersity. Following infusion, the net effect depends on the type of colloid, the concentration, the distribution of its molecular weight (MW), and the crystalloid carrier.

Large molecules have restricted movement across the capillary wall. By acting as effective osmoles, they keep water in the intravascular space and prevent free movement into the interstitial space (oncotic pressure) (see **Table 2**). In contrast, small solutes move rapidly into the extravascular space in response to a concentration gradient and/or hydrostatic pressure. In health, a low concentration of protein is also found in the interstitium, which exerts a small tissue oncotic pressure.

The barrier between the intravascular compartment and the interstitium consists of multiple components, including the endothelial cell wall, tight junctions between cells, extracellular matrix in the interstitial space, and the endothelial basement membrane (EBM). Now recognized for its crucial importance is the endothelial glycocalyx layer (EGL). The EGL is located on the apical surface coating the luminal side of the vascular endothelium and consists of a matrix of glycosaminoglycans and proteoglycans, which have a negative charge. It creates a largely impermeable physical and electrochemical barrier to negatively charged macromolecules, such as albumin. In addition to maintaining the oncotic effects of albumin, the EGL also acts as an important reservoir of noncirculating plasma volume (700–1000 mL).[9]

IMPORTANT PROPERTIES OF COLLOIDS
Molecular Weight

Large molecules have a greater oncotic effect and may take longer to be metabolized and eliminated and, therefore, lengthen the duration of action. Smaller molecules may be cleared faster and are also more permeable across the capillary wall. The oncotic effects are dynamic as larger molecules may be broken down to smaller molecules with differing properties.[10]

Oncotic Pressure

The oncotic pressure generated by a colloid is primarily determined by the MW and concentration (**Table 3**). Hyperoncotic preparations (eg, albumin 20%) expand the plasma volume by more than the volume infused.[11]

Metabolism, Elimination, and Duration of Effect

The body handles each type of colloid differently, and the plasma half-lives vary greatly (see **Table 3**). In general, larger molecules take longer to be metabolized and have a longer duration of action, especially if their metabolites are also osmotically active. Smaller molecules less than the glomerular threshold of 60 kDa are excreted in the urine, provided the renal function is intact.

Carrier Fluid

All colloids are carried in a crystalloid solution. Commonly this is NaCl based, although balanced colloids are available (see **Table 3**). The carrier solution has similar effects to when infused alone (eg, hyperchloremic metabolic acidosis in the case of 0.9% NaCl). The degree to which this occurs depends on the volume, rate, and underlying physiology.

Table 1
Composition of commonly used crystalloids compared with plasma

Parameter	Plasma	NaCl 0.9%	NaCl 0.18%/ Glucose 4%	NaCl 0.45%/ Glucose 4%	Glucose 5%	Hartmann's solution	Ringer Lactate	Ringer Acetate	Plasma-Lyte	Sterofundin	Isolyte S	NaHCO₃ 1.26%	NaHCO₃ 1.4%	NaHCO₃ 8.4%
Na⁺ (millimole per liter)	135–145	154	31	77	—	131	130	130	140	145	141	150	167	1000
K⁺ (millimole per liter)	3.5–4.5	—	—	—	—	5	4	5	5	4	5	—	—	—
Cl⁻ (millimole per liter)	95–105	154	31	77	—	111	109	112	98	127	98	—	—	—
HCO₃⁻ (millimole per liter)	24–32	—	—	—	—	29 (as lactate)	28 (as lactate)	27 (as acetate)	(as acetate + gluconate)	(as acetate + malate)	(as acetate + gluconate)	150	167	1000
Lactate (millimole per liter)	1	—	—	—	—	29	28	—	—	—	—	—	—	—
Acetate (millimole per liter)	—	—	—	—	—	—	—	27	27	24	27	—	—	—
Gluconate (millimole per liter)	—	—	—	—	—	—	—	—	23	—	23	—	—	—

Component														
Malate (millimole per liter)	—	—	—	—	—	—	—	—	5	—	—	—	—	—
Ca²⁺ (millimole per liter)	2.2–2.6	—	—	—	2	—	1.5	1	1.5	2.5	—	—	—	—
Mg²⁺ (millimole per liter)	0.8–1.2	—	—	—	—	—	1	1.5	1	1	—	3	—	—
Phosphate (millimole per liter)	0.8–1.2	—	—	—	—	—	—	—	—	—	1	—	—	—
Glucose (millimole per liter)	3.5–6.0	—	236	278	252	—	—	—	—	—	—	—	—	—
pH	7.35–7.45	4.5–7.0	3.5–5.5	3.5–6.5	5.0–7.0	6.0–7.5	6–8	4.0–6.5	—	5.1–5.9	7.0–7.8	7.0–8.5	7.0–8.5	7.0–8.5
Osmolarity (milliosmole per liter)	275–295	308	284	406	278	279	273	277	294	309	295	301	333	2000
In vivo estimated SID (millimole per liter)	0	0	0	0	0	28[a]	27[a]	50	27	29	50	0	0	0

Abbreviations: Ca, calcium; Cl, chloride; K, potassium; Mg, magnesium; Na, sodium; SID, strong ion difference.
[a] Assumes stable plasma lactate concentration of 1 mmol/L.

Table 2	
List of common terminology	
Term	**Description**
Crystalloid	Solution of electrolytes, glucose, and/or organic anions (lactate, acetate, gluconate, bicarbonate, or maleate) in water
Colloid	Dispersion of large molecules or noncrystalline particles in a carrier crystalloid that exert an oncotic pressure; can be divided into synthetic (starches, gelatins, and dextrans) and natural (albumin)
Balanced solution	Solution with a composition more similar to plasma than sodium chloride 0.9%
Osmolarity	Measure of solute concentration, defined as the number of osmoles of solute per liter of solution; affected by changes in water content, temperature, and pressure
Osmolality	Measure of the osmoles of solute per kilogram of solvent; independent of changes in temperature and pressure
Osmotic pressure	Hydrostatic pressure that would be required to resist the diffusion of water across a semipermeable membrane from a higher solute concentration to a lower solute concentration
Oncotic pressure	Portion of osmotic pressure that is caused by large molecular weight particles, especially proteins; dependent on molecular weight and concentration of particle; depends on both the integrity of the barrier and the difference in concentration of oncotic particles across the barrier between the intravascular compartment and the interstitium
Tonicity	Effective osmolality of a solution (ie, comparison of the osmolality of a particular fluid to that of plasma)
Strong ion difference	Net electrical charge difference of the infusate strong cations minus the anions

Types of colloid

Human albumin solution Albumin is the most abundant protein in human plasma contributing 50% to 60% of the total. At 66 to 68 kDa, it has negligible renal excretion in intact glomeruli and contributes 80% of the oncotic pressure.[12]

Human albumin solution (HAS) is manufactured from cryo-depleted human plasma. Its physiochemical properties (highly water soluble, highly negatively charged, resistant to denaturing at extremes of heat and pH) make it relatively easy to separate and treat (ie, pasteurization to prevent transmission of viruses). Modern processing techniques have minimized impurities, such as endotoxin and prekallikrein activator, which have historically been associated with febrile reactions and hypotension.[13] Octanoate and N-acetyltryptophanate are added as stabilizers against heat and oxidization.

Products available for therapeutic use may be iso-oncotic (4%–5%) or hyperoncotic (20%) (see **Table 3**). Hyperoncotic albumin is often referred to as salt poor as the Na concentration is reduced at 130 mmol/L.

Gelatin-based colloid Gelatins are derived from the hydrolysis of collagen in cattle bones. Because of their relatively small size, they are rapidly excreted by the kidneys so that the effective plasma half-life is relatively short (~2.5 hours). Modern gelatins are modified by processes that limit the MW so that they do not solidify during storage.

Gelofusine and geloplasma contain gelatin treated by succinylation, which results in stretched and negatively charged polypeptide chains up to 30 kDa.[14] Gelofusine is available in a NaCl solution albeit with a lower chloride content than 0.9% NaCl (see **Table 3**). Geloplasma is a balanced colloid with a solvent similar to Ringer lactate.

Polygeline (Haemaccel) is created from urea cross-linked gelatins. It also has a balanced solvent (see **Table 3**).

Dextran-based colloid Dextrans are large, complex carbohydrate polymers. They are synthesized from sucrose by the B-512F strain of *Leuconostoc mesenteroides* via the actions of the glucosyltransferase enzyme. The MWs generated are highly variable. A process of acid hydrolysis and ethanol fractionation allows separation of smaller molecules.

Referring to the average MW, dextran 40 kDa and dextran 70 kDa are commercially available. They have several differences. Dextran 40 is usually dissolved in 0.9% NaCl, whereas dextran 70 is available in 5% dextrose and 0.9% NaCl. In dextran 40, most of the molecules are small enough to be filtered by the kidneys or transported into the interstitial space. Consequently, the effective plasma half-life is much shorter, although some higher MW molecules may persist for several days. The larger weight components of dextran 70 are slowly metabolized by reticuloendothelial dextranases and may be present for several weeks. Renal excretion is very limited.[7]

Hydroxyethyl starch Hydroxyethyl starches (HES) are derivates of the glucose polymer amylopectin obtained from naturally occurring starch products, such as maize and potato. To avoid rapid hydrolysis by α-amylases in plasma and to increase the oncotic effect, therapeutic starch solutions undergo several modifications:

1. Hydroxylation at the C2 and C6 positions occurs. The degree of hydroxylation, also known as the molar substitution (MS), is indicated as a ratio of the number of hydroxyethyl residues on average per glucose subunit. Expressed as a number between 0 and 1, it gives rise to the Greek nomenclature (eg, hetastarch 0.7, pentastarch 0.5). The higher the degree of MS, the more resistant and the longer the plasma half-life.
2. Hydroxylation at C2 confers more resistance to α-amylases than C6. The higher the C2/C6 ratio, the longer the plasma half-life.

HES types are physicochemically characterized by their MS, mean MW, and C2/C6 ratio. For instance, hetastarch 130/0.4 stands for MS 0.7, mean MW 130 kDa, and an average of 4 hydroxyethyl residues per 10 glucose subunits.

There is a range of HES solutions with differing properties (see **Table 3**). They are traditionally classified as high (450–670 kDa), medium (130–200 kDa), and low (≤70 kDa) MW starches. However, for a given mean MW, there will be a range of molecular size and weight particles present. More relevant than MW is the classification according to MS, which affects plasma half-life. An HES type with an MS of 0.62 to 0.75 is considered highly substituted; an MS of around 0.5 is medium; and HES types with MS of 0.4 or less are considered low substitution.

Clearance of HES solutions depends on their MW. Smaller MW starches less than 60 kDa undergo rapid renal excretion. The larger molecules are broken down to smaller ones by α-amylases, excreted in the bile, or deposited in tissues. The accumulation of HES within the reticuloendothelial system is implicated in adverse events and toxicity.[7,15]

PHYSIOLOGICAL EFFECTS OF DIFFERENT FLUIDS
Volume Expansion

Fluids vary in their ability to expand the plasma volume (**Table 4**). The effect of a fluid infused depends on the MW and half-life of the molecule, EGL function and

Table 3
Composition of plasma and commonly used colloids

Parameter	Plasma	Albumin 5%	Albumin 20%	Haemaccel	Gelofusine	Geloplasma	Dextran 40	Dextran 70 in NaCl	Tetraspan 6% HES 130/0.42	Hetastarch 6% HES 130/0.4	Hetastarch 6% HES 670/0.75
Colloid source	—	Human donor	Human donor	Bovine gelatin	Bovine gelatin	Bovine gelatin	Sucrose	Sucrose	Potato starch	Maize starch	Maize starch
Na+ (millimole per liter)	135–145	148	130	145	154	150	154	154	140	154	143
K+ (millimole per liter)	3.5–4.5	—	—	5.1	—	5	—	—	4	—	3
Cl− (millimole per liter)	95–105	128	77	120	120	100	154	154	118	154	124
HCO3− (millimole per liter)	24–32	—	—	—	—	30 (as lactate)	—	—	—	—	28 (as lactate)
Lactate (millimole per liter)	1	—	—	—	—	30	—	—	—	—	28
Ca2+ (millimole per liter)	2.2–2.6	—	—	6.25	—	—	—	—	2.5	—	2.5
Mg2+ (millimole per liter)	0.8–1.2	—	—	—	—	1.5	—	—	1	—	0.45
Glucose (millimole per liter)	3.5–6.0	—	—	—	—	—	—	—	—	—	5

Acetate (millimole per liter)	—	—	—	—	—	—	—	—	24	—	—
Malate (millimole per liter)	—	—	—	—	—	—	—	—	5	—	—
Octanoate (millimole per liter)	—	8	16	—	—	—	—	—	—	—	—
N-acetyltryptophanate (millimole per liter)	—	—	16	—	—	—	—	—	—	—	—
pH	7.35–7.45	6.4–7.4	7.4	7.4	7.4	7.4	3.0–7.0	4.5–7.0	5.6–6.4	4.0–55.0	5.9
MW (kilodalton)	—	69	69	30	30	30	40	63–77	130	130	670
Osmolarity (milliosmole per liter)	275–295	309	293	274–300	274	273	308–310	310	297	286–308	307
Oncotic potential	—	IO	HO	IO	IO	IO	HO	HO	HO	HO	HO
Effective half-life	—	Half-life 17–19 d Distribution half-life 15 h	Half-life 17–19 d Distribution half-life 15 h	5 h	2.5 h	2.5 h	12–24 h	12–24 h	12 h	6–12 h	24–48 h

Abbreviations: Ca, calcium; Cl, chloride; HES, hydroxyethyl starches; HO, hyperoncotic; IO, iso-oncotic; K, potassium; Mg, magnesium; Mw, molecular weight.

Table 4
Metabolic effects and plasma expansion of commonly used crystalloids

Parameter	NaCl 0.9%	NaCl 0.18%/ Glucose 4%	NaCl 0.45%/ Glucose 5%	Glucose 5%	Hartmann's solution	Ringer Lactate	Ringer Acetate	Plasma-Lyte	Isolyte S	NaHCO$_3$ 1.2%	NaHCO$_3$ 8.4%
Caloric content (kilocalorie per liter)	0	136	170	170	9	9	6	21	21	0	0
CO$_2$ generation per 1 L solution[a] (millimole)	0	1334	1668	1668	87	84	54	192	192	0	0
Plasma expansion from infusion of 1 L in milliliters	207	200	250	190	196–225	190–200	190–200	200	200	210–230	810

[a] Theoretic CO$_2$ production from complete oxidative metabolism of 1 mmol of organic anion. In vivo CO$_2$ production likely lower as part of the organic anions are metabolized via alternative pathways that produce less CO$_2$.[32]

endothelial integrity, as well as hydrostatic and osmotic pressure gradient between the intravascular and extravascular compartment. In acute volume loss or redistribution, low hydrostatic pressure prolongs the filling effect of both crystalloids and colloids. Therefore, they both perform well and the theoretic benefit of colloids is reduced.

Volume expansion is necessary in hypovolemia, especially in cases of associated hypoperfusion. However, there is increasing evidence that overzealous fluid resuscitation and fluid overload are associated with poor outcomes.[16,17] Recent data also suggest that the function of the EGL may be adversely affected by overexpansion of plasma volume with colloid.[18]

Renal Effects

- Use of NaCl 0.9% may result in hyperchloremia and metabolic acidosis. Studies in animals and human volunteers have shown an association between hyperchloremia and renal vasoconstriction and reduced glomerular filtration.[19–21] Observational studies in patients undergoing major surgery and during critical illness have shown a higher incidence of acute kidney injury in those treated with chloride-rich fluids.[22–24]
- Several randomized controlled trials (RCTs) comparing HES with Ringer acetate, Ringer lactate, and 0.9% NaCl have demonstrated an increased need for renal replacement therapy in the groups assigned to HES.[25–28]
- Recent observational data suggest that gelatin may be associated with the development of nephrotoxicity similar to that observed with HES.[29,30] However, this has not been demonstrated in the RCTs conducted to date.[31]
- The higher concentration of smaller molecules in dextran 40 may cause an osmotic diuresis.

Hematological Effects

- Significant reductions of factor VIII and von Willebrand factor are observed after infusion of dextrans, gelatins, and HES, with high-molecular HES and dextran having the greatest effect on hemostasis.
- Dextrans have an anticoagulant effect through platelet inhibition, profibrinolytic actions, and decreased factor VIII levels. This effect is more pronounced for dextran 70 when significant bleeding complications have been reported.
- Dextrans may interfere with blood cross matching.
- Solutions containing a significant Ca^{2+} concentration, such as Haemaccel, carry the risk of clotting infusion lines when co-infused with blood products.

Metabolic Effects

- Glucose and organic anions in crystalloid and colloid fluids provide calories[32] (see **Table 4**).
- Metabolism of glucose and organic anions results in CO_2 production[32] (see **Table 4**). For instance, 3 mmol CO_2 are produced from every metabolized millimole of lactate.
- HES infusion causes an occasional elevation of the serum amylase levels. Although this has no clinical implication, it may interfere with the diagnosis of acute pancreatitis.
- Human albumin has several functions beyond oncotic pressure, including as a carrier protein for electrolytes, hormones, and drugs. It is also a buffer for hydrogen ions and has antioxidant properties.[7]

Anaphylaxis

Anaphylactoid reactions have been reported with all classes of colloids, although this is rare with albumin. A systematic review including RCTs, cohort studies, and pharmacovigilance studies ranked the relative risk as gelatins >HES >dextrans >albumin.[33] However, a more recent systematic review limited to RCTs only concluded that there was no evidence that one colloid was safer than another.[34]

POTENTIAL INDICATIONS

The choice of fluid and rate of administration should be guided by the physiologic needs of patients. Given the differences in electrolyte composition, osmolality, and physiochemical characteristics, all fluids have particular indications when they are most suited.

0.9% Sodium Chloride

Saline 0.9% is the fluid of choice in conditions associated with hypovolemia and chloride loss, especially when metabolic alkalosis is present, for instance, severe vomiting.

Bicarbonate Solutions

Intravenous $NaHCO_3$ 1.2% and 1.4% can be used to correct hypovolemia and metabolic acidosis in conditions characterized by fluid and bicarbonate loss (ie, diarrhea or high-output ileostomy). It is also used in cases when urinary alkalinization is desired (ie, rhabdomyolysis), has a role in the treatment of certain drug intoxications (tricyclic antidepressant, salicylate), and is used to prevent contrast-induced acute kidney injury. Intravenous bicarbonate has no role in the treatment of respiratory acidosis and should be used with caution in patients with hypercapnia as the CO_2 produced from the dissociation of infused HCO_3^- may worsen the respiratory acidosis, especially if the ability to exhale CO_2 is already limited.

Administration of 8.4% $NaHCO_3$ can rapidly correct metabolic acidosis, which may be useful in the management of life-threatening hyperkalemia. Likewise, it should be avoided when metabolic acidosis occurs concurrently with hypokalemia as it can reduce the potassium concentration even further and precipitate arrhythmias.

Intravenous bicarbonate should not be mixed with calcium-containing solutions as they may precipitate.

Dextrose

Dextrose solutions provide water and glucose. They are indicated in hypoglycemia and in situations associated with severe water loss, for instance, hypernatremic hypovolemia.

Dextrose solutions are not suitable as resuscitation fluids but may be incorporated into maintenance regimes. The rationale is that adults require a daily water intake of 25 to 30 mL/kg but only approximately 1 mmol/kg/d of potassium, sodium, and chloride.[35] Therefore, regimens that include dextrose 5% avoid the inevitable sodium and chloride loading with continuous infusion of 0.9% NaCl or any balanced solutions.

Dextrose solutions provide some caloric support and may also be indicated if enteral nutrition is not possible and other means of nutritional support have not been established. They also serve as a diluent for injectable medications.

Balanced Crystalloid Solutions

The different types of balanced crystalloid solutions vary slightly in their electrolyte composition. They can be used for resuscitation and maintenance purposes. The individual choice depends on the characteristics of the patient, the type of fluid lost, and the availability.

Human Albumin Solutions

Human albumin is commonly used in situations when there is a desire to draw to, or keep, volume in the intravascular space without additional salt or volume loading, such as in liver cirrhosis or nephrotic syndrome or following large-volume paracentesis. HAS 5% leads to 80% initial volume expansion, whereas the 25% solution is hyperoncotic and leads to a 200% to 400% increase within 30 minutes.[10]

Hypoalbuminemia is common in a wide range of acute and chronic disease states. Regular infusion will increase the serum albumin level unless there is a profound protein-losing state. However, targeting hypoalbuminemia per se with HAS has not been shown to improve outcomes.[36] In states of endothelial dysfunction/capillary leak, significant quantities of albumin can enter the interstitial space and contribute to tissue edema.[37]

Hydroxyethyl Starches

HES were the most widely prescribed colloids, but the use is now restricted in several countries following evidence of nephrotoxicity. They are primarily used for acute intravascular volume expansion during surgery. There is no particular physiologic advantage of HES over any other colloid solution.

Gelatin-Based Colloids

Gelatins are used for acute volume expansion, but their duration is shorter than that of albumin or starches. They are not licensed worldwide.

Dextrans

Despite theoretic advantages in improving blood flow through reduced viscosity and anticoagulation, dextrans have no specific indication apart from acute volume expansion.

SUMMARY

The ubiquitous nature of intravenous fluid prescription in hospital belies the level of consideration that needs to be given when choosing the most suitable fluid, rate, and volume appropriate for individual patients. Iatrogenic disturbances in plasma volume, tissue edema, acid-base balance, and electrolytes may have a significant impact, which can be minimized with careful selection of the most appropriate type of fluid. However, without adequately powered RCTs, many fundamental questions, such as the true value of balanced versus unbalanced solutions and the optimal fluid regime, remain unanswered. The current evidence is leaning toward the judicious use of fluids to minimize fluid overload, a preference for balanced solutions over 0.9% NaCl and the avoidance of synthetic colloids.

REFERENCES

1. Myburgh JA, Mythen MG. Resuscitation fluids. N Engl J Med 2013;369:1243–51.
2. Edwards MR, Mythen MG. Fluid therapy in critical illness. Extrem Physiol Med 2014;3:16.
3. Raghunathan K, Murray K, Beattie WS, et al. Choice of fluid in acute illness: what should be given? Management strategies from the twelfth consensus conference

of the acute dialysis quality initiative (ADQI) London 2013. Br J Anaesth 2014;
113(5):772–83.

4. Severs D, Hoorn EJ, Rookmaaker MB. A critical appraisal of intravenous fluids:
   from the physiological basis to clinical evidence. Nephrol Dial Transplant 2015;
   30:178–87.

5. Lira A, Pinsky MR. Choices in fluid type and volume during resuscitation: impact
   on patient outcomes. Ann Intensive Care 2014;4:38.

6. Raghunathan K, McGee WT, Higgins T. Importance of intravenous fluid dose and
   composition in surgical ICU patients. Curr Opin Crit Care 2012;18:350–7.

7. Kaplan LJ, Kellum JA. Fluids, pH, ions and electrolytes. Curr Opin Crit Care 2010;
   16(4):323–31.

8. Greenfield RH, Bessen HA, Henneman PL. Effect of crystalloid infusion on hematocrit and intravascular volume in healthy, nonbleeding subjects. Ann Emerg Med
   1989;18(1):51–5.

9. Chappell D, Jacob M. Role of the glycocalyx in fluid management: small things
   matter. Best Pract Res Clin Anaesthesiol 2014;28(3):227–34.

10. Mitra S, Khandelwal P. Are all colloids same? How to select the right colloid? In-
    dian J Anaesth 2009;53(5):592–607.

11. Margarson MP, Soni NC. Changes in serum albumin concentration and volume
    expanding effects following a bolus of albumin 20% in septic patients. Br J
    Anaesth 2004;92(6):821–6.

12. Weil MH, Henning RJ, Puri VK. Colloid oncotic pressure: clinical significance. Crit
    Care Med 1979;7(3):113–6.

13. Matejtschuk P, Dash CH, Gascoigne EW. Production of human albumin solution: a
    continually developing colloid. Br J Anaesth 2000;85(6):887–95.

14. Saddler JM, Horsey PJ. The new generation gelatins. A review of their history,
    manufacture and properties. Anaesthesia 1987;42(9):998–1004.

15. Westphal M, James MF, Kozek-Langenecker S, et al. Hydroxyethyl starches:
    different products - different effects. Anesthesiology 2009;111(1):187–202.

16. Vincent JL, Sakr Y, Sprung SL, et al. Sepsis in European intensive care units: re-
    sults of the SOAP study. Crit Care Med 2006;34(2):344–53.

17. Boyd JH, Forbes J, Nakada TA, et al. Fluid resuscitation in septic shock: a pos-
    itive fluid balance and elevated central venous pressure are associated with
    increased mortality. Crit Care Med 2011;39(2):259–65.

18. Chappell D, Bruegger D, Potzel J, et al. Hypervolemia increases release of atrial
    natriuretic peptide and shedding of the endothelial glycocalyx. Crit Care 2014;
    18(5):538.

19. Hansen PB, Jensen BL, Skott O. Chloride regulates afferent arteriolar contraction
    in response to depolarization. Hypertension 1998;32(6):1066–70.

20. Chowdhury AH, Cox EF, Francis ST, et al. A randomized, controlled, double-blind
    crossover study on the effects of 2-L infusions of 0.9% saline and plasma-lyte (R)
    148 on renal blood flow velocity and renal cortical tissue perfusion in healthy vol-
    unteers. Ann Surg 2012;256(1):18–24.

21. Wilcox CS. Regulation of renal blood flow by plasma chloride. J Clin Invest 1983;
    71(3):726–35.

22. Shaw AD, Bagshaw SM, Goldstein SL, et al. Major complications, mortality, and
    resource utilization after open abdominal surgery: 0.9% saline compared to
    Plasma-Lyte. Ann Surg 2012;255(5):821–9.

23. Yunos NM, Bellomo R, Hegarty C, et al. Association between a chloride-liberal vs
    chloride-restrictive intravenous fluid administration strategy and kidney injury in
    critically ill adults. JAMA 2012;308(15):1566–72.

24. McCluskey SA, Karkouti K, Wijeysundera D, et al. Hyperchloremia after noncardiac surgery is independently associated with increased morbidity and mortality: a propensity-matched cohort study. Anesth Analg 2013;117(2):412–21.
25. Perner A, Haase N, Guttormsen AB, et al. Hydroxyethyl starch 130/0.42 versus Ringer's acetate in severe sepsis. N Engl J Med 2012;367:124–34.
26. Myburgh JA, Finfer S, Bellomo R, et al. Hydroxyethyl starch or saline for fluid resuscitation in intensive care. N Engl J Med 2012;367:1901–11.
27. Brunkhorst FM, Engel C, Bloos F, et al. Intensive insulin therapy and pentastarch resuscitation in severe sepsis. N Engl J Med 2008;358(2):125–39.
28. Serpa Neto A, Veelo DP, Peireira VG, et al. Fluid resuscitation with hydroxyethyl starches in patients with sepsis is associated with an increased incidence of acute kidney injury and use of renal replacement therapy: a systematic review and meta-analysis of the literature. J Crit Care 2014;29(1):185.e1–7.
29. Bayer O, Schwarzkopf D, Doenst T, et al. Perioperative fluid therapy with tetra-starch and gelatin in cardiac surgery–a prospective sequential analysis. Crit Care Med 2013;41(11):2532–42.
30. Bayer O, Reinhart K, Sakr Y, et al. Renal effects of synthetic colloids and crystalloids in patients with severe sepsis: a prospective sequential comparison. Crit Care Med 2011;39(6):1335–42.
31. Thomas-Rueddel DO, Vlasakov V, Reinhart K, et al. Safety of gelatin for volume resuscitation–a systematic review and meta-analysis. Intensive Care Med 2012; 38(7):1134–42.
32. Langer T, Ferrari M, Zazzeron L, et al. Effects of intravenous solutions on acid-base equilibrium: from crystalloids to colloids and blood components. Anaesthesiol Intensive Ther 2014;46(5):350–60.
33. Barron ME, Wilkes MM, Navickis RJ. A systematic review of the comparative safety of colloids. Arch Surg 2004;139(5):552–63.
34. Bunn F, Trivedi D. Colloid solutions for fluid resuscitation. Cochrane Database Syst Rev 2012;(7):CD001319.
35. Padhi S, Bullock I, Li L, et al. Intravenous fluid therapy for adults in hospital: summary of NICE guidance. BMJ 2013;347:f7073.
36. Caironi P, Tognoni G, Masson S, et al. Albumin replacement in patients with severe sepsis or septic shock. N Engl J Med 2014;370(15):1412–21.
37. Fleck A, Raines G, Hawker F, et al. Increased vascular permeability: a major cause of hypoalbuminaemia in disease and injury. Lancet 1985;1(8432):781–4.

Renal Replacement Therapy

Gianluca Villa, MD[a],*, Zaccaria Ricci, MD[b], Claudio Ronco, MD[c,d]

KEYWORDS

- Continuous renal replacement therapy • Timing • Dose • Citrate • Heparin

KEY POINTS

- Early renal support therapy may be more effective than late renal replacement therapy (RRT) to improve the outcomes of patients with acute kidney injury (AKI).
- Continuous RRTs should be preferred to intermittent therapies, mainly for hemodynamically unstable patients with AKI.
- The prescribed dose should be carefully evaluated for each patient and the delivered dose continuously monitored during the treatment.
- Citrate anticoagulation may be used for all patients without contraindications, particularly in high-expertise centers: heparin as a first choice is still feasible in nonbleeding patients, especially for units using RRT less frequently.

INTRODUCTION

Acute kidney injury (AKI) is a clinical syndrome characterized by a sudden decrease in kidney function resulting in accumulation of fluids, creatinine, urea, and other waste products.[1] The incidence of AKI widely ranges depending on the studied population and on the definition used. Through integration of the previous risk, injury, failure, loss, and end stage classification (RIFLE) and acute kidney injury network (AKIN) classifications, in 2012 the Kidney Disease: Improving Global Outcomes (KDIGO) guidelines defined AKI as an increase in the serum creatinine level of 0.3 mg/dL (26.5 μmol/L) or more within 48 hours, a serum creatinine level that has increased by at least 1.5 times the baseline value within the previous 7 days, or a urine volume of less than 0.5 mL/kg of body weight per hour for 6 hours.[2]

The authors declare no disclosures.

[a] Section of Anaesthesiology and Intensive Care, Department of Health Science, University of Florence, Florence, Italy; [b] Pediatric Cardiac Intensive Care Unit, Department of Cardiology and Cardiac Surgery, Bambino Gesù Children's Hospital, IRCCS, Piazza Sant'Onofrio 4, CAP 00165, Rome, Italy; [c] Department of Nephrology, Dialysis and Transplantation, San Bortolo Hospital, Viale Ferdinando Rodolfi 37, CAP 36100, Vicenza, Italy; [d] International Renal Research Institute, San Bortolo Hospital, Vicenza, Italy

* Corresponding author. Section of Anesthesiology and Intensive Care, Department of Health Sciences, University of Florence, Largo Brambilla 3, Florence 50134, Italy.
E-mail address: gianlucavilla1@gmail.com

Crit Care Clin 31 (2015) 839–848
http://dx.doi.org/10.1016/j.ccc.2015.06.015
0749-0704/15/$ – see front matter © 2015 Elsevier Inc. All rights reserved.

criticalcare.theclinics.com

Approximately 5% to 7% of hospitalized patients develop AKI during their hospital length of stay; this incidence is further increased to 25% among critically ill patients in the intensive care unit (ICU).[1,3] A mortality rate more than 50% has been reported for patients with AKI and multiorgan failure.[3] In the absence of any effective pharmacologic therapies, AKI is usually managed through supportive treatments focused on optimization of fluid balance, prevention or treatment of electrolyte and acid-base disturbances, adjustment of the dosing of medications that are excreted by the kidney, and avoidance of secondary hemodynamic and nephrotoxic renal injuries. Beyond these conservative therapies, renal replacement therapy (RRT) is essentially the only effective method for the management of the critically ill patients with severe AKI.[1,3]

Even if it is currently a matter of debate if RRT optimization may reduce the mortality of patients with AKI,[4] it is reasonable to remark that avoidance of renal support in an oligo-anuric critically ill patient is not acceptable. Furthermore, an accurate evaluation of the most important issues on RRT, such as timing, modality, and dose of treatment, may be quintessential to improve renal and nonrenal outcomes in these patients.

TIMING OF INITIATION

The adequate timing for the RRT initiation in patients with AKI has not been exactly defined, so far. In current practice, the decision to initiate an RRT is often based on clinical or biochemical features of fluid overload and/or solutes imbalances (azotemia, hyperkalemia, severe acidosis).[2] However, these emergency indications characterize a rescue therapy for renal substitution in which the initiation of the treatment forestalls an imminent death. More reasonably, current practice should be based on the preemptive initiation of RRT, well before the development of these advanced complications; the aim is to early support the renal function during early phases of organ dysfunction instead of completely replacing kidney function in the late phases of organ insufficiency (**Table 1**).

An early onset of RRT is usually considered to be associated with an improved outcome in patients with AKI, even if no significant evidence supports this notion in current literature; however, indications of RRT and timing of RRT initiation are currently 2 of the fundamental questions listed among the top priorities in research in this field.[4] The levels of evidence that guide current practice primarily derive from retrospective and observational cohort studies and small, underpowered prospective trials.[5] With not-graded recommendations, the KDIGO guidelines currently suggest to emergently initiate an RRT when life-threatening changes in fluid, electrolyte, and acid-base

Table 1
Examples of possible indications for a late RRT aimed to completely substitute the kidney function and for an early renal support therapy aimed to promptly maintain homeostasis, to reduce organs dysfunction, and the further renal insult

RRT	Renal Support Therapy
Absolute Indications (Life-Treating Conditions)	**Relative Indications**
Acid-base control	Volume removal in patients with fluid overload
Ions alterations	Immunomodulation in sepsis
Solutes control	Allowing to reach an adequate nutrition support
	Blood purification during cancer chemotherapy

balance exist and to further consider, in the broader clinical context, the presence of conditions that can be modified with RRT for clinical decision making to start RRT (**Fig. 1**).[2]

The association between early RRT and survival was first suggested by case series with historical controls conducted in the 1960s and 1970s[6]; in these studies, levels of blood urea or blood urea nitrogen (BUN) were used to define the early and late start of dialysis. Similarly, a recent prospective multicenter observational cohort study performed by the Program to Improve Care in Acute Renal Disease (PICARD) analyzed the RRT initiation, defined according to the predialysis BUN concentrations. In this study, a late onset of RRT resulted statistically associated with an increased risk of death in a multivariate analysis.[7] Similar results were also obtained by other studies comparing early versus late onset of RRT when BUN or blood urea were considered to define them.[7]

Timing between the extracorporeal therapy initiation and the ICU admission is another issue that should be taken into account for classification purposes of early and late RRT. Data available from the Beginning and Ending Supportive Therapy (BEST) for the kidney registry[8] reveal that when timing was analyzed in relation to ICU admission, the late RRT was associated with greater crude mortality, covariate-adjusted mortality, RRT requirement, and hospital length of stay.[8]

As pointed out by Shiao and colleagues,[9] the staging of AKI at the RRT initiation, evaluated through clinical classifications, may be used to identify early and late treatments. In an observational study on surgical patients with AKI, these investigators have showed a statistical correlation between late RRT and worst renal and nonrenal outcomes.[9]

Although several studies have suggested a possible positive role of early RRT among patients with AKI, contrasting results are available in literature. In 2002 Bouman and colleagues[5] showed no differences for ICU or hospital mortalities and for renal recovery among patients treated with an early or late RRT. However, if cumulatively considered in systematic review or meta-analysis, independently by parameters used to define the onset, an early initiation of RRT seems to be associated with an improved outcome.[10] In a recent meta-analysis, including 15 unique studies published until 2010 on comparison between early and late initiation of renal

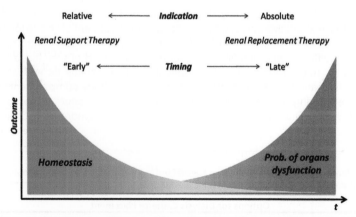

Fig. 1. If compared with a late RRT, an early renal support therapy seems to allow a prompt maintenance of systemic homeostasis, mainly if the treatment prescription fulfills the concept of *adequacy* and it is specifically oriented to patients' relative indications. As a consequence, the renal support therapy seems to be associated with a reduced probability of organ dysfunction and progression of kidney disease.

support, Karvellas and colleagues[10] have calculated an odds ratio for 28-day mortality of 0.45 associated with an early RRT. Similar results were obtained by Wang and Yuan[11] in 2012 in a meta-analysis encompassing data from 2955 patients; the results of this study have clearly demonstrated that an early initiation of both continuous and intermittent RRT may reduce the mortality of patients with AKI compared with late treatments.

Once identified, the conditions are potentially improvable through an early renal support therapy; once an early initiation of RRT has been decided, physicians must address the vascular access placement and the prescription phases in which the modality and the dose of the treatment should be decided.

VASCULAR ACCESS

A large-bore, double-lumen, noncuffed, nontunneled dialysis catheter is typically used for RRT in critically ill patients with AKI. The vein used for the catheter insertion should be chosen taking into account the patients' clinical characteristics (eg, the risk to evolve forward chronic kidney disease) and the instrumental features (eg, vein thrombosis or ratio between vein and catheter diameter). Ceteris paribus, the international KDIGO guidelines suggest a specific order for catheter placement (**Table 2**).[2]

The rationale is mainly based on the evaluation of the incidence of catheter-related complications (eg, infection or thrombosis) related to each site as well as taking into account the relative high frequency of chronic renal disease in patients with AKI, the long-term RRT requirements, and the need of a vascular access for chronic dialysis such us an artero-venous fistula.

The catheter should be inserted with the use of ultrasonographic guidance and with adherence to infection-control policies.[1] No evidences exist in literature about the most effective lumen dispositions within a dialytic catheter to reduce recirculation and improve clearance of the treatment.

TREATMENTS AND MODALITIES

The most adequate treatment of RRT for patients with AKI was not defined in literature for several years; the initial setting for RRT was usually chosen according to treatment availability in the center, technical skills of the operators, and patients' hemodynamic status.

Intermittent hemodialysis (IHD) was proposed as the treatment of choice for the management of critically ill patients with AKI. During IHD, solute and fluid control are mainly achieved by diffusion and ultrafiltration over a limited period of time (usually hours); consequently, major repercussions on patients' volemic status as well as a rapid change of fluid and solute components among different body compartments may all be expected during the treatment. Systemic hypotension occurs in approximately 20% to 30% of IHD treatments[12] as well as disequilibrium syndrome.[13] On the other

---

Table 2
In accordance with KDIGO guidelines, a specific order for catheter placement should be adopted if clinically acceptable and technically feasible

Options for Dialysis Catheter Placement	
First choice	Right jugular vein
Second choice	Femoral vein
Third choice	Left jugular vein
Last choice	Subclavian vein with preference for the dominant side

hand, continuous RRT (CRRT) includes a spectrum of treatments developed in the 1980s specifically for the management of critically ill patients with AKI who could not undergo traditional IHD because of hemodynamic instability or in whom IHD could not control the volume or metabolic derangements.[14] During CRRT, the lesser solute clearance and the slower removal of fluid per unit of time than IHD is thought to allow for better hemodynamic tolerance (**Table 3**).[1] Finally, experience with peritoneal dialysis (PD) in AKI is limited, except in the pediatric setting and in regions with limited resources.[2]

Although several randomized clinical trials have compared CRRT with IHD in patients with AKI, most of them have excluded hemodynamically unstable patients for the analysis. As a consequence, meta-analyses currently available on this topic have failed to demonstrate a clear superiority of continuous treatments over intermittent ones among critically ill patients with AKI.[15,16] Differently, in large observational studies including all patients receiving RRT, CRRT resulted an independent predictor of renal recovery among patients who survived to the acute illness.[2,17] Currently, CRRT is strongly suggested for hemodynamically unstable patients with AKI and for patients with acute brain injury or other causes of increased intracranial pressure or generalized brain edema in which large fluctuations of solute concentration and fluid shifts should be avoided.[2]

One last aspect may be relevant: if short-term hard outcomes are not impacted by RRT modality, it may not be the case for long-term ones. As a matter of fact, IHD has been suspected to cause long-term chronic kidney disease in patients with AKI. Two recent studies (a meta-analysis and a retrospective analysis) remarked that[18,19] compared with CRRT, IHD prescription for AKI treatment is significantly and strongly associated with a lower possibility of recovery of renal function. If these data were further confirmed, IHD should be abandoned for the treatment of AKI.

There are currently insufficient data to recommend a specific extracorporeal modality over another. In continuous veno-venous hemodialysis, solute removal is mainly achieved by diffusion; ceteris paribus, it is negatively related to the solute

Table 3
Advantages and disadvantages for IHD, prolonged, and CRRT

Treatments	Advantages	Disadvantages
IHD	• Rapid removal of toxins circulating solutes • Reduced downtime for diagnostic and therapeutic procedures • Reduced exposure to anticoagulation • Lower cost than CRRT	• Rapid fluid removal and frequent hypotension • Dialysis disequilibrium and risk of cerebral edema • Technically complex
Prolonged (e.g. sustained low-efficiency daily dialysis)	• Slower volume and solute removal than IHD • Faster solutes clearance than CRRT • Reduced downtime than CRRT • Reduced exposure to anticoagulation than CRRT	• Faster volume and solute removal than CRRT (increased risk for hypotension and disequilibrium syndrome in prone patients) • Technically complex
CRRT	• Continuous removal of toxin and solutes (avoid concentration rebound) • Hemodynamic tolerability • Easy control of fluid balance • Avoid disequilibrium syndrome • User-friendly machines	• Slower solutes clearance than IHD • Need for prolonged anticoagulation • Reduced possibility of patients' mobilization • Hypothermia • Increased costs than IHD

molecular weight. On the other hand, in continuous veno-venous hemofiltration (CVVH), solute removal is achieved by convection and strongly influenced by intrinsic properties of membrane as the ultrafiltration coefficient. The extracorporeal removal of small molecular weight molecules, as urea and creatinine, are of scarce interest during the early renal support therapy in the ICU; for this reason, many clinicians prefer to use CVVH for critically ill patients with AKI in the belief that convection can more effectively reduce the effects of the systemic inflammatory response syndrome by removing cytokines, most of which are middle molecular weight molecules. However, most controlled studies have not shown a clinically significant and sustained effect on cytokine plasma concentrations or an improvement in outcome. Therefore, the selection of a specific method is primarily based on institutional experience and preference.

DOSE

Because initial studies demonstrated a direct relationship between dose and survival, both for intermittent and continuous RRT,[20,21] great attention has been paid to identify the optimal dose of RRT in the last 10 years.

Dose may be represented by the efficiency (or clearance) of the treatment, which identifies the amount of blood cleared of waste products and toxins by the extracorporeal circuit over a given period of time.[22] The concept of clearance needs to be referred to a particular solute; urea, usually considered a uremic toxin marker, is most commonly used to quantify dose. Considering that CRRT is usually performed over several days or weeks, it is important to provide information about the total time during which the treatment clearance is delivered. The intensity of treatment is, thus, expressed as the product between the clearance and the effective time of treatment.[22] Including the downtime (the amount of time in which the treatment is interrupted), a significant difference could be found between the prescribed and the actual delivered doses. Finally, considering the whole pool of solute that needs to be cleared, it is possible to express the efficacy of the treatment as the ratio between the intensity and the volume of distribution of the marker solute.[22] All these concepts should be taken into consideration during the prescription phase of the treatment.

The demonstration of a direct correlation between dose and patients' outcomes prompted clinicians to carefully evaluate the initial RRT prescription. The *target prescribed dose* is the amount of clearance required for the specific patient in his or her specific clinical condition, and it represents the amount of clearance that the practitioner desires to actually deliver to the patient. During the treatment, considering the instantaneous flows in the extracorporeal circuit, a *current dose* may be identified. During downtime, when the machine treatment is stopped, the current dose is zero; the total amount of downtime during the treatment strongly influences the *delivered dose*.

In patients with AKI who are treated with CRRT in the ICU, the dose may be grossly estimated considering the effluent flow rate set in the CRRT machine[23] and then by indexing it over the patient body weight (ie, if a 60-Kg patient is treated with 1200 mL/h of isovolumic postdilution hemofiltration, the dose of its treatment may be indicated as 20 mL/kg/h). As for every simplification, with this method a relatively broad level of error should be accepted, especially when continuous predilution hemofiltration or continuous hemodialysis are delivered. Furthermore, it cannot obviously take into consideration the progressive decrease of membrane performance observed in the prolonged session (especially after the first 24 hours). As a matter of fact, the ease of this calculation may be very useful on the practical side.[24]

Several efforts have been made in the literature in order to define the most adequate dose; the idea is that CRRT delivery may imply a dose-dependent range, whereby the treatment efficiency does correlate with outcomes and a dose-independent range in which further improvements will not result in further benefits for these patients. Consequently, during the last decade, several attempts have been made in order to confirm the first dosage proposal (35 mL/k/h) that showed a direct correlation between CRRT efficiency and patients' outcomes.[21] However, the randomized evaluation of normal vs. augmented level (RENAL)[20] and the acute renal failure trial network (ATN)[25] studies seemed to definitely confute this evidence. These 2 large multicenter, randomized controlled trials did not show an improved outcome with a "more intensive dose" (40 and 35 mL/kg/h respectively) with respect to a "less intensive dose" (25 and 20 mL/kg/h respectively).[26] Based on these findings, the current KDIGO guidelines recommend delivering an effluent volume of 20 to 25 mL/kg/h for CRRT in patients with AKI.[2]

In addition, by comparing 2 multicenter CRRT databases, Uchino and colleagues[27] found that patients with AKI treated with low-dose CRRT were not associated with worse short-term outcomes compared with patients treated with the currently considered standard dose. In particular, comparing patients from The BEST study[3] and from The Japanese Society for Physician and Trainees Intensive Care (JSEPTIC) Clinical Trial Group,[28] the investigators observed no differences between groups of patient treated with a dosages of 14.3 mL/kg/h and 20.4 mL/kg/h.

Finally, considering that high-dose CRRT could lead to electrolyte disorders, removal of nutrients and drugs (eg, antibiotics), and high costs[29] and low-dose CRRT may expose patients to undertreatment resulting in worsening outcomes, seeking the range of an adequate treatment dose is currently a crucial issue. Nowadays, a delivered dosage (without downtime) between 20 and 35 mL/kg/h may be considered clinically acceptable.[27] In particular, a CRRT dosage prescription less than 20 mL/kg/h and more than 35 mL/kg/h may be definitely identified as the *dose-dependent range*, whereby the dialytic intensity is likely known to negatively affect outcomes (both caused by underdialysis and overdialysis). On the other hand, the prescriptions laying between these 2 limits can be considered as *practice-dependent*; variables such as timing, patient characteristics, comorbidities, or concomitant supportive pharmacologic therapies may have a significant role for patients' outcomes and should trigger a careful prescription and a closest monitoring of dose delivery (**Fig. 2**).

ANTICOAGULATION

Anticoagulation (and filter patency) is a fundamental issue strictly related to dialysis delivery and to the personalized prescription of an adequate CRRT treatment. Systemic and regional anticoagulation, as well as heparin grafting membranes, are potentially able to reduce the filter clotting and consequently the membrane fouling. Analyzing data from the PICARD study, Claure-del Granado and colleagues[30] evaluated the association of an anticoagulation strategy used on solute clearance efficacy and circuit longevity. In particular, the investigators showed that, if compared with heparin or no anticoagulation, the use of regional citrate for anticoagulation in CRRT significantly prolonged the filter life and increased its efficacy in terms of delivered dose.[30] De Vriese and colleagues[31] clearly demonstrated membrane dysfunction affected solute clearance during CRRT treatment. Unfortunately, this predictable mechanism is not simply quantifiable in clinical practice. When the membrane fouling occurs and clearance of urea (a 60-Da non–protein-bound molecule) decreases by 20%, the clearance of larger solutes may have already been impaired in the CRRT circuit life span.[32] In this context, if middle molecular weight molecules are the solute target to be removed, an accurate

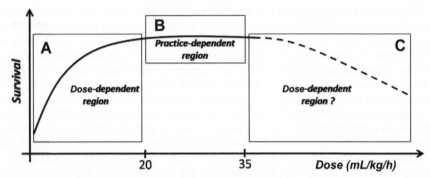

Fig. 2. Relationship between delivered dosage and patients' survival. Increasing the dosage to 20 mL/kg/h (*A*), the higher the dosage obtained during RRT, the higher the patient survival observed (dosage-dependent region). Further increase in dosage prescription to 35 mL/kg/h (*B*) may not influence patients' survival. On the other hand, other variables, such as the time of treatment, the optimization of blood perfusion, or drug adjustments, may influence the outcome (practice-dependent region). With further increase of prescribed dosage (more than 35 mL/kg/h) (*C*), patients may be prone to electrolyte disorders and removal of nutrients and drugs (eg, antibiotics), potentially reducing the survival.

anticoagulation should be performed also to ensure that an adequate sieving coefficient for these molecules is maintained for a long period of time.

Despite the most recent guidelines suggest using regional citrate anticoagulation in all patients without contraindications and with either high or low risk of bleeding, the administration of unfractionated heparin into the CRRT circuit remains the most used anticoagulation during CRRT. On the other hand, unfractionated or low-molecular-weight heparin, rather than other anticoagulants, are suggested for patients with a low risk of bleeding who present an absolute contraindication to citrate administration. Other anticoagulants are finally recommended in patients with heparin-induced thrombocytopenia; in particular, in these patients, all heparin must be stopped and direct thrombin inhibitors (such as argatroban) or factor Xa inhibitors (such as danaparoid or fondaparinux) rather than other anticoagulants or no anticoagulation should be adopted during RRT.[2]

SUMMARY

An early RRT aimed to support the residual kidney function during the early phases of organ dysfunction may improve the renal and nonrenal outcomes of patients with AKI with respect to late treatments. For critically ill patients in the ICU, and mainly for patients who require a slower fluid removal and a more gentle solute control, continuous treatments should be preferred. Vascular access placement as well as the treatment modalities should be carefully evaluated for each patient. The adequacy of the treatment should finally take into consideration the amount of clearance required for the treatment. The prescribed dose should be continuously evaluated for each patient, and the delivered dose should be monitored during the treatment. Mainly reducing downtime and membrane fouling, anticoagulation is able to reduce discrepancies between the prescribed and the actual delivered dose.

REFERENCES

1. Tolwani A. Continuous renal-replacement therapy for acute kidney injury. N Engl J Med 2012;367:2505–14.

2. Kidney Disease: Improving Global Outcomes (KDIGO) Acute Kidney Injury Work Group. KDIGO clinical practice guideline for acute kidney injury. Kidney Int Suppl 2012;2:1–138.

3. Uchino S, Kellum J, Bellomo R, et al. Acute renal failure in critically ill patients: a multinational, multicenter study. JAMA 2005;294(7):813–8.

4. Kellum JA, Mehta RL, Levin A, et al. Development of a clinical research agenda for acute kidney injury using an international, interdisciplinary, three-step modified Delphi process. Clin J Am Soc Nephrol 2008;3:887–94.

5. Bouman CS, Oudemans-Van Straaten HM, Tijssen JG, et al. Effects of early high-volume continuous venovenous hemofiltration on survival and recovery of renal function in intensive care patients with acute renal failure: a prospective, randomized trial. Crit Care Med 2002;30(10):2205–11.

6. Palevsky P. Renal replacement therapy in AKI. Adv Chronic Kidney Dis 2013; 20(1):76–84.

7. Liu KD, Himmelfarb J, Paganini E, et al. Timing of initiation of dialysis in critically ill patients with acute kidney injury. Clin J Am Soc Nephrol 2006;1(5): 915–9.

8. Bagshaw SM, Uchino S, Bellomo R, et al. Timing of renal replacement therapy and clinical outcomes in critically ill patients with severe acute kidney injury. J Crit Care 2009;24(1):129–40.

9. Shiao CC, Wu VC, Li WY, et al. Late initiation of renal replacement therapy is associated with worse outcomes in acute kidney injury after major abdominal surgery. Crit Care 2009;13(5):R171.

10. Karvellas CJ, Farhat MR, Sajjad I, et al. A comparison of early versus late initiation of renal replacement therapy in critically ill patients with acute kidney injury: a systematic review and meta-analysis. Crit Care 2011;15(1):R72.

11. Wang X, Yuan WJ. Timing of initiation of renal replacement therapy in acute kidney injury: a systematic review and meta-analysis. Ren Fail 2012;34(3): 396–402.

12. Selby NM, McIntyre CW. A systematic review of the clinical effects of reducing dialysate fluid temperature. Nephrol Dial Transplant 2006;21:1883–98.

13. Ronco C, Bellomo R, Brendolan A, et al. Brain density changes during renal replacement in critically ill patients with acute renal failure. Continuous hemofiltration versus intermittent hemodialysis. J Nephrol 1999;12(3):173–8.

14. Cerdá J, Ronco C. Modalities of continuous renal replacement therapy: technical and clinical considerations. Semin Dial 2009;22(8):114–22.

15. Pannu N, Klarenbach S, Wiebe N, et al. Renal replacement therapy in patients with acute renal failure. JAMA 2008;299(7):793–805.

16. Bagshaw SM, Berthiaume LR, Delaney A, et al. Continuous versus intermittent renal replacement therapy for critically ill patients with acute kidney injury: a meta-analysis. Crit Care Med 2008;36(2):610–7.

17. Bell M, Granath F, Schön S, et al. Continuous renal replacement therapy is associated with less chronic renal failure than intermittent haemodialysis after acute renal failure. Intensive Care Med 2007;33:773–80.

18. Schneider AG, Bellomo R, Bagshaw SM, et al. Choice of renal replacement therapy modality and dialysis dependence after acute kidney injury: a systematic review and meta-analysis. Intensive Care Med 2013;39(6):987–97.

19. Wald R, Shariff SZ, Adhikari NKJ, et al. The association between renal replacement therapy modality and long-term outcomes among critically ill adults with acute kidney injury: a retrospective cohort study. Crit Care Med 2013;42(4): 1–10.

20. RENAL Replacement Therapy Study Investigators, Bellomo R, Cass A, et al. Intensity of continuous renal-replacement therapy in critically ill patients. N Engl J Med 2009;361(17):1627–38.

21. Ronco C, Bellomo R, Homel P, et al. Effects of different doses in continuous veno-venous haemofiltration on outcomes of acute renal failure: a prospective rando-mised trial. Lancet 2000;356(9223):26–30.

22. Ricci Z, Bellomo R, Ronco C. Dose of dialysis in acute renal failure. Clin J Am Soc Nephrol 2006;1(3):380–8.

23. Uchino S, Bellomo R, Morimatsu H, et al. Continuous renal replacement therapy: a worldwide practice survey. The beginning and ending supportive therapy for the kidney (B.E.S.T. kidney) investigators. Intensive Care Med 2007;33(9): 1563–70.

24. Ricci Z, Salvatori G, Bonello M, et al. In vivo validation of the adequacy calculator for continuous renal replacement therapies. Crit Care 2005;9(3):R266–73.

25. VA/NIH Acute Renal Failure Trial Network, Palevsky P, Zhang J, et al. Intensity of renal support in critically ill patients with acute kidney injury. N Engl J Med 2008; 359(1):7–20.

26. Ricci Z, Ronco C. Timing, dose and mode of dialysis in acute kidney injury. Curr Opin Crit Care 2011;17(6):556–61.

27. Uchino S, Toki N, Takeda K, et al. Validity of low-intensity continuous renal replacement therapy. Crit Care Med 2013;41(11):2584–91.

28. Kawarazaki H, Uchino S, Tokuhira N, et al. Who may not benefit from continuous renal replacement therapy in acute kidney injury? Hemodial Int 2013;17(4): 624–32.

29. Rimmelé T, Kellum JA. Clinical review: blood purification for sepsis. Crit Care 2011;15(1):205.

30. Claure-del Granado R, Macedo E, Soroko S, et al. Anticoagulation, delivered dose and outcomes in CRRT: the program to improve care in acute renal disease (PICARD). Hemodial Int 2014;18:641–9.

31. De Vriese A, Colardyn F, Philippé J, et al. Cytokine removal during continuous hemofiltration in septic patients. J Am Soc Nephrol 1999;10(4):846–53.

32. Pasko DA, Churchwell M, Salama N, et al. Longitudinal hemodiafilter perfor-mance in modeled continuous renal replacement therapy. Blood Purif 2011; 32(2):82–8.

Understanding Acid Base Disorders

Hernando Gomez, MD, MPH, John A. Kellum, MD, FACP*

KEYWORDS

- Acid base • Hydrogen • Stewart • Henderson–Hasselbalch • pH • Base excess
- Strong ion difference

KEY POINTS

- There are currently 3 methods to assess acid base balance in the clinical setting, the Henderson-Hasselbalch equation, the standard base excess, and the Stewart approach, all of which are approximations to represent physiologic behavior of aqueous solutions.
- All 3 methods provide the means to arrive at similar conclusions in daily clinical practice, because they are all fundamentally based on equilibrium equations.
- The Stewart approach conceived aqueous solutions as systems, and thus, attempted to explain the behavior of pH by including every possible mechanism (ie, the Henderson–Hasselbalch's proposed evaluation of the HCO_3–pCO_2 base pair).
- These methods should be conceived as complementary, and not substitutive.

INTRODUCTION

Although most ion concentrations exist naturally in the millimolar range in people, the concentration of the hydrogen ion is regulated within a narrow margin at the nanomolar range, between 16 and 160 nmol/L, with a physiologic value approaching 40 nmol/L in human whole blood.[1] Such rigorous regulation is not by chance, as hydrogen is a highly reactive ion that can interact with hydrogen bonds, proteins, and enzymes, and can alter protein structure and function,[2] compromising thereby biochemical processes and even cell survival. It is not surprising then that the correct assessment of acid–base balance and the adequate management of its alterations are of major importance in clinical medicine.

Disclosure Statement: The authors have no disclosures.
Department of Critical Care Medicine, Center for Critical Care Nephrology, The CRISMA Center, University of Pittsburgh, 3550 Terrace Street, Pittsburgh, PA 15261, USA
* Corresponding author. Department of Critical Care Medicine, Center for Critical Care Nephrology, University of Pittsburgh School of Medicine, Room 604, Scaife Hall, 3550 Terrace Street, Pittsburgh, PA 15261.
E-mail address: kellumja@ccm.upmc.edu

Crit Care Clin 31 (2015) 849–860
http://dx.doi.org/10.1016/j.ccc.2015.06.016   criticalcare.theclinics.com

Before 1923, acids and bases were conceived as anions and cations, respectively. Although Humphrey Davy had already observed and reported the association of acidity with the presence of hydrogen ions in the early 19th century, it was not until the seminal work by Arrhenius, Brønstead and Lowry, and Lewis, that clarity was brought to the field with the establishment of the hydrogen ion as the centerpiece of acid base analysis, and the concept that what determines acidity of a solution is the chemical potential of hydrogen ions. This paradigm shift also established the modern definitions of acids and bases as substances able to release, or accept hydrogen ions at a given pH, respectively,[3] and of buffer pairs as weak acids that enter in equilibrium with their complementing weak bases, also at a given pH.[3]

Relative consensus was achieved in terms of the effect of partial pressure of carbon dioxide (P_{CO_2}), as an independent variable, on the concentration of hydrogen ions in solution by virtue of the following chemical reaction,

$$CO_2 + H_2O \leftrightarrow H_2CO_3 \leftrightarrow H^+ + HCO_3^- \tag{1}$$

where CO_2 denotes carbon dioxide, H_2O water, H_2CO_3 carbonic acid, H^+ hydrogen ion, and HCO_3^- bicarbonate.

There are currently 3 widely recognized approaches to assess changes in acid–base status, which essentially differ in their method to quantify the nonrespiratory (or metabolic) component:

1. The traditional Henderson–Hasselbalch approach, also called the physiologic approach, which uses the relationship between HCO_3^- and P_{CO_2}
2. The standard base excess (SBE) approach based on the Van Slyke equation
3. The quantitative or Stewart approach, which uses the strong ion difference (SID) and the total weak acids (A_{Tot})

In essence, all methods to quantify acid base disorders are simply increasingly accurate (and more complex) approximations to the estimation of the equilibrium of carbonate and noncarbonate buffers,[4–6] and as shall be seen, all methods are readily compatible with each other when assessed from a multicompartment modeling standpoint.[7] Despite this apparent interchangeability, and the potential benefit of conceiving these methods as complementary rather than mutually exclusive, intense discussions rage on between advocates and detractors of each of these models. Indeed, the controversy raised by Stewart's relatively novel postulates is reminiscent of the intense discussions between advocates of the bicarbonate-based approximations (conceptually centered on the Henderson-Hasselbalch approach and geographically located mainly in Boston) and the supporters of the SBE approach (led essentially by Siggaard-Andersen from Copenhagen, Denmark), which was immortalized by Bunker in his famous editorial entitled the "Great trans-Atlantic acid–base debate".[8]

This article explores the origins of the current concepts framing the existing methods to analyze acid base balance, to demonstrate that despite having differences, these approaches can all be used to improve the understanding of acid–base derangements in the clinical setting. The unification of concepts will also provide clarity to the debate and provide the clinician with the necessary tools to better assess these alterations at the bedside.

THE CONCEPT OF EQUILIBRIUM AND THE EVOLUTION OF THE ANALYSIS OF ACID–BASE PHYSIOLOGY

Every method to qualitatively or quantitatively describe the chemical transactions associated with significant changes in hydrogen ion concentration in biological fluids is anchored on the concept of chemical equilibrium. Equilibrium is the chemical state in which reactants and products are present in concentrations that have no further tendency to change with time.[9] However, most biological systems implicated in acid–base balance never reach true equilibrium because of the complexity of chemical interactions and mechanisms. Yet the application of thermodynamic equilibrium equations seems to perform well to describe–acid base physiology regardless of the specific method employed. This explains why a set of master equations can derive all variables regardless of the method employed, and why there is commonality between such approximations. For instance, the total concentration of proton acceptor sites in a solution, which we will call C_B, is given by

$$C_B = C + \sum_i C_i \cdot \bar{e}_i - D \tag{2}$$

where C is the total concentration of proton acceptor sites in carbonate species including HCO_3^-, CO_3^2, and $PrNHCOO^-$ (carbamine), C_i is the concentration of non-carbonated species I; $\bar{e}_i$ is the average number of proton acceptor sites per molecule of species i, and D is Ricci's difference function ($D = [H^+] - [OH^-]$)

The Physiologic Approach and the Henderson–Hasselbalch Equation

The use of thermodynamic equilibrium equations as first proposed by Henderson has represented not only one of the earliest, but also one of the most common methods of acid–base analysis for decades. Taking into account that at physiologic pH the contribution of CO_3^{2-} and $PrNHCOO^-$ is negligible, and assuming that the solution does not contain noncarbonate buffers, equation 2 can be simplified to

$$C_B = HCO_3^- \tag{3}$$

Henderson, applying the law of mass action, derived an equation relating the concentration of hydrogen ions $[H^+]$ to the concentrations of the base pair CO_2-HCO_3^-:

$$[H^+] = \frac{k \times [CO_2]}{[HCO_3^-]} \tag{4}$$

Finally, Hasselbalch used Sorensen's convention, and expressed $[H^+]$ in terms of the base 10 logarithm or pH, putting together the well-known Henderson–Hasselbalch equation,

$$pH = pK + \log\frac{[HCO_3^-]}{S \times PCO_2} \tag{5}$$

where K is the dissociation constant, and S is the solubility of CO_2. The Henderson–Hasselbalch equation then is based on the isohydric principle, under the construct that the balance between acid–base pairs, which in this case includes both the respiratory (PCO_2) and metabolic (HCO_3^-) components, is related to the concentration of free hydrogen ions in solution, expressed as its negative logarithm, or pH

According to the Henderson–Hasselbalch approach, changes in pH in serum are only dependent on the PCO_2 - HCO_3^- buffer pair. This approach is also based on the theory that the regulation of the concentration of this specific buffer pair determines the ratios of all other buffer pairs, because it fixes the pH, thus making the assessment and inclusion of other noncarbonic or intracellular buffers unnecessary.

The Henderson–Hasselbalch equation results in an adequate model to characterize the acid–base status of plasma in the presence of several conditions[10]:

1. The system is fully equilibrated with the atmosphere or completely controlled by a ventilator system, so that P_{CO_2} remains constant (open system)
2. Bicarbonate does not change form, so that its analytical and equilibrium concentrations remain identical.
3. The logarithm of the ratio of plasma $[HCO_3^-]$ to P_{CO_2} has a direct, linear relation with pH, according to Equation 5.
4. The $[HCO_3^-]/P_{CO_2}$ is assumed as the master buffer system, setting the concentrations of all other carbonate and noncarbonate conjugate buffer pairs.
5. The effects of CO_3^{2-}, albumin and other noncarbonate buffers may safely be omitted from Equation 2.

When the previously mentioned conditions are satisfied, dissolved CO_2 in plasma is a function of the P_{CO_2} (which is controlled and held constant by ventilation), thus providing a descriptive tool with a simple conceptual separation between the respiratory (pCO_2^-) and metabolic (HCO_3^-) components for the assessment of acid–base disorders. The usefulness of any model can be characterized by evaluating its predictions and how well it conforms to experimental data. The predicted linear relationship between log P_{CO_2} and pH by the Henderson–Hasselbalch equation fails to reproduce actual experimental data, describing such relationship as nonlinear.[11] Although changes in plasma HCO_3^- are useful to establish the direction of the change and thus the type of acid–base status alteration, it fails to quantify the magnitude of such a change unless P_{CO_2} is held constant. Further attempts to solve this and the problem of interdependence between P_{CO_2} and $[HCO_3^-]$ included methodological modifications of the quantification of bicarbonate by measuring it after equilibration of blood to a P_{CO_2} of 40 Torr or 5.33 kPa (the so-called standard bicarbonate) and by applying different approaches leading to the concepts of buffer base, base excess, and SBE.

Buffer Base, Base Excess, and Standard Base Excess

Singer and Hastings submitted a different approach in 1948, when they proposed the Buffer Base (B_B^+) concept. Stepping back into the old definition of acids and bases as cations and anions, they defined the B_B^+ as the sum of the products of the concentrations (cAl) and charges (zAl) of strong acids (aprotes [ie, lacking protons], nonbuffer cations or strong cations) minus the concentrations (cBl) and charges (zBl) of strong bases (aprotes, nonbuffer anions or strong anions) and conceived it in the context of the principle of electroneutrality, as a stoichiometric reflection of the accumulation of a strong acid or base. Under this concept then, the sum of the products of strong ions (ie, strong cations and anions, or cAl x zAl) would equal the negative sum of the products of the buffer or weak ions (ie, cBl × zBl):

$$B_B^+ = \sum (cAl \times zAl) - \sum (cBl \times zBl) = 0 \qquad (6)$$

Although B_B^+ was independent of changes in P_{CO_2} (as elevations of HCO_3 due to P_{CO_2} increments, would be matched by a decrease in other buffer anions such as albumin), at the time of its development, it was difficult to calculate given the need to include all strong ions in the solution. An easier way is to express it in terms of the counterpart of the equality (cBl x zBl), which is the sum of HCO_3^- and nonvolatile weak buffer anions like hemoglobin and albumin (A$^-$):

$$B_B^+ = HCO_3^- + A^- \qquad (7)$$

Given that the normal mean value of B_B^+ depends entirely on the concentration of other buffers like hemoglobin and albumin, Singer and Hastings recommended using the change in B_B^+ (ΔB_B^+) to denote metabolic acid–base disturbances.

Further refinement of the methods to measure the B_B^+ led to the development of the concept of the base excess (BE). In a physicochemical system the 2 quantities that describe a chemical component are the chemical potential and the stoichiometric amount of substance.[12] In terms of hydrogen, the chemical potential is expressed as the pH (which is inversely proportional to the chemical potential). The stoichiometric amount of H^+ in solution is accounted for by the concentration of titratable ion.[3] Thus BE is the amount of acid or base that needs to be added to a sample of whole blood in vitro to restore a pH of 7.4 while P_{CO_2} is held at 40 mm Hg (5.33 kPa) and temperature at 37°C, and represents the quantification of present acidosis or alkalosis. Interestingly, BE is numerically equal to Singer and Hastings' ΔB_B^+, and perhaps the most common formula to calculate it is the equation developed by Siggaard-Andersen and named after Donald D. Van Slyke in recognition of his contributions to the understanding of acid–base physiology[6] – the Van Slyke equation:

$$BE = \left(HCO_3^- - 24.4 + [2.3 \times Hb + 7.7]\right) \times (1 - 0.023 \times Hb) \tag{8}$$

Despite the fact that in vitro BE remains stable when P_{CO_2} is changed and reproduces experimental data for separated plasma and whole blood, it fails to reproduce the experimental CO_2 titration curve in vivo in people. The reason for this is thought to be that just as the plasma compartment is in equilibrium with the erythrocyte compartment, the plasma of whole blood is also in equilibrium with the interstitial compartment. Indeed in vivo P_{CO_2} equilibrates with all compartments including blood and interstitial fluid, and thus increments in P_{CO_2} will result in differential changes in pH in compartments that have differential buffering. For instance, this will result in a decrease in pH in the interstitial fluid that is poorly buffered, whereas will result in a slight increase in blood that is well buffered by hemoglobin.[3] Hydrogen ions then flow from the interstitium to the blood to be buffered inside the erythrocytes, ultimately producing a slight decrease in whole blood BE, and a slight increment in plasma BE. For this reason, Siggaard-Andersen modeled the BE of what he called the extracellular fluid (a combination of plasma, erythrocytes, and interstitium) by diluting blood in its own plasma at a 2:1 ratio. He called this BE of the extracellular fluid,[3] also known as SBE.

In an attempt to improve accuracy in vivo, the BE equation was standardized to the effect of hemoglobin on CO_2 titration, resulting in a common version of the SBE equation:

$$SBE = 0.9287 \times \left([HCO_3^- - 24.4 + 14.83] \times [pH - 7.4]\right) \tag{9}$$

Despite providing better accuracy than BE, SBE remains relatively unstable in vivo upon changes in P_{CO_2}.[13] Furthermore, SBE assumes that nonvolatile weak acids (A^-) are constant and normal, which is unlikely, particularly in the acutely ill patient, in whom albumin and phosphate concentrations commonly change. Thus, Wooten[14,15] developed a correction for the SBE based on the levels of albumin and phosphate to describe changes in acid–base balance now in the context of a multicompartment model:

$$SBE_c = \left(HCO_3^- - 24.4\right) + \left([8.3 \times Albumin \times 0.15]\right) \\ + [0.29 \times phosphate \times 0.32] \times [pH - 7.4] \tag{10}$$

where SBE_c is the SBE corrected; albumin is considered in g/dL, and phosphate is considered in mg/dL.

With this, it has been shown that the equations developed for single-compartment models share mathematical relationships with those developed for multicompartment models. In this same way, Kellum and colleagues[16] showed that SBE is equal to the quantity of strong acid or base required to restore the SID to a baseline, at which pH is 7.4, and Pco_2 is 40 mm Hg, and that a change in SBE is equivalent to a change in SID (assuming constant A_{Tot}).

THE STEWART APPROACH

Peter Stewart described a different approach in 1981. He reasoned that the quantitative analysis of ionic solutions by application of physicochemical principles, limited in the past because of the complexity of the required calculations, was possible now in the era of computers. Stewart also departed from the conventional paradigm by conceiving solutions as systems. This is an important shift, because in a system, the resulting effect of multiple interacting, independent mechanisms can only be fully and quantitatively explained by the behavior of all such interacting mechanisms, and not by the behavior of any single one of these mechanisms in isolation. The genius of the well-known Henderson–Hasselbalch equation and its accompanying rules is that although still limited by relying on a single mechanism (ie, the behavior of the base pair Pco_2/HCO_3^-), it provided a simple method that proved safe and useful in the clinical setting. Nevertheless, in the absence of such procedural constraints, a more complete analysis of the system seemed not only possible, but also necessary. Thus, in his seminal papers in the early 1980s,[17] Stewart described experiments in 4 types of solutions—pure water, strong ion solutions, weak acid or buffer solutions, and solutions containing CO_2—to discuss and identify the determining factors of hydrogen ion concentration in aqueous solutions and as the basis of his proposed methodology.

Stewart applied the principle of electrical neutrality and conservation of charge to identify the species present in the system (ie, aqueous solutions), find the equilibrium constants relating the concentrations of such species, and define a set of mass balance equations.[17] As described in detail by Corey and colleagues,[10] Stewart established several features:

1. Conceived human plasma as composed of fully dissociated ions (or strong ions), partially dissociated weak acids (like albumin and phosphate),and volatile buffers (carbonate species) to frame his theory
2. Set the concentration of carbonate species or CT as a nonfixed value, to improve in vivo conditions
3. Included the equilibrium constant for HCO_3^-, K3 in the model
4. Used concentrations instead of chemical activities
5. Weak acids in plasma (ie, proteins and phosphate ion) can be modeled as a single pseudomonoprotic acid (or HA)
6. Ignored temperature, pressure, and ionic strength dependencies of various equilibrium constants[10]

He defined 6 equilibrium equations that included all the mechanisms involved in the system (incorporating the Henderson–Hasselbalch equation), and that thus would accurately explain the behavior of the hydrogen ion in aqueous solutions as shown below:

1. Water dissociation equilibrium

$$[H^+] \times [OH^-] = K'_W \tag{11}$$

2. Weak acid dissociation equilibrium

$$[H^+] \times [A^-] = K_A \times [HA] \tag{12}$$

3. Conservation of mass for "A"

$$[HA] + [A^-] = [A_{Tot}] \tag{13}$$

4. Bicarbonate ion formation equilibrium (Henderson–Hasselbalch relationship)

$$[H^+] \times [HCO_3^-] = K_c \times pCO_2 \tag{14}$$

5. Carbonate ion formation equilibrium

$$[H^+] \times [CO_2^{3-}] = K_3 \times [HCO_3^-] \tag{15}$$

6. Electrical neutrality

$$[SID] + [H^+] - [HCO_3^-] - [A^-] - [CO_2^{3-}] - [OH^-] = 0 \tag{16}$$

The inclusion of these 6 equations ultimately led to the quadratic equation that defines the relationships of all the interacting mechanisms with the concentration of hydrogen ions in aqueous solutions, and that has been known as the Stewart equation:

$$\begin{aligned}
[H^+]^4 &+ ([SID] + K_A) \times [H^+]^3 + (K_A \times ([SID] - [A_{TOT}]) - K'_W - K_c \times pCO_2) \\
&\times [H^+]^2 - (K_A \times (K'_W + K_c \times pCO_2) - K_3 \times K_c \times pCO_2) \times [H^+] - K_A \\
&\times K_3 \times K_c \times pCO_2 = 0
\end{aligned} \tag{17}$$

and, the Stewart equation can be further simplified to the following:

$$pH = pK_1 + \log \frac{[SID] - K_a - [A_{Tot}]/[K_a + 10^{-pH}]}{SPCO_2} \tag{18}$$

where K_1 is the equilibrium constant for the Henderson–Hasselbalch equation; K_a is the weak acid dissociation constant, and S is the solubility of CO_2 in plasma.

This simplified Stewart equation now has the form of Equation 5, which mathematically describes the buffer curve, but now pH is also a function of A_{Tot}. Importantly, Equation 18 also shows how the addition of parameters describing the difference between strong cations and anions like the SID, and the behavior of nonvolatile weak acids (A_{Tot}) to the Henderson–Hasselbalch equation, allows it now to fit experimental data as demonstrated by Corey[18] and Constable.[11] This also raises 2 important points:

The HCO_3^- – P_{CO_2} relationship described by the Henderson–Hasselbalch equation is not sufficient to explain the behavior of hydrogen ions in biologic solutions because it only incorporates one of the many mechanisms at play.

This relationship is necessary to fully explain the behavior of hydrogen ions in biologic solution, because it is one of the fundamental mechanisms.[10]

A Closer Look at the Strong Ion Difference

Plasma ions can be classified into 2 different categories: strong ions (or nonbuffer ions), which fully dissociate, and weak ions (or buffer ions), which partially dissociate at a plasma physiologic pH. The SID is defined as the difference between all strong (completely dissociated) cations and anions, which do not participate in proton transfer reactions (ie, strong ions are neither H+ acceptors, nor donors). Weak acids and CO_2 balance the difference between strong ions according to the principle of electrical neutrality. Electrical neutrality means that the sum of all the charges in any solution must equal to zero. Thus, SID can be expressed either as Equation 19, also known as SID apparent or SIDa, or in terms of CO_2 and weak acids as in Equation 20, also known as the effective SID or SIDe.[19] Is important to note here that SIDe is identical to the $B_B{}^+$, and from this, it is also evident that changes in SBE will represent changes in SID.[13,16] This interchangeability is important, because as has been mentioned, the Stewart approach is mathematically related to other methodologies described in the past, including the Henderson–Hasselbalch equation.

$$SID_a = \sum[\text{strong cation charge concentration}]$$
$$- \sum[\text{strong anion charge concentration}] \tag{19}$$

$$SID_a = [Na^+]+[K^+]-[Cl^-]-[\text{Lactate}]-[\text{Other Strong Ions}] \tag{20}$$

$$SID_e = HCO_3^- + A_{Tot} = B_B^+ \tag{21}$$

The advantage of using SID is that all components can be measured without any reference to pH, and valence and the behavior of chemically reactive species can be safely ignored. When all plasma cations are accounted for, $SID_e = SID_a$. However, if unmeasured anions are present, SID_a will differ from SID_e, giving rise to the strong ion gap (SIG) as shown in the equation below:

$$SIG = SID_a - SID_e \tag{22}$$

This approach, and specifically this term, has been criticized because of its focus on electrical charges rather than proton transfer reactions.[20] However, Figge and others demonstrated how SID can be also obtained in terms of the summation of proton donor and acceptor sites of each buffer group (like albumin) incorporating pK values of individual histidine residues on human albumin, and when knowing the values for pH P_{CO_2} and the concentrations of albumin and phosphate.[21]

Leaving aside the contribution of histidine residues demonstrated by Figge and colleagues, it is possible to equate SID to the total concentration of proton acceptor sites (C_B) when albumin is assumed to act as a single monoprotic acid. Accordingly, Equation 2 can be rewritten as follows:

$$C_B = SID = [HCO_3^-]+2[CO_3^{2-}] + [A^-] + [OH^-] + [H^+] \tag{23}$$

These associations demonstrate that the Stewart equation can be understood from the context of a variety of approaches including the consideration of electrical charge or proton acceptor and donor sites,[10] and are also meant to point out to the reader that the Stewart approach includes all of the traditional approximations to describe acid–base equilibrium:

The Henderson–Hasselbalch equation (pH and P_{CO_2})
The Van Slyke equation or titratable base ($C_B = SID$ vs pH)
The Van Slyke buffer formula (β_A vs pH)

Thus, rather than alternative, the Stewart approach should be regarded as complementary to the current knowledge on the topic.[10] Finally, the fact that the Stewart equation is inclusive of all other modalities of acid–base evaluation explains why similar results can be attained by using any one of these models, but also underscores why only the Stewart equation can accurately reproduce experimental data and thus explain fully the behavior of hydrogen ions in biologic solutions.

Weak Nonvolatile Acids

In contrast to strong ions, weak ions (buffer ions) are derived from weak acids and bases in plasma, and by definition are not fully dissociated at plasma pH. The dissociation equilibrium of the weak acid (HA) – conjugate base (A-) pair follows the formula, $HA \leftrightarrow H^+ + A^-$, with a dissociation constant (K_a) given by, $K_a = [H^+][A^-]/[HA]$. In order for a weak acid to act as buffer, its pK_a ($= -\log K_a$) must be within pH $\pm$ 1.5.[22] At the physiologic pH of 7.4, phosphate and plasma proteins act as effective weak acids (buffer ions), because their pKa lays between 5.9 and 8.9. In addition, weak acids can be further divided into volatile (HCO_3^-, which is an open buffer system in equilibrium with P_{CO_2}) and nonvolatile (non-HCO_3^- or A^-, which acts as a closed-system buffer).

A NOTE ON THE STEWART MECHANISM

Stewart conceived water dissociation as the key mechanistic element to explain changes in the [H^+] in different compartments of the body. He departed from the notion that different cells in the body, especially in the kidney, reclaim or excrete acid or hydrogen ions to regulate pH. Instead, he proposed that the highly ionizing power of water, that through its high dielectric constant causes substances to dissociate once dissolved in it, can also dissociate to increase [H^+]. He further proposed that such dissociation would be dependent on the interplay of 3 so-called independent variables, notably SID, A_{Tot}, and P_{CO_2}, and demonstrated how [H^+] would change with variations in these variables in different ways to the classic pH titration curve using increasingly complex aqueous solutions.[10] Autoionization of water has been recognized by others as a key mechanism to explain changes in [H+] in aqueous solutions.[23] For instance, it is known that an intact water molecule can dissociate in liquid water, yielding hydronium (H_3O^+) and hydroxide (OH^-) ions in roughly 10 hours.[24]

Geissler and colleagues[24] studied the autoionization of water and demonstrated that long-range electric fields drive the dissociation of hydrogen bound to oxygen, and that usually hydrogen ions produced in this way rapidly recombine, because the initiating electric field fluctuation disappears very rapidly (ie, tens of femtoseconds). Interestingly, these transiently dissociated ions seem to persist anchored to oxygen by hydrogen bond wires, and can recombine with other oxygen molecules distant from the parent molecule. However, they also noted that if such initiating electric field fluctuation is coincident with breaking of the hydrogen bond wire, rapid recombination is not possible, and this signature is amenable of observation and quantification. Once dissociated, nascent ions are separated from each other by 2 to 3 molecules of water that eventually re-unite.

Despite this experimental evidence, there are no clinical data suggesting that this mechanism is at play in the regulation of acid–base balance in biologic solutions. Stewart extrapolated this finding directly to conceive SID, A_{Tot}, and P_{CO_2} as those solutes responsible for the dissociation of water, and attributed [H^+] regulation to this mechanism. Despite this being the case, the absence of support for this mechanism does not preclude it as a possible explanation, and certainly does not invalidate the virtues of Stewart's methodology and attempt to better characterize changes in acid–base.

SUMMARY

The understanding, evaluation, and adequate assessment of the pathophysiologic processes that circumscribe acid–base balance in clinical medicine are important, because these premises directly motivate treatment. Furthermore, several clinical studies have shown that regardless of the model used to assess them, acid–base derangements are predictive of outcome, thus representing an appealing area of effective intervention. Historically, the evaluation of acid–base models has seen many developments, mostly driven by the limitations of the immediate antecessor. For instance, the limitations of the Henderson–Hasselbalch equation motivated the development of the buffer base and the SBE concepts. Similarly, Stewart's reappraisal of the assessment of acid–base balance in biologic solutions found motivation in the fact that in the modern era, computers permitted complex calculations that were not possible before, and thus sought to identify a unique equation that could describe and explain the fluctuations of the entire system.

Stewart made compromises in the development of his model, including the choice of selecting a charge-centered rather than a proton transfer-centered approach. However, this methodology provides equivalent results compared with other methods utilizing quantification of proton acceptor sites like base excess approach, or proton number quantification. In addition, he chose to model weak acids as a monoprotic entity, rather than as its true poliprotic nature.[10] Finally, Stewart emphasized both the independent nature of SID, A_{Tot}, and P_{CO_2}, and the link of these independent variables to the water dissociation mechanisms, for which he has been highly criticized. Nevertheless, even in the absence of evidence for a mechanism, the Stewart approach provides an alternative explanation to acid–base derangements.

Although Stewart's theory has re-energized the polarity of opinions regarding this controversial area, his approach provides mathematical unity to the different available methods for the assessment of acid base derangements. As such, by establishing the 6 equilibrium equations and computing them into a master equation, Stewart incorporated the virtues of the classic approach by Henderson–Hasselbalch and the base excess-based approaches, overcame the individual limitations of each of these models, and provided for the first time, a real quantitative tool to assess acid–base derangements in clinical situations. For this reason, it is not surprising that these distinct methods perform similarly when utilized to assess acid–base derangements. It is thus equivocal and unnecessary to think of these methods as mutually exclusive. These methods should be thought of as complementary, and should be used to further the understanding of the mechanisms governing acid–base biology.

REFERENCES

1. Berend K, de Vries AP, Gans RO. Physiological approach to assessment of acid–base disturbances. N Engl J Med 2014;371(15):1434–45.
2. Morris CG, Low J. Metabolic acidosis in the critically ill: part 1. Classification and pathophysiology. Anaesthesia 2008;63(3):294–301.
3. Siggaard-Andersen O, Fogh-Andersen N. Base excess or buffer base (strong ion difference) as measure of a non-respiratory acid–base disturbance. Acta Anaesthesiol Scand Suppl 1995;107:123–8.
4. Corey HE. Stewart and beyond: new models of acid–base balance. Kidney Int 2003;64(3):777–87.
5. Roos A, Boron WF. The buffer value of weak acids and bases: origin of the concept, and first mathematical derivation and application to physico-chemical systems. the work of M. Koppel and K. Spiro (1914). Respir Physiol 1980;40:1–32.
6. Siggaard-Andersen O. The van Slyke equation. Scand J Clin Lab Invest Suppl 1977;146:15–20.
7. Wooten EW. The standard strong ion difference, standard total titratable base, and their relationship to the Boston compensation rules and the Van Slyke equation for extracellular fluid. J Clin Monit Comput 2010;24(3):177–88.
8. Bunker JP. The great trans-atlantic acid-base debate. Anesthesiology 1965;26:591–4.
9. Atkins P, de Paula J. Physical chemistry for the life sciences. By Peter Atkins and Julio de Paula. 8th edition. Oxford University Press; 2006. p. 200–2.
10. Corey HE, Kellum JA, Wooten WE. Stewart's acid-base theory: trends in comparative. Comp Biochem Phyisol 2009;14:35–54.
11. Constable PD. A simplified strong ion model for acid–base equilibria: application to horse plasma. J Appl Physiol 1997;83(1):297–311.
12. Siggaard-Andersen O, Durst RA, Maas AH. International Federation of Clinical Chemistry, Scientific committee, analytical section: and approved recommendation (1984) on physico-chemical quantities and units in clinical chemistry with special emphasis on activities and activity coefficients. J Clin Chem Clin Biochem 1987;25(6):369–91.
13. Kellum JA. Determinants of plasma acid-base balance. Crit Care Clin 2005;21(2):329–46.
14. Wooten EW. Calculation of physiological acid-base parameters in multicompartment systems with application to human blood. J Appl Physiol 2003;95(6):2333–44.
15. Wooten EW. Science review: quantitative acid-base physiology using the Stewart model. Crit Care 2004;8(6):448–52.
16. Kellum JA, Bellomo R, Kramer DJ, et al. Splanchnic buffering of metabolic acid during early endotoxemia. J Crit Care 1997;12(1):7–12.
17. Stewart PA. Modern quantitative acid-base chemistry. Can J Physiol Pharmacol 1983;61(12):1444–61.
18. Corey HE. Bench-to-bedside review: fundamental principles of acid-base physiology. Crit Care 2005;9(2):184–92.
19. Figge J, Mydosh T, Fencl V. Serum proteins and acid-base equilibria: a follow-up. J Lab Clin Med 1992;120(5):713–9.
20. Kurtz I, Kraut J, Ornekian V, et al. Acid-base analysis: a critique of the Stewart and bicarbonate-centered approaches. Am J Physiol Renal Physiol 2008;294(5):F1009–31.

21. Figge J, Rossing TH, Fencl V. The role of serum proteins in acid-base equilibria. J Lab Clin Med 1991;117(6):453–67.
22. Constable PD. Clinical assessment of acid-base status: comparison of the Henderson–Hasselbalch and strong ion approaches. Vet Clin Pathol 2000;29(4): 115–28.
23. Siwick BJ, Bakker HJ. On the role of water in intermolecular proton-transfer reactions. J Am Chem Soc 2007;129(44):13412–20.
24. Geissler PL, Dellago C, Chandler D, et al. Autoionization in liquid water. Science 2001;291(5511):2121–4.

Index

Note: Page numbers of article titles are in **boldface** type.

A

Acid base analysis, Henderson-Hasselbalch equation in, physiologic approach to, 851–852
Acid base disorders, due to kidney injury, 753
    plasma ions and, 856
    Stewart approach to, 854–858
    strong ion difference and, 856–857
    understanding of, **849–860**
    weak nonvolatile acids and, 857
Acid base physiology, analysis of, equilibrium and, 850–854
    buffer base, base excess, and standard base excess, 852–854
Acid base status, approaches to assess, 850
Albumin, in cirrhosis, 743
Albumin solutions, human, 835
Anticoagulation, for treatment of acute kidney injury, 845–846

B

Bicarbonate solutions, indications for, 834
Blood pressure, systemic, in septic acute kidney injury, 652–653
Brain, acute kidney injury and, 755

C

Cardiac surgery, acute kidney injury associated with, 635–638
Cardiorenal syndrome, acute, biomarkers in, 686–690
        clinical approach to, **685–703**
        clinical assessment of, 691–692
        epidemiology of, 686
        pathophysiology of, 690–691
        treatment of, 692–696
Cirrhosis, acute kidney injury in, **737–750**
    albumin in, 743
    renal dysfunction in, assessment of, 739–741
Colloids, 824–825
    anaphylactic reactions to, 834
    carrier fluid of, 825, 830–831
    for fluid management, 792–794
    gelatin-based, 835
    metabolism, elimination, and duration of effect of, 825, 830–831
    molecular weight of, 825
    oncotic pressure of, 825, 830–831

Crit Care Clin 31 (2015) 861–866
http://dx.doi.org/10.1016/S0749-0704(15)00069-X
0749-0704/15/$ – see front matter © 2015 Elsevier Inc. All rights reserved.

criticalcare.theclinics.com

Colloids (*continued*)
  properties of, 825–829
  types of, 828–829
Contrast agents, acute kidney injury associated with, **725–735**
  causing acute kidney injury, 729
Creatinine, baseline, estimated, 625–626
  serum, and urine output, 623, 626–628
Critical illness, and sepsis, acute kidney injury associated with, 638–641
  fluid overload and adverse outcomes in, 803–806
Crystalloids, balanced, 824, 834–835
  composition of, 826–829
  for fluid management, 791–792
  unbalanced, 824
Cytokine homeostasis, acute kidney injury and, 755–756

D

Dextrans, 835
Dextrose solutions, 834
Disseminated intravascular coagulation, and acute kidney injury, 666–667
  management of, 667
  tissue factor in, 666
Diuretic therapy, in acute heart failure, 693–694
Drug-induced acute kidney injury, **675–684**

E

Electrolyte disturbance, due to kidney injury, 752–753
Extracorporeal volume removal, in acute cardiorenal syndrome, 694–695

F

Fluid composition, and effects of, **823–837**
Fluid intake, controlling of, 810–811
Fluid management, and central venous pressure, in septic acute kidney failure, 654
  and drug prescription, analogy of, 786
  colloids for, 792–794
  crystalloid solutions for, 791–792
  de-escalation of, 789
  fluid accumulation in, mitigation of, 795–797
  history of, 786–787
  monitoring and reassessment of, 789, 790
  optimization in, 788
  phases of, 787–789
  principles of, **785–801**
  quantitative toxicity of, 792–794
  rescue phase of, 788
  stabilization in, goals of, 788–789
  types of, 789–791
Fluid overload, **803–821**
  and adverse outcomes, in critical illness, 803–806

changes in, in critically ill patients, assessment of response to, 813–814
development of, patient-physician interaction in, 806–807
due to kidney injury, 754
in organ systems, pathologic sequelae of, 804, 805
management of, 810–815
pathogenesis of, 807–810
prevention and treatment of, clinical approach to, 811, 812
Fluid(s), hematological effects of, 833
    indications for, 834–835
    metabolic effects of, 833
    physiological effects of, 829–834
    plasma volume expansion by, 829–833
    removal of, diuretics, ultrafiltration, and monitoring of, 811
    renal effects of, 833
    therapeutic effects of, 823–824
    types of, 824–825

G

Gastrointestinal tract, acute kidney injury and, 755

H

Heart, acute kidney injury and, 755
Heart failure, acute, diuretic therapy in, 693–694
Hemodialysis, intermittent, for treatment of acute kidney injury, 842–843
Hemolytic uremic syndrome, 664–666
    and acute kidney injury, 665
    complement pathway in, shiga toxins and, 665
    management of, 665–666
Henderson-Hasselbalch equation, in acid base analysis, physiologic approach to, 851–852
Hepatorenal syndrome, extracorporeal liver support in, 745
    pathophysiology of, 738–739
    renal replacement therapy in, 745
    therapies in, 743
    vasoconstrictor therapy in, 743–744
Hydroxyethyl starches, 835

I

Immune system, innate, acute kidney injury and, 755–757
Intravenous fluids, to prevent contrast-associated kidney injury, 730

K

Kidney, response to sepsis, 650–651
Kidney disease, global outcomes of, improving of, 742
Kidney failure, acute, renal replacement therapy in, 654–655, 779–780, **839-848**, 654
Kidney injury, acute, and innate immune system, 755–757
    animal studies in, 756

Kidney (*continued*)
    associated with cardiac surgery, 635–638
    associated with critical illness and sepsis, 638–641
    biomarkers of, **633–648**
        at emergency room presentation, 641–642
        characteristics and physiologic action for, 636–637
        discriminatory function of, 642–643
        novel, 628–630
    causes of, 746
    classification of, 773–774
    clinical studies in, 756–757
    contrast-associated, **725–735**
        incidence of, 727
        outcomes associated with, 727–729
        prevention of, 729–731
        risk factors for, 726–727
    conventional markers of, limitations of, 765
    criteria for, 622, 634
        standardized, purpose of, 622–624
    definition of, 633
    diagnostic criteria for, **621–632**
    disseminated intravascular coagulation and, 666–667
    drug-induced, **675–684**
        epidemiology of, 675–676
        future directions in, 680–681
        management of, 680
        prevention of, 679–680
        risk assessment in, 677–679
        risk factors for, 676–677
    established, interactions for, 779
    etiology of, affecting outcome, 767
    global burden of disease study and, 775–776
    hemolytic uremic syndrome and, 665
    impaired neutrophil function in, 756–757
    in cirrhosis, **737–750**
        epidemiology of, 738
        inflammation and, 738
        novel biomarkers of, 741–743
        pathophysiology of, 738–739
    in liver disease, diagnosis and definitions in, 741–743
    in surgical patient, **705–723**
        clinical prediction scores and, 712–713
        imaging techniques and, 710–711
        risk factors for, 707–709
        risk stratification for, 710
        urine and plasma biomarkers used in, 711–712
    increasing awareness of, 775
    long-term follow-up of, **763–772**
    long-term risks of, 766
        identification of patient with, 767–769
    management of, long-term, 769

reducing variations in, 776–780
markers of, role of, 765–766
natural history of, pretransplant and posttransplant, 746
pathophysiology of, 650–651
patient monitoring in, 768, 769
perioperative, definitions, epidemiology, and outcomes associated with, 706–707
    prevention and treatment of, 713–715
prevention of, **773–784**
    identification of high-risk individuals for, 777
    initiative goals of, 774
    prompt diagnosis for, 777–779
    strategies for, 774–780
proinflammatory changes in, 755–756
recovery from, defining of, 764–766
rehabilitation in, 780
renal replacement therapy in, 779–780
sepsis-induced, **649–660**
    future therapies in, 655–656
    glomerular hemodynamics of, 651–652
    management of patients with, 652–655
    therapeutic targets in, 653
short-term effects of, **751–762**, 754–757
    conventional perspective on, 752–754
    new perspective on, 754–757
surviving of, course of, 763
thrombocytopenia-associated, with multiple organ failure, **661–674**

L

Liver disease, acute kidney injury in, diagnosis and definitions in, 741–743
Lungs, acute kidney injury and, 755

M

Midodrine, in hepatorenal syndrome, 744
Multiple organ failure, thrombocytopenia-associated, 667–668
    and acute kidney failure, 668
    management of, 668

N

Noradrenaline, in hepatorenal syndrome, 744

O

Octreotide, in hepatorenal syndrome, 744

P

Pharmacologic agents, to prevent contrast-associated kidney injury, 729–730

R

Red blood cell transfusion, in septic acute kidney failure, 654
Renal dysfunction, assessment of, 739–741
    in cirhosis, assessment of, 739–741
Renal function, baseline, 624–626
Renal replacement therapy, in acute kidney failure, 654-655, 779-780, **839-848**, 654
    in acute kidney injury, 779–780
        initiation of, indications for, 840–841
            timing of, 840–842
            treatments for, 842–844
            vascular access for, 842
        optimal dose of, 844–845
    in hepatorenal syndrome, 745
    to prevent contrast-associated kidney injury, 729

S

Sepsis, kidney response to, 650–651
Sepsis-induced acute kidney injury, **649–660**
Sodium chloride, 824, 834
Stewart approach, to acid base disorders, 854–858
Surgical patient, acute kidney injury in, **705–723**

T

Thrombocytopenia-associated multiple organ failure, in acute kidney failure, **661–674**
Thrombocytopenia purpura, thrombotic, 662–664
        acute kidney injury and, 663–664
        management of, 664
        Von Willebrand factor and ADAMTS-13 in, 662–63
Transjugular intrahepatic portosystemic shunt, 744–745

U

Uremia, due to kidney injury, 753
Urine output, serum creatinine and, 623, 626–628

V

Vasoactive drugs, in acute cardiorenal syndrome, 694–695
Vasoconstrictor therapy, in hepatorenal syndrome, 743–744
Vasopressin analogues, in hepatorenal syndrome, 743–744
Vasopressor therapy, in septic acute kidney failure, 654
Veno-venous hemofiltration, continuous, for treatment of acute kidney injury, 843–844

United States Postal Service

Statement of Ownership, Management, and Circulation
(All Periodicals Publications Except Requestor Publications)

1. Publication Title Critical Care Clinics	**2. Publication Number** 0 0 0 0 - 7 0 0 8	**3. Filing Date** 9/18/15
4. Issue Frequency Jan, Apr, Jul, Oct	**5. Number of Issues Published Annually** 4	**6. Annual Subscription Price** $210.00

7. Complete Mailing Address of Known Office of Publication (*Not printer*) (*Street, city, county, state, and ZIP+4®*)

Elsevier Inc.
360 Park Avenue South
New York, NY 10010-1710

Contact Person
Stephen R. Bushing
Telephone (*Include area code*)
215-239-3688

8. Complete Mailing Address of Headquarters or General Business Office of Publisher (*Not printer*)

Elsevier Inc., 360 Park Avenue South, New York, NY 10010-1710

9. Full Names and Complete Mailing Addresses of Publisher, Editor, and Managing Editor (*Do not leave blank*)

Publisher (*Name and complete mailing address*)

Linda Belfus, Elsevier Inc., 1600 John F. Kennedy Blvd., Suite 1800, Philadelphia, PA 19103

Editor (*Name and complete mailing address*)

Patrick Manley, Elsevier Inc., 1600 John F. Kennedy Blvd., Suite 1800, Philadelphia, PA 19103-2899

Managing Editor (*Name and complete mailing address*)

Adrianne Brigido, Elsevier Inc., 1600 John F. Kennedy Blvd., Suite 1800, Philadelphia, PA 19103-2899

10. Owner (*Do not leave blank. If the publication is owned by a corporation, give the name and address of the corporation immediately followed by the names and addresses of all stockholders owning or holding 1 percent or more of the total amount of stock. If not owned by a corporation, give the names and addresses of the individual owners. If owned by a partnership or other unincorporated firm, give its name and address as well as those of each individual owner. If the publication is published by a nonprofit organization, give its name and address.*)

Full Name	Complete Mailing Address
Wholly owned subsidiary of	1600 John F. Kennedy Blvd, Ste. 1800
Reed/Elsevier, US holdings	Philadelphia, PA 19103-2899

11. Known Bondholders, Mortgagees, and Other Security Holders Owning or Holding 1 Percent or More of Total Amount of Bonds, Mortgages, or Other Securities. If none, check box ▶ ☐ None

Full Name	Complete Mailing Address
N/A	

12. Tax Status (*For completion by nonprofit organizations authorized to mail at nonprofit rates*) (*Check one*)
The purpose, function, and nonprofit status of this organization and the exempt status for federal income tax purposes:
☐ Has Not Changed During Preceding 12 Months
☐ Has Changed During Preceding 12 Months (*Publisher must submit explanation of change with this statement*)

PS Form 3526, July 2014 (Page 1 of 3 [Instructions Page 3]) PSN 7530-01-000-9931 **PRIVACY NOTICE:** See our Privacy policy in www.usps.com

---

13. Publication Title	14. Issue Date for Circulation Data Below
Critical Care Clinics	July 2015

15. Extent and Nature of Circulation			Average No. Copies Each Issue During Preceding 12 Months	No. Copies of Single Issue Published Nearest to Filing Date
a. Total Number of Copies (*Net press run*)			802	673
b. Legitimate Paid and/Or Requested Distribution (By Mail and Outside the Mail)	(1)	Mailed Outside County Paid/Requested Mail Subscriptions stated on PS Form 3541. (*Include paid distribution above nominal rate, advertiser's proof copies and exchange copies*)	403	322
	(2)	Mailed In-County Paid/Requested Mail Subscriptions stated on PS Form 3541. (*Include paid distribution above nominal rate, advertiser's proof copies and exchange copies*)		
	(3)	Paid Distribution Outside the Mails Including Sales Through Dealers And Carriers, Street Vendors, Counter Sales, and Other Paid Distribution Outside USPS®	180	171
	(4)	Paid Distribution by Other Classes of Mail Through the USPS (e.g. First-Class Mail®)		
c. Total Paid and/or Requested Circulation (*Sum of 15b (1), (2), (3), and (4)*) ▶			583	493
d. Free or Nominal Rate Distribution (By Mail and Outside the Mail)	(1)	Free or Nominal Rate Outside-County Copies Included on PS Form 3541	66	66
	(2)	Free or Nominal Rate In-County Copies included on PS Form 3541		
	(3)	Free or Nominal Rate Copies mailed at Other classes Through the USPS (e.g. First-Class Mail®)		
	(4)	Free or Nominal Rate Distribution Outside the Mail (Carriers or Other means)	66	66
e. Total Nonrequested Distribution (Sum of 15d (1), (2), (3) and (4)) ▶			66	66
f. Total Distribution (Sum of 15c and 15e) ▶			649	559
g. Copies not Distributed (See instructions to publishers #4 (page #3)) ▶			153	114
h. Total (Sum of 15f and g) ▶			802	673
i. Percent Paid and/or Requested Circulation (15c divided by 15f times 100) ▶			89.83%	88.19%

* If you are claiming electronic copies go to line 16 on page 3. If you are not claiming Electronic copies, skip to line 17 on page 3

16. Electronic Copy Circulation	Average No. Copies Each Issue During Preceding 12 Months	No. Copies of Single Issue Published Nearest to Filing Date
a. Paid Electronic Copies ▶		
b. Total paid Print Copies (Line 15c) + **Paid Electronic copies** (Line 16a) ▶		
c. Total Print Distribution (Line 15f) + **Paid Electronic Copies** (Line 16a) ▶		
d. Percent Paid (Both Print & Electronic copies) (16b divided by 16c X 100) ▶		

☐ I certify that 50% of all my distributed copies (electronic and print) are paid above a nominal price

17. Publication of Statement of Ownership
☐ If the publication is a general publication, publication of this statement is required. Will be printed in the __October 2015__ issue of this publication.

18. Signature and Title of Editor, Publisher, Business Manager, or Owner

Stephen R. Bushing – Inventory Distribution Coordinator
Stephen R. Bushing – Inventory Distribution Coordinator

Date: September 18, 2015

I certify that all information furnished on this form is true and complete. I understand that anyone who furnishes false or misleading information on this form or who omits material or information requested on the form may be subject to criminal sanctions (including fines and imprisonment) and/or civil sanctions (including civil penalties).

PS Form 3526, July 2014 (Page 3 of 3)

Printed and bound by CPI Group (UK) Ltd, Croydon, CR0 4YY

03/10/2024

01040485-0007